DEBT FINANCING AND CAPITAL FORMATION IN HEALTH CARE INSTITUTIONS

Contributors

Thomas Arthur
Frederick R. Blume
Robert G. Donnelley
John Fenner
William D. Gehl
Harvey J. Gitel
William J. Gray

Thomas E. Lanctot
Robert C. Liden
Earl L. Metheny
Arthur J. Simon
James J. Unland
Donna S. Wetzler
James R. Wyatt

DEBT FINANCING AND CAPITAL FORMATION IN HEALTH CARE INSTITUTIONS

Edited by
Geoffrey B. Shields

Gardner, Carton & Douglas
Chicago, Illinois

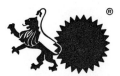

AN ASPEN PUBLICATION®
Aspen Systems Corporation
Rockville, Maryland
London
1983

Library of Congress Cataloging in Publication Data
Main entry under title:

Debt financing and capital formation in health care
institutions.

Bibliography: p. 307
Includes index.
1. Hospitals—Finance.   2. Credit.   I. Shields,
Geoffrey B.
RA971.3.D36   1982   362.1'1'0681   82-11407
ISBN: 0-89443-662-7

Publisher: John Marozsan
Editorial Director: Michael Brown
Managing Editor: Margot Raphael
Editorial Services: Scott Ballotin
Printing and Manufacturing: Debbie Collins

Library of Congress Catalog Card Number: 82-11407
ISBN: 0-89443-662-7

Printed in the United States of America

1   2   3   4   5

To
My Father,
John W. Shields

Table of Contents

Chapter 9—   **Equipment Financing**
      Geoffrey B. Shields

Foreword

Since World War II there have been four main sources of financing for health care construction and equipment: gifts; government grants; retained earnings; and borrowing. Beginning in the mid-1960s, while the first two sources of funds have diminished to a trickle, borrowing has developed as the primary source of capital financing for most health care institutions.

Hand-in-hand with the emergence of borrowing as the primary source of financing for capital projects has come a dramatic increase in the complexity of health care finance and in the variety of financing techniques. During this period:

- Tax-exempt financing has convincingly replaced taxable financing as the primary mode of brick and mortar borrowing for health care facilities.
- The dollar volume of hospital borrowing for capital projects has tripled, from less than $2 billion in 1972 to $6 billion in 1981.
- A wide variety of credit pooling and credit enhancing techniques have been and are being developed, including multihospital, systemwide financing, letters-of-credit-backed bonds, insured bonds, and pooled equipment bond trusts.
- The sophistication of debt documents has greatly increased— recognizing the special nature of health care institutions.
- The number of investment bankers, feasibility consultants, lawyers, and other professionals specializing in health care finance has mushroomed.

Today the health care provider faces a wide range of choices among forms of financing, document terms, and the experts it can employ to prepare and market its borrowing. Board and administration decisions on which choices to make have been based primarily on the oral advice of investment bankers, feasibility consultants, and lawyers. The literature on health care finance has consisted primarily of magazine articles on narrow subjects of current interest. There has been a need for a single, comprehensive reference book addressing the whole field of health care finance.

This is the first such book.

Debt Financing and Capital Formation in Health Care Institutions provides an overview of the financing process for trustees, hospital administrators, and others interested in health care financing. It explains the long-term planning steps health care providers should initiate *now* to assure the availability of financing in the future. It discusses in detail the various financing alternatives available to a health care corporation, comparing the merits and drawbacks of each method of financing.

This book presents sound suggestions for selecting the best team of experts for a particular financing.

No book can answer all the questions that arise on a particular financing, but by reading this book and having it available as a reference source, health care administrators and involved board members will be able to ask the right questions of investment bankers and other experts involved in financing. This book provides both an overview of the financing alternatives available to health care institutions and detailed information on how to make the appropriate decisions at each step of a financing.

Richard J. Brashler, Jr.
President, Ziegler Securities, Inc.

Preface

Financing health care facilities and equipment is a multifaceted field. Experts from the fields of investment banking, accounting, hospital consulting, and law were generous in offering advice while the outline for the book was being developed. Many of these same people, and others, reviewed various chapters while they were in draft form and offered valuable advice leading to modifications from early drafts.

Because several authors have contributed to this book, the style varies from chapter to chapter, and there is some redundancy of material. It is hoped that the wide range of experts who contributed to the book will compensate for the inevitable drawbacks of a multi-author book.

Among those who must be thanked are some who were not involved with the development of this book, but who taught me and many of the other authors so much while "doing deals." They include Richard J. Brashler, Sr., John R. Burrell, Lynn L. Coe, Theodore L. Dehne, Philip J. Dorman, C. Robert Foltz, Arthur J. Guastella, Thom W. Harrow, Arthur J. Henkel, Bruce Mansdorf, David Miller, Manly W. Mumford, David Nelson, L. Patrick Oden, George C. Phillips, Jr., George Pitt, Lee Ponder, Nancy Rapoport, and Edward F. Reifsnyder.

Among those who gave advice on the book from time to time are Francis J. Byrnes, David Beemer, John Glidden, and David Winston of Blyth Eastman Paine Webber Health Care Funding, Inc.; Dennis R. Rognerud and Donald A. Carlson, Jr., of Ziegler Securities, Inc.; Timothy Schwertfeger of John Nuveen & Co.; Terry Hiduke of the accounting firm of Main Hurdman, Inc.; David Shanahan of Ernst & Whinney; John E. Gilchrist of A. G. Becker, Incorporated; and John W. Shields, past chairman of the board of Ziegler Securities, Inc.

The research assistance of Ann Morris, the chief librarian of Gardner, Carton & Douglas, was very helpful. Several people contributed to the typing and proofreading of the book as it developed, including Debbie

Rosenwinkel, Jean Provenzano, Pat Agema, Laura Bernardo, Mary Redmond, Renee Robinson, and Lauretta McMillan.

Mary K. Klauck's assistance in coordinating the flow of information among the various authors and her organizational initiative have been invaluable. Without her help this book could not have been completed. Michael Williams and Lucille Allen were of great assistance in preparing the manuscript.

Finally, Mike Brown and Scott Ballotin of Aspen Systems have been patient and effective editors whose skills are greatly appreciated.

Geoffrey B. Shields
October 1982

Chapter 1

The Financing Team

Geoffrey B. Shields

A major debt financing is one of the most important and complicated transactions in which a chief financial officer and chief executive officer of a hospital will ever engage. It involves drafting hundreds of pages of legal documents which require a hospital to adhere to scores of convenants over the life of the bond issue—often 30 years or longer. The transaction requires coordination of the efforts of a large number of experts who bring differing skills to the structuring of the borrowing. The hospital should carefully select each of these experts, realizing that it is important to have experienced participants in each role. An experienced accountant cannot make up for inexperienced hospital counsel and vice versa.

A few years ago the "quarterback" of every financing team was the investment banker. Once selected by the hospital the investment banker set the financing schedule, decided on the terms of the financing (in consultation with the hospital), and coordinated all aspects of processing, pricing, and selling the bond issue. Today the underwriter is still usually the quarterback, although in some cases this role has been assumed by the staff of state health facilities authorities, sophisticated hospital administrators, or even special counsel to the hospital. Over the last decade the number of participants taking an active role in a financing has increased substantially.

While the primary role of each participant in a financing can be characterized, in most "deals" the roles overlap somewhat, and the best structure and terms for the transaction result from full participation and solicitation of the views of all the parties.

Descriptions of the various participants and their roles in structuring and drafting a major borrowing follow.

1

THE HOSPITAL STAFF

There should be at least three participants from the hospital staff involved in the preparation for the bond issue: the chief executive officer; the chief financial officer; and the hospital's in-house reimbursement expert.

The chief executive officer should be involved in selecting the team members for the transaction and in making the major decisions with regard to the borrowing, such as the term of the borrowing, the selection of the investment bankers, the property to be mortgaged (if any), and the major covenants in the documents limiting the hospital's ability to engage in various kinds of activities (the merger covenant, the transfer to affiliates provisions, the sale and transfer of assets, the rate covenant, the additional borrowing covenants, etc.). Sometimes, the chief executive officer will wish to attend all financing team meetings, maintaining a "hands-on" position with regard to all decisions. At other times, the chief executive officer will wish to delegate the day-to-day responsibility for the advancement of the preparations for the issuance of bonds to the hospital's chief financial officer.

The chief financial officer, working closely with outside accountants and the hospital's attorney and special counsel, must get involved in the day-to-day preparation of the debt documents. Frequently, the chief financial officer will be the hospital's "strawboss," seeing that the transaction moves forward quickly and that all parties are doing their assigned tasks on schedule. The chief financial officer will have to live with the provisions of the debt documents: meeting the debt payment schedule; borrowing additional debt only under the conditions allowed in the debt documents; making periodic reports to the trustee and to the major bondholders as provided in the debt documents; making sure that the rates charged by the hospital are sufficient to meet the rate covenants in the debt documents; and investing money in the various bond funds as permitted in the documents. In order to understand these provisions fully, it is almost essential that the chief financial officer be involved in the drafting of the documents.

In addition, the chief financial officer will wish to structure many provisions to accommodate the hospital. He or she will want to make sure that the debt documents are sufficiently flexible to accommodate the hospital's plans for expansion and future borrowing, for the creation of affiliated corporations or a foundation, and for the hospital's short-term borrowing needs. In addition, the chief financial officer will want to structure the documents to provide for the best possible treatment of the earnings on the various bond funds by the reimbursement agencies and by the rate-setting agency in the state, if one exists. In these considerations, the chief financial officer will want to work closely with the reimbursement expert from the hospital and with the outside accountants and lawyers expert in reimbursement.

The structure of the debt documents may have a major impact on whether or not there is a Medicare/Medicaid reimbursement offset for earnings on the debt service reserve fund and other funds established under the indenture, and on reimbursement treatment of any extinguishment of debt, whether through a defeasance or prepayment. In addition, the structure of the documents, including rate covenants and provisions with regard to debt repayment, may have an impact on the rates which the state rate-setting entity will allow to be charged. Thus, the hospital's reimbursement expert, whether a full-time employee of the hospital or an outside consultant, should be charged with reviewing the early drafts of the debt documents to assure that they adequately provide for the best reimbursement treatment for the hospital.

INDEPENDENT CERTIFIED PUBLIC ACCOUNTANTS

The hospital's accountants should be involved from the very beginning of the drafting process. They should review carefully the financial covenants of the debt documents and advise on changes that would be advantageous to the hospital. They will be asked to provide comparative financial statements covering the last three to five years for inclusion as an appendix to the official statement. In addition, they will be asked to discuss the hospital's financial condition and any footnotes to their financial reports as part of the "due diligence" review conducted by the underwriters and their counsel.

FINANCIAL FEASIBILITY CONSULTANTS

The marketability of hospital bonds is dependent, in large part, upon the financial feasibility study that projects both the demand for hospital services (the "demand analysis") and the financial position of the hospital (the "financial projections") two to three years after completion of the construction project. There are now at least 20 firms with substantial experience in preparing financial feasibility studies. These include both major accounting firms and hospital consulting firms.

Conflicts of Interest

Some authorities issuing hospital bonds have established guidelines which provide that it is a conflict of interest for the hospital's accountants to act as feasibility consultants. However, in most instances there is no externally imposed prohibition against the hospital retaining its own accountants to act as feasibility consultants.

Choosing a Financial Feasibility Consultant

There are many factors to be considered in choosing a financial feasibility consultant, and it is generally worthwhile for a hospital to interview several firms before deciding on which one it wishes to use. Factors to be considered include the experience of the particular team of people conducting the study (not just of the firm) in preparing financial feasibility studies, the turnaround time for preparing the feasibility study (making sure that it will be prepared in a timely manner to allow the hospital to go to market with its bonds on schedule), and the cost of the feasibility study (in some instances the hospital can establish a fixed price for the feasibility study based on set specifications for the study). Because this is often a very expensive item it may be desirable to negotiate a fixed price contract for it. In addition, some hospitals will want to use the feasibility study as a management tool to help assess how to increase occupancy rates in the future and to determine what additional services should be provided. Also, experience in using the feasibility study as a basis for consulting recommendations should be discussed with prospective feasibility consultants.

INVESTMENT BANKERS

Until a few years ago there were only a handful of investment banking firms that financed hospitals. Today there are at least 20 investment banking houses with broad experience in publicly issued, tax-exempt bonds for hospitals. Several major banks have experience in financing teaching hospitals, though at publication of this book they were still barred by the Glass-Steagall Act from underwriting tax-exempt revenue bonds for nonteaching hospitals. The number of investment banking firms regularly engaged in taxable financings for hospitals is considerably smaller, although if tax-exempt bonds for hospitals should be ended through federal legislation, it is likely that many of the firms currently engaged in tax-exempt financing for hospitals would move into the taxable financing area.

Frequently the hospital will have had an ongoing relationship with an investment banking house which it deems to be satisfactory. The investment bankers (also referred to as the "underwriters") may have periodically helped provide financial information for certificate-of-need applications and counseled the hospital with regard to borrowing at various times. This kind of relationship is valuable for a hospital and the facility may decide that it is best to continue to do all of its financings through one investment banker without opening each financing to general competition. But even when this is done, it is valuable for the hospital to insist that its investment bankers provide detailed comparative information about other bond issues coming to market at the same time as the hospital's. This information should include a description of all the important terms used in a range of other financings and a description of the types of third-party security (letters of credit, guaranties, insurance, etc.). In addition, prior to the signing of the bond purchase agreement the hospital should receive information on interest rates and discounts (the underwriter's "spread" or "fee") for similar deals that are going to market at approximately the same time. This rigorous review of other pending bond issues in the market will help both the regular underwriter and the hospital to realize the very best structure for the hospital's financing and assure that the hospital receives a competitive interest rate and underwriter's discount.

If the hospital does not have a regular investment banker, then it may wish to open the negotiations for the underwriting to three or four investment banking firms. It is probably best for a hospital to look very carefully at a small number of investment banking firms rather than to open the competition so widely that only a casual review of a large number of underwriters is undertaken. When interviewed, each underwriter will suggest the criteria that it thinks is most important for selection. Obviously, underwriters will discuss criteria in which they excel. The following is a list of criteria against which any underwriter may be judged. Each hospital may wish to add to it.

Experience

While it is important that the underwriting firm chosen by the hospital be experienced in both structuring a bond issue and marketing hospital bonds, it is also important that the individual from the investment banking house working on the particular financing be experienced. Occasionally, there will be a "bait and switch" in which the investment banking house will have a very attractive senior member of its firm make the "pitch" for the hospital business. Then a junior, inexperienced member of the firm will be assigned to work with the hospital through the financing. The hospital should insist on knowing exactly who will be working with the hospital on a day-to-day basis and should also make sure that that person's credentials with regard to specific financings on which he or she worked are reviewed thoroughly.

Expertise in Structuring

The investment banker selected should have significant expertise in structuring bond issues with regard to both financial considerations and health care planning and regulatory considerations. The financial considerations include such things as third-party credit arrangements (letters of credit, guaranties, insurance, etc.), the impact of debt provisions, additional borrowing provisions, redemption provisions, the interest rate obtainable on the bonds, and other such considerations. In addition, the underwriter should show demonstrated knowledge and expertise in structuring a bond issue to respond to the peculiar reimbursement, regulatory, and planning framework in which hospitals must function today. These considerations include the hospital's ability to maximize Medicare/ Medicaid reimbursement, the hospital's ability to obtain rates which will permit it to easily repay the debt being incurred in the bond issue, the hospital's ability to engage in corporate reorganization without having to refinance its debt, and other considerations which are peculiar to the hospital industry and of which investment bankers who do not specialize in health care will generally be unaware.

Marketing Capabilities

The investment banker should demonstrate a capability to market bonds to both institutions and individuals. In bond issues larger than $5 million to $10 million, the investment banker will frequently put together a "syndicate" of investment banking houses to assist in selling bonds. The investment banker's experience in syndicating hospital bond issues should be reviewed.

Local Comanager

Sometimes the hospital will want to select a local investment banking house to act as comanager on its bond issue in order to take advantage of local sales capability. The advisability of selection of a local comanager should be discussed with potential lead manager candidates.

The Investment Banker's Fee

The investment banker receives its compensation through a "bond discount." Most frequently, this "discount" or "spread" will be represented as the difference between the face value stated on the bonds (the "par value") and the purchase price at which it purchases the bonds from the issuer. The discount will be allocated to at least four different functions. These include the manager's fee, which it receives for putting together the financing and structuring the bond issue; the expenses of the investment banker, which include not only its own out-of-pocket expenses, but also generally the cost of underwriters' counsel (sometimes the blue sky (state securities authorities) registration fees are paid directly by the hospital and at other times by the investment banker); the "takedown" fee, which is available to the syndicate to cover the risk of purchasing bonds; and the sales fee, which is paid to the bond sellers as an incentive for each bond sold by them. In recent years, the discount normally has ranged between 2.5 percent and 3.5 percent of the total bond issue for financings rated "A" or better. For lower rated or unrated financings the discount generally is somewhat higher to account for the fact that almost all sales of such bonds are made to individuals rather than institutions. Each sale to an individual tends to be considerably smaller in dollar amount than institutional sales, and, therefore, bond issues sold primarily to individuals require a greater sales effort than institutional sales.

Today, the market "risk" factor for investment bankers in hospital bond issues is relatively small. This is because hospital financings are almost always "negotiated" financings in which the investment banker has an opportunity to "presell" the bonds prior to entering into a bond purchase agreement with the hospital. This "preselling" takes place from the time the official statement in preliminary form (the "red herring" or the "preliminary official statement") is distributed. Once the investment bankers in the selling syndicate have sufficient orders for all or most of the bonds being issued, a price recognizing those orders will be offered by the lead manager (the hospital's investment banker) to the hospital in the bond purchase agreement. Thus, the investment banker is not "at risk" if the market for bonds deteriorates after it has purchased the bonds because it has a commitment for purchase for all or most of the bonds prior to buying them from the hospital.

The selling capability of the investment banker during the "preselling" period is very important to the hospital because the bonds are priced on a marginal basis rather than on an average basis. That is, for each maturity of the bonds of the hospital the underwriter will price all of the bonds of that maturity at the interest rate it is able to receive for the last bond it is able to sell of the bonds of that particular maturity. For example, assume that there are $10 million of 30-year term bonds offered in a bond issue. Of those, $9 million can be sold at 10 percent, and the remaining $1 million could only be sold at an interest rate of 10.2 percent. All of the bonds will be priced at 10.2 percent. Thus, since the marginal rate is the rate at which the bonds will be purchased, it can be very important to the hospital, especially in a large bond issue, to have an investment banker who can sell to the widest possible market in order to bring down the marginal rate on the bonds to the lowest possible level.

Negotiations of Discount

It may be to the hospital's advantage to allow the underwriter a generous discount in return for its efforts to price the bonds at an interest rate which is most advantageous to the hospital under current market conditions. If a bond seller can make $20.00 for each $1,000 of bonds sold on a particular hospital's bond issue and only $17.50 on another hospital issue that is pending at the same time, the seller will normally choose to promote the issue which is out at $20.00.

The trade-off between higher discount and lower interest rate should be discussed carefully with the investment banker. The hospital should insist on seeing examples of other recently priced bond issues, showing both the net interest cost on the bonds and the underwriter's discount for the particular bond issue. It may be possible for the hospital to push the underwriter to offer a slightly better interest rate than first offered, and the hospital should be very much involved in the pricing of the bonds.

Issuing Authority's Selection of Investment Bankers

In certain states the statewide issuing authority will select the investment banker to be used by the hospital. In other instances the authority will recommend an investment banker but leave the final decision to the hospital. Although investment bankers who are members of the regular rotating lead management group used by "closed underwriting group authorities" are generally highly competent and reputable investment banking firms, they may not be the best firm for the hospital to use. Thus, even though the authority may recommend a particular investment banking house, it is important that the hospital, whenever possible, make the final decision with regard to its investment banker and feel comfortable that the investment banker's allegiance is primarily to it rather than to the issuing authority. This will give the hospital an advocate to argue over deviations from the authority's standard terms, methods of processing a financing, and timing of the hospital's bond issue. In addition, it will permit the hospital to get certain ongoing free services from the investment banker that may not, as a matter of course, be provided by the investment banker recommended by the authority.

THE LAWYERS

Putting together a major hospital financing requires legal expertise of several different kinds. During the last decade a specialty in health care financing has developed for lawyers, and there are now a number of law firms that specialize in various aspects of health care financing transactions. The hospital administration should be sure that experienced and competent lawyers are selected to represent the hospital and to act as bond counsel. Generally, the hospital's local counsel will not have adequate experience to represent the hospital, and special hospital counsel should be retained. In addition, the hospital administration should insist that the underwriters' counsel is a law firm experienced in both health finance work and general representation of hospitals.

Hospital Counsel

If the hospital's regular counsel has not been involved in a number of previous health care financings, it is advisable for the hospital to seek out special counsel to represent it in negotiation of the financing documents. The hospital's regular counsel, the feasibility consultant, the Hospital Financial Officer's Association, the state hospital association, and the underwriter can advise the hospital about selection of a competent firm of lawyers with wide experience in representing hospitals on health care transactions. The cost of special counsel to a hospital will be small in comparison to the probable dollar savings and the greater flexibility of the debt documents which the hospital will be able to achieve by using an experienced firm. Even if special counsel is selected to help the hospital in negotiating debt documents, the hospital's regular outside counsel will be involved in various aspects of the financing.

The tasks performed by the hospital's counsel and special counsel will include the following:

- assistance with disclosing information to the underwriters with regard to pending litigation and other legal problems which the hospital may be having;
- assistance with certificate-of-need and Section 1122 applications;
- negotiation of construction contracts for the hospital;
- drafting of certain sections of the official statement dealing with disclosure of legal matters and litigation matters;

- negotiation on outstanding debt to be retired prior to the issuance of the bonds;
- participation in the negotiation with the bond trustee with regard to the trustee's fees and services to be rendered by the trustee;
- negotiation of all of the covenants in the debt documents;
- review of various zoning, property, and title matters and obtaining all necessary building permits; and
- delivery of an opinion with regard to the binding effect of the debt documents upon the hospital and various other legal matters (see Appendix 1-A hereto for a form of hospital counsel's opinion).

Bond Counsel

If the bond issue is done in a tax-exempt, rather than taxable way, bond counsel will have to be employed and paid by the hospital. In taxable bond issues, because there is no tax-exemption opinion rendered, there is no bond counsel. Instead, the underwriter's counsel will be the principal draftsman of legal documents. The bond counsel is the "high priest" of tax-exempt financing. Some issuers have a regular bond counsel that they use on all of their transactions, but in most hospital financings the hospital has a choice of which bond counsel firm to use. Bond counsel not only gives opinions with regard to the tax exemption of the hospital bonds and the legality of the bonds under state authorizing legislation, but it also takes primary responsibility for drafting most of the loan documents, including the indenture, the loan agreement, and, if there is one, the mortgage and security agreement or lease and lease-back agreement.

Since bond counsel firms differ in their interpretations of state authorizing legislation and federal tax law, it may be important before selecting the bond counsel to discuss whether bond counsel will render an approving legal opinion on various aspects of the bond issue's structure.

In selecting bond counsel it is important that, at a minimum, the following criteria be met:

1. The bond counsel should have significant experience in acting as bond counsel on hospital financing transactions.
2. If the transaction involves defeasance of outstanding debt, the bond counsel should have had experience in defeasance transactions.
3. The bond counsel should be a firm with which the underwriter feels comfortable.

4. The bond counsel should be a firm that is acceptable to the issuer of the bonds.

Issuer's Counsel

In tax-exempt transactions there frequently will be a counsel for the issuing entity, which is generally an authority, a city, or a county. The role of the issuer's counsel is to give legal opinions stating that the issuer is bound by the documents and that there is no litigation pending against the issuer which would bar it from issuing the bonds.

Underwriters' Counsel

The underwriters' counsel is responsible for representing the underwriter(s) in negotiating the documents, qualifying the bonds for sale in the various states in which the bonds will be marketed ("blue sky work"), and drafting certain of the financing documents, including the bond purchase agreement, the agreement among underwriters (which sets out the contractual relationship among the syndicate members), the blue sky memorandum, and the legal investment survey. Frequently, the underwriters' counsel will be responsible for coordinating the drafting of the official statement. In other instances, this job is done by an employee of the underwriter or an employee of the issuing authority. In taxable bond issues the underwriters' counsel will draft the main legal documents, including the loan agreement, indenture, and, if there is one, a mortgage and security agreement.

The hospital should insist that the underwriters' counsel be experienced in health care financing work. It is helpful to have an underwriters' counsel who understands general hospital representation and is up to date on the various regulatory requirements that affect hospitals, including certificate of need, Section 1122, licensing, rate review, and Medicare/ Medicaid reimbursement questions. All of these are important questions of disclosure for the official statement and also will affect the structure of legal documents. Although the underwriter is responsible for choosing the underwriters' counsel, if the hospital is anxious that a particular experienced underwriters' counsel be hired, frequently the underwriter will acquiesce in hiring that counsel. The legal fees for the underwriters' counsel are paid by the underwriter, except in certain instances where the blue sky registration legal fees are paid by the hospital. This is a matter of negotiation between the hospital and the underwriter and should be established early in the negotiations on the financing.

ISSUING UNIT

In a tax-exempt bond issue (except with "63-20" issues) there has to be a governmental issuer for the bonds. The possible governmental issuers vary from state to state. In many states there is an opportunity to issue bonds not only through statewide health facilities authority, but also through local entities such as counties or cities. In other states bonds are generally issued through a local authority which will generally have powers within either city or county jurisdictional lines.

Some authorities are very experienced and have done many financings. These generally will have their own bond counsel and documents which have standard terms. Often these terms are not as advantageous to the borrowing hospital as the terms it can negotiate with a local issuer, but, even in these situations, the hospital, aided by an experienced counsel, should be able to modify the documents and terms to meet the special needs of that hospital. The larger authorities, particularly statewide authorities, frequently have a financial adviser who will assist in preparing the official statement and give advice with regard to the structure of the bond issue. Generally, the authority's fee and that of its financial adviser will be paid by the hospital, and the fees charged by each available issuer should be discussed before a hospital decides what issuer to use in issuing its bonds.

In those states where a choice of issuers exists the hospital should compare fees and consult with its underwriter and special counsel on which issuer to use.

PRINTERS

In public issues a legal printer will print the official statement, which is used in offering the bonds for public sale. The hospital should consult the underwriter about ways in which to hold down printing costs. The easiest way to accomplish this is to type the first several drafts of the official statement. After the form and substance of the official statement are agreed upon and the statement has been edited two or three times, the final copy should be sent to the printer. Printing fees are very substantial and are paid by the hospital. The investment banker is the best source of information about the financial printers best suited to do the work on a particular issue.

Appendix 1-A

Sample Hospital Counsel Opinion

[Date]

County of Cook
Chicago, Illinois

  Re: $_____ Cook County, Illinois
     Hospital Revenue Bonds, Series 1982
     (Hospital Project)

Gentlemen:

 As counsel to the "Hospital" of Chicago, an Illinois not-for-profit corporation (the "Corporation"), we have examined the proceedings had and taken by the Corporation in connection with the issuance by the County of Cook in the State of Illinois (the "County") of $_____ in aggregate principal amount of its Hospital Revenue Bonds Series 1982, dated June 1, 1982 (the "Series 1982 Bonds"), for the purpose of rendering this opinion pursuant to Section 8(c)(3) of the Purchase Contract dated July 7, 1982 (the "Purchase Contract") between and among the several underwriters named therein, the County, and the Corporation.

 For purposes of this opinion, reference is made to the Purchase Contract, the Indenture of Mortgage and Deed of Trust dated as of July 1, 1982 (the "Indenture") by and between the County and a Bank and Trust Company of Chicago, Illinois (the "Trustee"), the Lease dated as of July 1, 1982 by and between the County and the Corporation (the "Lease"), the Guaranty and Supplemental Agreement dated as of July 1, 1982 by and between the Corporation and the Trustee (the "Guaranty"), the Escrow

Agreement dated July 25, 1982 by and between the Corporation and an Illinois National Bank and Trust Company of Chicago, Chicago, Illinois (the "Escrow Agreement"), and a warranty deed in which the Corporation conveys title to Land and Existing Facilities (such terms as defined in the Indenture) to the County (the "Deed").

In connection with this opinion, we have examined such documents, certificates, records, and corporate proceedings of the Corporation and such other information, documents, and related matters of law as we have deemed necessary to enable us to render this opinion. On the basis of the foregoing, we are of the opinion that:

1. The Corporation has been duly incorporated and is validly existing as a not-for-profit corporation in good standing under the laws of the State of Illinois, with full power and authority to own its properties and conduct its business as described in the Official Statement dated July 7, 1982 (the "Official Statement"), and is duly qualified to do business in each jurisdiction, if any, where its ownership or leasing of property or conduct of business requires such qualification;

2. The Corporation is an organization described in Section 501(c)(3) of the Internal Revenue Code of 1954, as amended (the "Code"), is exempt from Federal income taxes under Section 501(a) of the Code, and is not a "private foundation" as that term is defined in Section 509(a) of the Code; and the application of the proceeds of the Series 1982 Bonds in the manner described in the Official Statement does not constitute a use by the Corporation with respect to a trade or business which is an unrelated trade, or business determined by applying Section 513(a) of the Code;

3. Except for authorizations, consents, approvals, and reviews that may be required under state securities laws, no authorization, consent, approval, or review of any court or public or governmental body or regulatory authority was or is required for the authorization, execution, and delivery by the Corporation of the Purchase Contract, the Lease, the Guaranty, the Deed, or the Escrow Agreement, or for any action by the Corporation taken in connection with the transactions contemplated thereby or by the Official Statement, which has not been obtained or effected;

4. The Purchase Contract, the Lease, the Guaranty, the Deed, and the Escrow Agreement have each been duly authorized, executed, and delivered by the Corporation and each is a legal, valid, and binding instrument of the Corporation, enforceable in accordance with its terms, except as such enforcement may be limited by bankruptcy,

reorganization, insolvency, moratorium, or similar laws affecting the enforcement of creditors' rights generally and except that the availability of the remedies of specific performance and injunction may be subject to the discretion of the court;

5. The Corporation has duly approved the provisions of the Indenture, the Preliminary Official Statement, dated June 26, 1982 (the "Preliminary Official Statement"), and the Official Statement and has duly authorized the use of the Official Statement as provided in the Purchase Contract;

6. Nothing has come to our attention, after due inquiry, which would lead us to believe that the information contained in the Official Statement (excluding therefrom financial statements, statistical data, and the Feasibility Study, but including particularly and without limitation the information contained under the captions "The Project," "Estimated Sources and Uses of Funds," and "The Hospital") contains an untrue statement of a material fact or omits to state a material fact necessary to make the statements therein, in light of the circumstances under which they were made, not misleading;

7. To the best of our knowledge, after due inquiry, there is no action, suit, proceeding, or investigation at law or in equity before or by any court, public board or body, pending or threatened against the Corporation, or to which the Corporation is a party or its property is subject, wherein an unfavorable decision, ruling, or finding would materially adversely affect the transactions contemplated hereby or by the Official Statement, or the validity or enforceability of the Purchase Contract, the Series 1982 Bonds, the Lease, the Indenture, the Guaranty, the Deed, or the Escrow Agreement or, except with respect to one suit as to which litigation counsel for the Corporation has given its opinion that the possibility of an adverse determination in a material amount is remote, upon which opinion we believe the Purchasers (as defined in the Purchase Contract) may reasonably rely, the financial conditions or operations of the Corporation;

8. The execution and delivery of the Purchase Contract, the Lease, the Guaranty, the Deed, and the Escrow Agreement, and the other agreements contemplated thereby and by the Official Statement, the approval by the Corporation of the Indenture, the Series 1982 Bonds, the Preliminary Official Statement, and the Official Statement, and compliance with the provisions thereof, do not and will not conflict with or constitute on the part of the Corporation a breach of or default under (a) Articles of Incorporation or Bylaws

of the Corporation, (b) to the best of our knowledge, after due inquiry, any resolution adopted by the Corporation or any agreement or instrument to which the Corporation is a party or by which it or its property is bound or (c) to the best of our knowledge, after due inquiry, any law, regulation, court order or consent decree to which the Corporation or its property is subject; and, to the best of our knowledge, after due inquiry, the Corporation is in compliance with all material laws and regulations applicable to it and its business;

9. To the best of our knowledge after due inquiry, the current use of the Land and Existing Facilities, the intended use of the Hospital Facilities, and the undertaking of the Project are in compliance with all laws, ordinances, agreements, or restrictions affecting land use and development;

10. The contracts described in the Official Statement under the caption "The Project" have been duly and validly authorized, executed, and delivered by the Corporation and are in full force and effect as of the date hereof;

11. Appropriate financing statements have been duly filed in all necessary offices with respect to the Gross Receipts (as defined in the Indenture), in order to perfect a first security interest in the County in such Gross Receipts to the extent possible under Illinois law;

12. The Lease creates a valid assignment to the County of the Corporation's Gross Receipts to the extent permitted by applicable law;

13. Except as set forth above, there is no requirement to record, rerecord, file or refile any document or other instrument to maintain the security interest purported to be created by the Lease except for the filing from time to time of continuation statements with respect to the financing statement described above, as may be required by law;

14. The Corporation has all approvals, licenses, and permits required under federal, state, or local laws or regulations (a) to enable it to carry on its business and operate its properties, (b) to construct, improve, or otherwise undertake the Project, except certain building and occupancy permits and other similar approvals, which we have no reason to believe cannot be obtained in due course, and (c) to qualify the Project for inclusion in the reimbursement base recognized by Medicare, Medicaid and Blue Cross for purposes of reimbursement under such programs; and the Corporation is in compliance with all requirements and conditions for the continued effectiveness of such approvals, licenses, and permits;

15. The Corporation has conveyed the County good and marketable title to the real estate specifically described in Exhibit A to the Indenture, free of all liens, charges, and encumbrances except Permitted Encumbrances (as defined in the Indenture); and
16. All of the Hospital Facilities are or will be located on the Land.

In rendering our opinion, we have relied upon title insurance policies dated July 6, 1982 issued by Chicago Title Insurance Company to the County and the Trustee and plats of survey of the Land and Existing Facilities (as defined in the Indenture) dated as of January 20, 1982, prepared by _____.

Very truly yours,

[Name of Counsel]

Chapter 2

The Capital Markets*

Geoffrey B. Shields

THE NEED TO BORROW

A number of factors have led to a voracious appetite among health care institutions for debt financing. Demographic factors including population growth, the increase in the median age of the population, and shifts of the population to the suburbs, the "sun-belt," and the "energy-belt" have created a long-term need for new health care facilities. New technology and the aging of physical plant and equipment dictate that there is a regular cyclical need for replacement financing. Various estimates of new health care construction costs in 1985 range from $6.5 billion to $11 billion.

In addition to new construction and equipment financing, administrators frequently refinance outstanding debt. Sometimes this is to take advantage of lower interest rates. At other times outstanding debt documents do not permit the issuance of the additional parity debt needed to finance construction or acquisition projects. In these cases, the old debt must be retired or defeased. Generally, this is done with money raised through borrowing. Changing management practices, the desire to accomplish a corporate reorganization, and the desire to merge or acquire new facilities have in many instances led to refinancing or advance refunding of outstanding debt in order to free the hospital of onerous restrictive covenants.

Debt financing is often the only viable means for many health care institutions to finance new physical plants. Construction financed with charitable contributions has been on the decline for a decade, and new tax laws further decrease the incentive of the charitable deduction.[1] Rate

---

* Donald A. Carlson, Jr., Executive Vice President and Director of Sales of Ziegler Securities, Inc., was of special help in preparing this chapter.

review, decreased Medicaid and Medicare reimbursement rates, and, in some cases, management and board decisions to hold down hospital room rates mean that few health care facilities accumulate sufficient surpluses to finance construction projects internally. Nor can not-for-profit institutions turn to the equity markets, although recent corporate reorganizations have meant that not-for-profit health corporations more and more frequently include for-profit affiliates in their "families" of corporations.[2] Eventually, some of these for-profit affiliates may sell stock to the public.

As the need for debt financing has increased, so has the availability, variety, and innovation of debt financing techniques. Until 1963, with the advent of the "63-20" method of tax-exempt financing, not-for-profit health care facilities borrowed at taxable rates, generally through banks

Table 2-1 Hospital Bond Issuers

	State	Local		State	Local
Alabama		X	Montana		X
Alaska	X	X	Nebraska		X
Arizona	X	X	Nevada	X	X
Arkansas		X	New Hampshire	X	
California	X	X	New Jersey	X	
Colorado	X	X	New Mexico		X
Connecticut	X		New York	X	
Delaware	X		North Carolina	X	X
District of Columbia	X		North Dakota		X
Florida		X	Ohio		X
Georgia		X	Oklahoma		X
Hawaii	X		Oregon		X
Idaho	X		Pennsylvania		X
Illinois	X	X	Rhode Island	X	
Indiana		X	South Carolina		X
Iowa		X	South Dakota	X	X
Kansas		X	Tennessee		X
Kentucky	X	X	Texas		X
Louisiana	X	X	Utah		X
Maine	X		Vermont	X	
Maryland	X	X	Virginia		X
Massachusetts	X		Washington	X	
Michigan	X	X	West Virginia		X
Minnesota		X	Wisconsin	X	X
Mississippi		X	Wyoming		X
Missouri	X	X	Total	27	38

Source: Legal Survey by Gardner, Carton & Douglas.

and insurance companies, or the handful of investment banking firms willing to underwrite hospitals in the era before Medicare and Medicaid reimbursement gave, or appeared to give, hospitals the assurance of a dependable source of cash flow.

Since 1970, every state has passed enabling legislation permitting local, county, or statewide entities (generally referred to as "authorities") to issue tax-exempt bonds to finance private not-for-profit health care facilities. Many states have multiple issuing entities which give a not-for-profit hospital and its investment bankers a choice of issuer through which to borrow tax-exempt funds.[3]

Table 2-1 shows the current availability of local and statewide issuers.

For-profit health care facilities now frequently borrow up to $10 million per project at tax-exempt rates through industrial development bonds. Recently, nursing home and life care facilities have turned frequently to tax-exempt financing for funds. The availability of tax-exempt financing for proprietary health care facilities is discussed in a later chapter.

Table 2-2 shows the approximate volume of hospital financing from 1975 to 1981.

THE CREDIT MARKETS

Long-term publicly offered health care issues are typically structured to appeal to one of more of several categories of purchasers.

Purchasers of tax-exempt bonds are usually one of four types of investors: commercial banks, insurance companies, bond funds, or individuals. On the other hand, taxable health care facility bonds are typically purchased by either individuals, life insurance companies, or, occasionally, pension funds.

The mix of the potential purchasers of health care bonds has varied significantly over time. During the 1970s, particularly as it relates to tax-exempt financings, there was an increase on the part of certain institutional investors in their purchasing health care credits. However, because of the unique nature of hospital finance, there is still a certain reluctance on the part of some institutions to purchase hospital bonds. This in part stems from the difficulty they perceive in evaluating and analyzing different hospital credits as well as the uncertainty of government programs that could affect the underlying credit worthiness of hospital operations.

Since 1980, there has been a dramatic decrease in the purchases of all tax-exempt bonds by institutional investors. Commercial banks have developed a large number of tax shelters, thus decreasing their appetite for

Table 2-2 Hospital Financing Volume 1975–1981

(In Millions of Dollars)

	Public Tax-Exempt Offerings	Private Placements*	Public Taxable Offerings	Government-Sponsored Programs	Mortgages with Commercial Banks	Total
1975						
Dollar Volume	1,959	44	275	350	100	2,728
Market Share (%)	71.8	1.6	10.1	12.8	3.7	100.0
1976						
Dollar Volume	2,726	214	300	500	200	3,940
Market Share (%)	69.2	5.4	7.6	12.7	5.1	100.0
1977						
Dollar Volume	4,731	381	350	600	250	6,312
Market Share (%)	75.0	6.0	5.5	9.5	4.0	100.0
1978						
Dollar Volume	3,122	339	275	290	200	4,226
Market Share (%)	73.9	8.0	6.5	6.9	4.7	100.0
1979						
Dollar Volume	3,517	253	325**	250**	200**	4,545
Market Share (%)	77.4	5.6	7.2	5.4	4.4	100.0
1980						
Dollar Volume	3,558	283	325**	225**	150**	4,541
Market Share (%)	78.4	6.1	7.2	5.0	3.3	100.0
1981						
Dollar Volume	5,045	330***	300**	175**	150**	6,000
Market Share (%)	84.1	5.5	5.0	2.9	2.5	100.0

* The source for private placement does not differentiate between taxable and tax-exempt. Currently, almost all private placements are tax-exempt.
** Estimated, based upon discussions with investment banking firms.
*** Estimated, based on first six months' figures.

Sources: For tax-exempt public offerings, *The Bond Buyer;* for private placements, *Investment Dealer's Digest;* for government-sponsored programs, U.S. Department of Housing and Urban Development and *National Journal.*

tax-exempt securities. Insurance companies have been almost completely out of the tax-exempt bond market because of their own underwriting losses and, therefore, lack of cash flow to be channeled into tax-exempt bonds. However, while the institutional investor has lost its appetite for tax exemption, the "household sector" (consisting of direct purchases by individuals and purchases by individuals through various types of bond funds and trust investment departments) has taken up much of the slack. Until the recent Reagan Administration tax cuts were imposed, individuals had steadily increased their purchases of tax-exempt securities, including health care issues. The tax-exempt bond funds, both unit trusts and managed funds, have steadily increased their purchases of health care bonds in the past few years, and about 80 percent of all tax-exempt health care issues are now being sold to the "household sector" whereas, in the late 1970s, institutions accounted for a much larger percentage of purchases.

HOUSEHOLD SECTOR

Individuals currently account for an increasingly significant percentage of health care bonds purchase—both taxable and tax-exempt. In fact, without the "household sector," including bond funds and trust investment departments, there really would be no viable market for health care bonds.

During 1981 and 1982, the usual percentage gap between the interest rates available on taxable and tax-exempt securities narrowed significantly. This was, in part, because of the uncertainty created by the impact of tax-cut legislation in combination with a very large volume of tax-exempt bonds available for sale. However, in more normal market conditions, investors with a marginal tax rate on investment income of 35 percent or higher improved their after-tax return by investing in tax-exempt rather than taxable securities. During the period from 1975 to 1980, the normal interest rate on a tax-exempt bond issue was about 65 percent of the interest rate on an equivalently rated taxable bond issue. A tax-exempt bond paying 12 percent to the investor in the 39 percent tax bracket would be worth a 19.68 percent yield if the buyer had to pay taxes on it. The 1981 tax cuts reduce the maximum marginal tax rate on unearned income of individuals from 70 percent to 50 percent as of 1982. The tax brackets are pushed considerably higher for the years 1982 through 1984. In addition, the Economic Recovery Tax Act of 1981 provides that after 1984 tax brackets will be adjusted to account for inflation. In addition, the "all savers certificate" plan will permit individuals through 1983 to receive up to $1,000 per person in tax-exempt interest from deposits with banks and savings and loans. The overall impact of these tax reforms is to diminish the attractiveness to individuals of investing in tax-exempt bonds, thereby tending to decrease the yield or interest rate spread between tax-exempt and taxable bonds.

COMMERCIAL BANKS

Although major buyers of tax-exempt bonds, commercial banks have never purchased a proportionate amount of health facilities bonds. Commercial banks must be more concerned with liquidity of investments than insurance companies and, therefore, do not purchase health care bonds because they provide a less viable secondary market than general obligation bonds. Insurance companies, on the other hand, are less concerned about liquidity than about the credit aspects of a given health care issue. Commercial banks tend to buy hospital bonds when loan demands and interest rates are low, continuing well into the business cycle expansion. Demand for business loans generally increases late in a business cycle. At this phase of the business cycle, banks slow their purchases of tax-exempt bonds, and some sell a portion of their holdings. This pattern has prevailed since the late 1940s.

While commercial banks increased their percentage of total purchase of tax-exempt bonds during the 1960s, this pattern was reversed during the 1970s. Leasing operations, through which banks could take advantage of the investment tax credit, permitted commercial banks an alternative method by which to lower their tax payments significantly. Still more favorable investment tax credit provisions in the Economic Recovery Tax Act of 1981 may further decrease commercial banks' appetites for tax-exempt bonds.

Commercial banks generally invest in maturities of tax-exempt bonds of 15 years or less, the so-called "serial bond" maturities, to assure themselves of liquidity and generally are reluctant to purchase bonds rated below an "A" rating. The trust departments of commercial banks also invest in tax-exempt health care bonds for their trust accounts. Generally, they will purchase bonds rated "A" or better for these accounts.

NONLIFE INSURANCE COMPANIES

Casualty insurance company profits are cyclical, depending upon the premium rates state insurance regulators permit companies to charge. In the mid-1970s insurance company purchases of tax-exempt bonds were particularly strong, reflecting premium rate increases authorized by the state insurance commissions. Since then, rate increases have generally not kept up with inflation. However, property and casualty companies have continued to increase the percentage of their assets held in tax-exempt bonds. By 1980, assets of property and casualty insurance companies held in tax-exempt bonds equalled about 50 percent of their total assets compared with 33 percent in 1970 and 25 percent in 1960. During 1981, the interest of nonlife insurance companies in tax-exempt bonds decreased as they sought to diversify their portfolios.

The accelerated depreciation provisions of the Economic Recovery Tax Act of 1981 may decrease the appetite for tax-exempt bonds of insurance companies as well as commercial banks.

TAXABLE BONDS

Taxable health care bonds have accounted for a decreasing portion of health care capital financing in recent years. As more and more states have passed enabling legislation permitting the issuance of tax-exempt health facility bonds and as concerns of the hospitals over having a governmental issuer have diminished, the lower interest rates and longer terms available for tax-exempt bonds have proved sufficiently attractive to convince most health care borrowers to use the tax-exempt borrowing route.

However, recent federal government initiative to end or curtail tax-exempt financing has increased interest in the availability of taxable financing.[4] Also, the narrowing of the spread between taxable and tax-exempt bonds and the high and volatile interest rates of recent years have increased the interest in medium-term (five- to ten-year), balloon-taxable bonds, callable at any time without penalty, as a way to borrow quickly with a minimum of refinancing cost once rates decline.

Sales of taxable health facility bonds (including public taxable bonds, government guaranty programs, and conventional institutional notes or mortgage placements) are made primarily to commercial banks, life insurance companies, pension funds (rather than nonlife insurance companies), individuals, and taxable bond funds.

Most sales to individuals and substantial bond fund sales are made through public sales by underwriters specializing in taxable health care bonds. These underwriters have built up a client base interested in purchasing taxable hospital bonds.

Sales of bonds to insurance companies are generally made on a direct placement basis. Banks are most interested in the shortest maturities while other institutional investors, such as insurance companies and bond funds, are more interested in longer-term maturities that provide the highest interest rate available.

NOTES

1. K. Schaner, "Tax Act Tosses Crumb to Nonprofits," *Modern Healthcare*, November 1981, p. 110; G. Shields, "Tax-exempt Ax Won't Work," *Modern Healthcare*, November 1981, p. 112.

2. Illinois Institute for Continuing Legal Education, *Representing Health Care Institutions and Professionals* (Chicago: The Institute, 1980), chap. 7.

3. Tax-exempt bonds for health care facilities are issued under a wide variety of statutory and constitutional authority. Bond counsel should be consulted about the applicable statutory authority for a particular financing.

4. D.L. Yanish, "Threat to Tax-exempt Bonds Forces Hospitals to Consider Alternatives," *Modern Healthcare*, November 1981, p. 106.

SUGGESTED READINGS

Changing Conditions in the Market for State and Local Government Debt. Joint Economic Committee, Congress of the United States, 1976.

Comprehensive Bond Values Tables. Boston: Financial Publishing Co, 1981.

E.F. Hutton Public Finance Group. *Selling Municipal Bonds.* New York: E.F. Hutton & Co., 1978.

Public Securities Association. *The Bond Guide.* Municipal Finance Statistics. New York: PSA, 1979.

Public Securities Association. *Tax Exempt Securities, An Investor's Guide.* New York: PSA, 1979.

Chapter 3

Debt Capacity, Credit Analysis, and the Rating Agencies

William J. Gray

DEBT CAPACITY

This discussion will concentrate upon debt capacity with respect to tax-exempt financing for nonprofit hospitals. Different financing approaches and for-profit status can alter an institution's debt capacity, but the principles of the analysis remain the same. Similarly, the assessment of debt capacity for nursing homes, retirement centers, clinics, and other health care institutions involves variations in analytical techniques, but, once again, the underlying principles are comparable.

Purpose

The purpose of the debt capacity analysis can best be described within the context of the long-range planning process. The textbook approach to developing a hospital's long-range plan often begins with the role and program study. This phase consists of identifying the health care needs in the hospital's service area and determining which of those needs to satisfy and what programs are required to do that. The second phase typically involves the identification of the resources required to implement those programs. Those resources include staff, facilities, and capital. It is at this stage that the debt capacity analysis comes into play.

Prior to expending the considerable time, effort, and money necessary to develop a detailed functional and space program and proceeding on to schematics, an assessment of the source of funds for the project is in order. When debt is contemplated as one of those sources, the debt capacity analysis becomes an appropriate step at this juncture in the planning process. In effect, the debt capacity analysis can serve as an early-warning mechanism to prevent the expenditure of time and money on a plan that runs a risk of being financially infeasible. In a sense, the purpose of the debt capacity analysis is to make the subsequent financial feasibility study an assessment of the extent to which the project is feasible, rather than whether it is feasible at all.

Scope and Approach

Unlike the financial feasibility study, the debt capacity analysis is an internal management tool and is not used to obtain financing. Consequently, its contents are not as formally defined as are those of a feasibility study which is subjected to the scrutiny of the rating agencies and potential lenders.

This lack of formal definition of content implies a degree of flexibility in scope, which is the case. The debt capacity analysis, as a checkpoint in the planning process, should be designed to provide comfort to the hospital in making the decision to proceed to the next phase of project planning. Each institution may have a different comfort level, so the depth of analysis will also differ from hospital to hospital. The analysis described in this chapter represents a scope that is effective in providing the degree of comfort required for most hospitals that have reached the above-described juncture in the planning process.

The analysis consists of two components, ratio analysis and analysis of nonfinancial factors. As the components suggest, the analysis of debt capacity is not a formula that will yield a specific number. Rather, it is a mix of numerical analyses and nonquantifiable considerations. The former provides a picture of the financial impact of incurring a specified level of debt, and the latter is intended to gauge the prudence of absorbing that impact.

Ratio Analysis

The ratio analysis component of the debt capacity assessment is conducted in two parts—historical and projected. The historical analysis is intended to provide a picture of the institution's relative financial health and to reveal trends, both positive and negative, which could enhance or restrict debt capacity, respectively. The projected analysis is intended to assess the impact that the debt will have upon financial operations as measured by certain key ratios.

Historical Analysis

The historical financial performance of the hospital will be carefully evaluated by the credit rating agencies and/or lenders. Operating results, ratios of income statement and balance sheet items, and degree of reliance on nonoperating income, among others, are examined with attention given to stability, positive growth, and existence of any negative or erratic patterns. For example, borrowing for cash flow purposes and high levels of accounts receivable are causes for concern.

The following ratios covering areas of liquidity, capital structure, activity, and profitability are helpful in assessing financial health.

- *Current ratio* measures the number of dollars held in current assets per dollar of current liabilities.

- *Quick ratio* is a more stringent test, measuring the number of dollars of liquid assets (cash plus marketable securities) plus accounts receivable per dollar of current liabilities.

- *Acid test ratio* is the most stringent test of liquidity, measuring the number of dollars in liquid assets (cash and marketable securities) available per dollar of current liabilities. This ratio provides a measure of ability to pay short-term obligations under the worst of all possible circumstances, that is, no collection of accounts receivable, normally the primary source of funds for payment of current liabilities.

- *Days in patient accounts receivable* provides a measure of the average time that receivables are outstanding, or the average collection period. A consistently high collection period value indicates required maintenance of a higher operating margin to provide the required level of permanent equity financing.

- *Average payment period* measures the average time that elapses before current liabilities are paid, that is, it measures the number of days of cash expenses not currently paid. High values may be an indication of liquidity problems.

- *Cash flow to total debt ratio* is an important indicator of possible future financial problems. Cash flow measures current funds available to retire debt, increase working capital or replace capital assets. Debt repayment is a nondiscretionary, contractual obligation with a priority in use of funds. Therefore, a decrease in this ratio may indicate a future debt repayment problem.

- *Equity financing ratio* measures the proportion of total assets financed with equity. High values imply that little debt financing has been used to acquire assets and may indicate that future debt financing is feasible and prudent.

- *Total asset turnover ratio* provides an index of the number of operating revenue dollars generated per dollar of asset investment. Higher values imply greater generation of revenues from a limited resource base. However, the ratio is affected by the age of the assets, placing a premium on operating with an old asset base.

- *Fixed asset turnover ratio* measures operating revenue dollars generated per dollar of fixed asset investment. High values imply good generation of revenue from a limited fixed asset base and are generally regarded as indicating efficient operation. The values can be distorted by age, older hospitals being more likely to attain higher values.

- *Current asset turnover ratio* measures the number of operating revenue dollars generated per dollar of investment in current assets. The lower the investment base in current assets, the more efficient the hospital and the higher the ratio value. A low ratio value may indicate an overinvestment in current assets.

- *Markup ratio* defines the multiple by which rates are set above expenses. High values imply higher rates or revenues per dollar of expenses and a greater likelihood of a favorable excess of revenues over expenses position.

- *Operating margin ratio* defines the proportion of operating revenue (net of deductions) retained as revenue. It is often used as the primary test of profitability.

- *Return on assets ratio* defines the amount of excess of revenues over expenses earned per dollar of investment. It provides a measure of the return on capital invested in operations. Adequate return is essential to continued viability and asset replacement. Values are affected by the average age of a hospital's plant.

- *Return on equity ratio* defines the amount of excess of revenues over expenses earned per dollar of equity investment. This is another primary test of financial viability. However, it is considered most significant where investors expect a return and is less important where debt is the financing vehicle.

- *Average age of plant ratio* measures in years the average age of fixed assets. High values indicate an older fixed asset base and the greater likelihood of a need for near-term replacement. This may indicate the need for financing, particularly where the excess of revenues over expenses has been minimal.

While trends in the financial performance of the hospital can be assessed in isolation by examining data over a five-year period, the results of the historical analysis are more meaningful when they are compared with other hospitals. This can be accomplished through the use of a database such as the Financial Analysis Service of the Hospital Financial Management Association. That particular database presents lower and upper quartiles and medians for these ratios for hospitals classified by bed size and region.

Projected Analysis

In gauging the financial impact of incurring a specified level of debt, the examination of a number of ratios can be revealing. Specifically, the following five ratios can provide an indication of ability to repay, debt burden, and leverage:

1. coverage of maximum debt service—maximum annual debt service divided into net income before interest, depreciation, and amortization
2. maximum debt service per patient day
3. maximum debt service as a percent of net operating revenue
4. long-term debt as a percent of long-term debt plus unrestricted fund balance
5. long-term debt per bed

Of the above ratios, the first one, debt service coverage, is the most critical, and the last one, debt per bed, the least. Debt service coverage is a straightforward test of the hospital's ability to repay the debt, with one exception. The ratio does not take into consideration the effect of working capital needs on the actual funds that would be available to service the debt. That is why a debt service coverage ratio of one, while appearing to be exactly sufficient, is in fact too little.

Debt per bed can be a useful rule of thumb, but it has several deficiencies which make it an unreliable measure by itself. First, it does not reflect the impact of the interest rate level. Debt per bed of $100,000 bearing interest at 10 percent is certainly a different proposition than the same level, but at 18 percent. Second, it does not take into consideration the differences among hospitals in revenue-generating capacity per bed. A hospital producing $500 of revenue per bed per day could very well service a higher level of debt per bed than a hospital producing $250. However, this ratio is popular with some investors and to some degree with the rating agencies, and it can be a useful measure of relative debt level when compared with a group of similar hospitals in terms of size and level of care.

These five ratios should be calculated for the first full year of debt service following project completion, when debt service must be paid from hospital operations rather than from bond proceeds. By making assumptions with regard to the levels of net operating revenue and net income for that year, all of the ratios can be calculated without constructing complete projected financial statements.

The issue again is one of comfort level. If the hospital is contemplating a major project that will affect its bed capacity and most of the ancillary departments, a pro forma operating statement may be necessary to proceed confidently to the next level of planning. On less ambitious projects, calculation of the ratios without projected financial statements may very well serve the planning needs at that decision level.

If a projected operating statement is done, the projections should be made in current dollars as well as inflated ones. In that way, the true financial impact of the proposed project can be isolated more easily and expressed in real terms. If, as is reasonable to expect, inflation affects other hospitals to approximately the same degree, it will be the real dollar impact of the project that will become the important factor in assessing whether there will be competitive or reimbursement problems with which to contend.

Database Comparison

The projected ratios carry meaning in their own right, particularly the debt service coverage ratio. However, as with the historical analysis, they take on added significance when compared to a database of the same ratios for other hospitals.

Table 3-1 presents ratio averages for 291 hospitals that incurred tax-exempt debt during 1979, 1980, and 1981. The data are arrayed according to the bond rating received from Standard & Poor's Corporation. The 291 hospitals represent a sample of those bond issues rated by Standard & Poor's during that period and do not necessarily reflect the actual averages for all bond issues so rated.

In making comparisons with the database, it should be remembered that the figures in the base are averages. The ranges for each ratio can be quite wide. For example, a hospital with $121,000 of debt per bed could receive an A− from Standard & Poor's while one with $38,000 of debt per bed might receive a BBB. Consequently, no single ratio should be viewed in isolation. Poor performance on one ratio may be more than made up by strong results on another. The hospital with the $121,000 debt per bed figure might also have had strong debt service coverage.

Sensitivity Analysis

Any projection involves making assumptions. The mathematics of calculating the projected ratios is not the area where errors are likely to

Table 3-1 Comparative Statistics for Standard & Poor's
Rating Categories

			Rating Category			
	BBB	*BBB+*	*A−*	*A*	*A+*	*AA*
Number of bond issues in the sample	22	25	66	106	62	10
Number of beds*	133	189	212	302	504	1,059
Percent occupancy*	71.7	75.6	76.2	79.9	81.0	83.4
Average age of active medical staff*	44.9	46.4	45.5	45.9	45.9	44.6
Percent of active staff board certified*	57.9	61.3	65.9	66.9	67.0	76.7
Percent of patient revenues from Medicare/Medicaid*	48.0	46.8	45.8	43.5	40.3	41.6
Net income as a percent of net operating revenue*	3.5	4.7	5.2	4.9	5.3	5.7
Coverage of maximum debt service**	1.6x	1.9x	2.2x	2.3x	2.7x	3.4x
Maximum debt service per patient day**	$38.00	$28.00	$27.00	$27.00	$19.00	$17.00
Maximum debt service as a percent of net operating revenue**	10.8	8.7	8.7	6.3	5.4	3.7
Long-term debt as a percent of long-term debt plus unrestricted fund balance**	86.2	73.3	70.6	64.8	58.2	42.3
Long-term debt per bed (in thousands of dollars)**	$94.9	$75.6	$76.0	$70.8	$67.8	$51.5

* As of the most recent fiscal year prior to bond sale.
** As projected for the first full fiscal year of debt service on the bonds.

Source: Blyth Eastman Paine Webber Health Care Funding Database.

occur. It is in the underlying assumptions that the risk lies. While the analyst attempts to make the most reasonable conservative assumption in each case, it is often useful to assess the impact that a change in any given assumption will have on the projection. This can be accomplished by performing a sensitivity analysis.

One of the key assumptions in the calculation of the debt service coverage ratio is the projected level of operating surplus or net income. The sensitivity of the coverage ratio to the net income assumption can be analyzed by calculating the ratio using a variety of net income levels. Similarly, the interest rate on the debt being contemplated can also affect several of the projected ratios. A sensitivity analysis assuming varying rates of interest will reveal the range of impact in this area. Utilization and revenue levels are also candidates for sensitivity analysis.

Competitive and Reimbursement Considerations

Strong performance on both a historical and a projected basis with regard to ratio analysis is an encouraging indication that the debt level under consideration is realistic. However, assessment of the impact that the project, the debt, and the attendant cost and charge increases will have on the hospital's competitiveness and ability to meet reimbursement constraints is also in order.

Competition among hospitals has typically manifested itself in efforts to attract and retain physicians and increase services more than in maintaining lower rates. While this may still be the case to a great extent, rate competition is taking on more importance in some areas of the country. If the intent of the Reagan Administration is realized, price competition will play a much greater role nationwide. Consequently, any assessment of debt capacity should logically include an analysis of the cost and rate impact of a project in relation to the costs and rates of the other hospitals in the service area.

The cost effect of the project can be analyzed by isolating the incremental costs that will result. These will include depreciation and interest expense in all instances where debt is used. If the plant size is increased, additional plant maintenance, housekeeping, and utility expense will occur. Other overhead costs, such as security and insurance, can be similarly identified by examining the components of the project and reviewing the detailed departmental cost center financial statement to determine which areas will incur additional costs. Even though these costs will not appear until the new areas are occupied, it is useful to calculate them on a current dollar basis without inflation. Once calculated, the costs can be allocated to the routine service, ancillary and outpatient revenue centers based upon the origin of the cost (that is, which department is being expanded or renovated), and the overhead allocation methodology utilized by the hospital. Once allocated, the incremental cost impact per unit of service can be calculated and assessed in light of the costs of competitors and of any reimbursement ceilings or rate review that may exist.

Analysis of Nonfinancial Factors

Hospitals have very good records as debtors. To date, the default rate on hospital loans, particularly tax-exempt bonds, has been very low. Most of the defaults that have occurred stemmed from either a failure to attain projected utilization or construction cost overruns. When construction has proceeded smoothly and utilization has attained or nearly attained projected targets, defaults have been virtually nonexistent.

One of the key assumptions made in the debt capacity analysis is projected utilization. At the stage in the planning process where the debt capacity analysis comes into play, the hospital has typically completed a role and program study which contains utilization projections. If such a study has been completed, presumably the utilization projections are based upon a somewhat rigorous analysis. If so, it is neither necessary nor useful for the debt capacity analyst to duplicate that effort. However, examination of the areas of market environment and medical staff can provide an indication of the overall strength or vulnerability of the utilization projections.

Market Environment

Market environment includes demographic, economic, and competitive factors. The utilization projections should be consistent with the demographic trend and pattern in the service area. Growth in utilization without population growth should be explained by aging, for example. The underlying economic trend in the service area can often provide a clue as to future demographic changes and resultant changes in utilization and reimbursement mix. With regard to competitive factors, Standard & Poor's Corporation explains its approach to analysis in the following manner:

> We also closely examine historical trends in utilization for the preceding five years. The important inpatient statistics are admissions, average length of stay, patient days, number of beds in service and occupancy. We look at ancillary services, outpatient and emergency room trends. These trends are considered within the context of the market in which the hospital is situated. We are particularly concerned with the competitive environment and credit will be given for market dominance or monopoly. Excess supply resulting from "overbedding" is a major concern, and the hospital's occupancy relative to the average area occupancy is considered. We also analyze service area use rates (admissions and patient days per thousand) to determine whether patients are

patronizing local hospitals or leaving the service area in favor, perhaps, of larger hospitals outside the service area. Conversely, the hospital may be capturing admissions and referrals from outside its immediate service area. In this part of the analysis, our focus is on the hospital's market share and on stability and trends thereof. Reasons for declining market share are examined in close detail and because of their potential impact on market share we also need information regarding any planned hospital expansions within the service area. The economic and demographic characteristics of the service area are also major considerations.

The utilization forecasts provided within the feasibility report should be consistent with historical performance. We are particularly concerned with the justification behind forecasts which assume increased market share or increased use rates reflecting greater penetration of the service area. Similarly, the base demographic projections to which use rates are applied should be reasonable and consistent with historical trends.[1]

Medical Staff

For most hospitals, the medical staff is still the major source of patients and therefore utilization. The strength or vulnerability of the utilization projections consequently hinges to a great extent upon the composition of the medical staff. Standard & Poor's Corporation again explains its analytical approach:

> Since the physician is the primary client of the hospital, a detailed analysis of the medical staff is probably the most important single component of our analysis.

> Our analysis seeks to determine the relative strengths and vulnerabilities of the staff relative to the size of the facility, the services offered, the area which it serves, and the availability of physicians in the area. We are particularly concerned with the number of physicians who utilize said hospital as the primary hospital for their admissions and the overlap between staffs of the hospital and competing hospitals. We look for gaps or potential weaknesses in the various specialties, particularly in the case of small facilities. Similarly, a medical staff with a high average age or one which is not sufficiently represented in the younger

age categories may be indicative of recruiting problems and may forewarn a potentially serious problem. Net additions to the staff in recent years provide an insight into the attractiveness of the hospital to physicians, the compatability of management and the medical staff, and the acceptance by the staff of new physicians. We are also interested in the reasons physicians may have left the staff. Staff allegiance is particularly important in highly competitive or overbedded areas. Board certification is more relevant in large institutions. Our concern here is that the staff's credentials are consistent with the role of the institution.[2]

Examination of the above factors by the debt capacity analyst may result in the use of more conservative projections in the analysis, or perhaps a sensitivity analysis of utilization indicating the impact at varying levels.

Summary

The debt capacity analysis is a step in the overall project planning process. It serves as an early warning mechanism to prevent the expenditure of time and money on a plan that runs a risk of being financially infeasible. The major purpose of the analysis is to provide a level of comfort to the hospital that will allow it to proceed to the next phase of planning. The scope of the analysis will vary with the degree of comfort sought, so no specific framework for the debt capacity assessment can be defined. The analytical outline presented in this chapter is based upon a scope of analysis which has proven effective in meeting the needs of most situations.

CREDIT ANALYSIS

The debt capacity assessment and the credit analysis are related with respect to general content and approach. They differ mainly in terms of timing and use. The debt capacity assessment is typically performed near the beginning of the long-range planning process and is used to estimate the feasible limits of the institution's ability to raise external debt capacity for a yet-to-be-defined project.

The credit analysis is performed just prior to the incurrence of debt. It assists potential lenders in deciding whether to lend to the institution. The debt capacity assessment is performed internally, usually by the institution's management and consultants. The credit analysis is performed by an independent party, usually a rating agency or institutional investors.

Content and Approach

Since the credit analysis is performed just prior to the incurrence of the debt, considerably more detailed information regarding the proposed project and its impact upon the institution's operations is available. In most instances, an independently conducted financial feasibility study is part of that information.

While the availability of additional specific information allows the credit analyst to perform a more detailed analysis than possible with the debt capacity assessment, the underlying principles and approach are similar. The following areas of investigation are critical to both:

- historical financial performance
- projected financial performance
- market characteristics
- reimbursement environment
- medical staff
- management

When the area of analysis deals with quantifiable aspects, such as financial ratios, comparisons can be more readily made. Table 3-2 presents such a comparison for hospitals that incurred tax-exempt debt during 1979, 1980, and 1981. The data are similar to that presented in Table 3-1, except that the information is arrayed according to the bond rating received from Moody's Investors Service rather than Standard & Poor's Corporation. The 200 hospitals compared in Table 3-2 represent a sample of those bond issues rated by Moody's during that period and do not necessarily reflect the actual averages for all bond issues so rated.

Appendixes 3-A and 3-B contain descriptions by the rating agencies of their approaches to performing the credit analysis for a hospital debt issue. A reading of those descriptions will indicate that the content and approach that characterize the credit analysis are indeed very similar to the debt capacity assessment.

Impact of the Credit Analysis

When the credit analysis results in a rating from the rating agency, as it frequently does in the case of hospital tax-exempt bonds, the impact is felt in the form of cost of debt capital. Specifically, the cost is manifested in two areas: the interest rate and the selling costs. In any given market, the lower the rating is the higher the interest rate and the selling costs will be.

Table 3-2 Comparative Statistics for Moody's Rating Categories

	Rating Category				
	Baa	*Baa-1*	*A*	*A-1*	*AA*
Number of bond issues in the sample	13	21	104	53	9
Number of beds*	184	198	282	441	957
Percent occupancy*	73.3	75.3	79.1	81.0	82.8
Average age of active medical staff*	45.7	45.8	46.0	46.0	45.7
Percent of active staff board certified*	51.2	57.5	66.1	66.7	72.1
Percent of patient revenues from Medicare/Medicaid*	45.7	45.0	44.1	41.7	37.3
Net income as a percent of net operating revenue*	3.4	4.7	5.1	5.6	6.0
Coverage of maximum debt service**	1.7x	2.0x	2.3x	2.7x	3.6x
Maximum debt service per patient day**	$27.00	$32.00	$27.00	$19.00	$13.00
Maximum debt service as a percent of net operating revenue**	8.8	8.9	7.4	5.2	3.7
Long-term debt as a percent of long-term debt plus unrestricted fund balance**	81.5	77.7	68.0	57.2	43.9
Long-term debt per bed (in thousands of dollars)**	$84.1	$88.2	$74.6	$65.6	$42.8

* As of the most recent fiscal year prior to bond sale.
** As projected for the first full fiscal year of debt service on the bonds.

Source: Blyth Eastman Paine Webber Health Care Funding Database.

Interest Rate

The rating's most obvious effect is on the interest rate. Table 3-3 presents conversion factors for assessing the impact upon interest rate resulting from different bond ratings from Standard & Poor's. The conversion factors are based upon 30-year hospital bond issues from 1979 and 1980, and are rules of thumb only.

The following example may prove helpful. If a recent 30-year maturity hospital tax-exempt bond rated A by Standard & Poor's carried an interest rate of 14 percent, the approximate rate on a similar maturity bond rated BBB+ would be (1.14/1.107)(14 percent) = 14.9 percent.

Table 3-3 Conversion Factors

Standard & Poor's Rating	Conversion Factor	30-year Interest Rate*
AA	1.00	13.32
A+	1.04	13.85
A	1.07	14.25
A−	1.11	14.78
BBB+	1.14	15.18

* Based upon the conversion factors and market conditions of early December 1981.

Source: Blyth Eastman Paine Webber Health Care Funding Database.

Selling Costs

The second area that the rating can affect is selling costs. Generally speaking, the lower the bond rating, the smaller the universe of prospective purchasers becomes, and the greater the expense is of selling to that diminished market. For example, the selling cost component of the bond discount for A rated, 30-year hospital tax-exempt bonds was approximately $18 per $1,000 of bonds in early December 1981. The selling cost for a BBB rated bond of the same maturity was approximately $28 per $1,000. On a bond issue of $10 million, the additional selling costs for the BBB rated issue were approximately $100,000 in December 1981.

Related Health Care Facilities

The volume of tax-exempt financing for nursing homes and life care centers has been rapidly increasing during the past several years, despite difficult market conditions. The underlying principles associated with performing a debt capacity assessment for a hospital are the same in the case of these other types of health care facilities. However, Standard & Poor's and Moody's do not presently perform credit analyses and issue bond ratings for these facilities. Consequently, any credit analysis would be performed by the underwriters and the potential investor.

Several aspects of the analysis for these facilities receive different emphasis than for hospitals. With nursing homes, added significance is placed upon utilization and reimbursement. Because of generally low levels of reimbursement from many third party payers, it often is essential that a nursing home maintain an extremely high occupancy, particularly when incurring debt. Consequently, the review of projected utilization and analysis of local reimbursement patterns and constraints become the most critical parts of the assessment.

With life care facilities, management and competition are of paramount importance. Management is critical because of the need to contain costs in order to remain competitive and to support an ongoing marketing effort. Because no certificate of need is required for the residential component of the life care center, no "franchise" exists to protect a facility from competing units being built nearby. Development of a facility with attractive location and features is therefore critical in face of the potential competition.

SUMMARY

Debt capacity assessment occurs early in the planning and constitutes an early warning system to guard against the development of a project plan that exceeds resources. Credit analysis, on the other hand, occurs at the end of the planning process and is a requirement for obtaining debt capacity. The debt capacity assessment is an internal management tool, and the credit analysis, while useful to management, is primarily an assistance to investors.

NOTES

1. Standard & Poor's Corporation, *Municipal and International Bond Ratings—An Overview* (New York: Standard & Poor's Corporation, 1981), pp. 41–42.
2. *Ibid.*, p. 42.

Appendix 3-A

Standard & Poor's Approach to Rating Hospital Revenue Bonds

OVERVIEW

The granting of tax exemption for bond issues involving health facilities has resulted in a steadily increasing volume of rating activity in recent years. Hospitals which had previously relied on philanthropy, federal funding, or conventional taxable financing have turned to the tax-exempt market. Numerous state health facility financing authorities have been established for the purpose of providing tax-exempt financing, and many local health authorities have been in existence for some time. Bond issues generally provide permanent and/or construction financing for individual institutions. Our involvement is generally limited to tax-exempt revenue bond issues for nonprofit hospitals, although we will accept rating applications for taxable bond offerings for nonprofit hospitals. We do not currently rate nursing home or life care center revenue bonds although these areas are under continuing surveillance.

APPROACH TO THE RATING

Standard & Poor's (S&P) will, upon written request, rate hospital revenue bond issues meeting our criteria. It is our policy not to rate start-up facilities, and similarly, we do not rate issues involving the relocation of a hospital unless a substantial portion of its patients are derived from the area to which the hospital is moving. There is no limitation as to minimum bed size as we believe that each situation must be evaluated on its merits regardless of size. However, small hospitals generally exhibit significantly greater vulnerability in a number of respects, and the issuer, therefore, should be prepared to address these concerns. It is our policy to assign

Source: Standard & Poor's Corporation, January 1982. Used by permission.

and to publish (with the exception of private placements) a rating whether or not the rating is "investment grade" ("BBB" category or above). This policy conforms to our general policy on debt ratings, and, simply stated, it means that once an application has been accepted for review, the application may not be withdrawn.

DOCUMENTATION REQUIREMENTS

The following outlines the documents we need to conduct our analysis. While we can initiate our analysis with draft documents, we should be apprised of any material changes in those documents as they are finalized. We must also be provided with final copies of all documents when they become available:

- official statement
- bond resolution or trust indenture
- feasibility study
- lease or loan agreement(s) (as applicable)
- audited financial statements for the five preceding fiscal years
- any other applicable legal documents

It may also be necessary to provide unaudited financial statements for the current year's interim period(s). If available, the auditor's management letter is also requested. It is also helpful to obtain examples of the hospital's internal control and budget variance reports.

MEETINGS AND FIELD TRIPS

As a component of our analysis, it is generally necessary to meet with representatives of the hospital's management and board of trustees, the feasibility consultant, the underwriter or financial adviser, and, as circumstances dictate, with the bond counsel or underwriter's counsel. This meeting is frequently held in our offices in New York, but if time permits and if it is deemed appropriate, this meeting could be more beneficially held at the hospital itself.

TIMING

The schedule should allow for our receipt of the required documentation at least three weeks prior to bond sale and at least one full week prior to any meeting or field trip. Our rating will be available approximately one week after the field trip or meeting, assuming everything is in order.

THE FEASIBILITY STUDY

The feasibility study is particularly important to our analysis of hospital revenue bonds. A well-prepared study presents an extensive amount of pertinent material in a concise, logical format; it states the explicit assumptions upon which the utilization and financial forecasts are based; and it is an indication of management's willingness to expose the hospital and the capital project to objective, independent scrutiny. The study should include two major components: a market and demand analysis, which defines the service area, examines demographic and utilization trends, and discusses competing institutions; and a financial analysis, which examines staffing parameters, reimbursement, operating costs, and pricing of services.

The forecasts should generally include five years, but should present at least two full fiscal years after completion of the project being financed with the bond proceeds. In the case of refunding or refinancings, where a project financing may not be involved, a shorter forecast period may be sufficient. The utilization forecasts should include the following patient statistics:

- admissions or discharges
- average length of stay
- patient days
- number of beds in service
- average occupancy
- emergency room visits
- outpatient visits

The utilization forecasts should also include other relevant outpatient and ancillary service statistics. The financial forecasts should include the following:

- statement of revenues and expenses
- balance sheet
- statement of changes in financial position (cash flow)
- statement of changes in fund balance

The statement should be prepared according to generally accepted accounting principles, or, if not so prepared, should be consistent with the hospital's historical method of preparation and presentation noting departures from GAAP. The forecasts should also clearly present any interfund transfers.

In our analysis we evaluate the reasonableness of the assumptions which support the forecasts, particularly in relation to historical performance. It is helpful to have a representative of the consulting firm present at the rating presentation to comment on the study and to answer questions regarding assumptions or methodology of preparation.

The feasibility study should be prepared by a nationally recognized firm with expertise in hospital consulting. In this respect, S&P cannot recommend firms nor does it publish a list of acceptable firms. Our concern is that the firm have sufficient resources and experience; if we are unfamiliar with the firm that has been retained, we will ask for a presentation to review the firm's credentials and to discuss the scope of the opinion and the methodology of preparation.

The feasibility study is a necessity in virtually all hospital revenue bond ratings because of the inherent complexities relating to cost accounting, third-party reimbursement and market position. Only in a very limited number of cases is it possible for us to rate without a feasibility study. These might involve refundings or refinancings or other situations where there is not a major capital project involved or hospitals we have previously rated. As a guideline, should the hospital show pro forma historical coverage of future maximum annual debt service (that is, the sum of the excess of revenues over expenditures, depreciation, and interest, divided by future maximum annual debt service) of at least 1.50 times for the two consecutive fiscal years immediately preceding issuance, it may be possible for us to rate the issue without a formal feasibility study prepared by an independent firm. However, even if a formal feasibility study is not required, the hospital would still have to furnish internal utilization and financial projections and support assumptions.

ANALYTICAL OUTLINE

The factors which are considered in our rating fall into five categories:

- legal provisions
- institutional characteristics and market position
- management factors
- medical staff characteristics
- financial factors

LEGAL PROVISIONS

As a part of hospital revenue bond analysis, we examine the legal documents underlying the transaction. These documents provide the structure of the financing, the security behind the bonds and for the bondholders, and a specified set of legally enforceable requirements.

Often, the actual issuer of the obligations is not the same party we are evaluating from a credit point of view when we are rating a hospital revenue bond issue. We rate the creditworthiness of the economic entity which is actually accountable for the payment of debt service, the identity of which is determined by a close examination of the various legal arrangements among the parties involved in the financing.

Generally, part or all of a hospital's revenue stream will be pledged to the payment of debt service; however, in our ratings we do not give added weight to a pledge of gross revenues (before operating expenses) versus a net (after operating expenses) revenue pledge. This is because we feel that a hospital must be able to pay its expenses in order to continue to operate and produce future revenues.

Often a hospital will mortgage all or part of its property, plant, and equipment in favor of the bondholders. Whether this enhances the creditworthiness of the bonds depends on the nature of the mortgaged assets. However, in all cases we will ascertain that a mortgage on the hospital facilities will not be available to other creditors.

An obligor will often unconditionally guarantee payment of debt service in connection with a lease agreement. While this betters the bondholders' position in the event of bankruptcy, we do not reflect this in a rating because when bankruptcy occurs the resultant disposition of assets is subject to action by the courts. This process does not normally ensure timely and full payment of debt service. We have also seen unconditional guaranties by corporate entities other than the obligor, generally a parent corporation of a multihospital system. In most cases, the parent corporation has greater strengths and resources than the direct obligor, and our rating is therefore based on the creditworthiness of the parent, as guarantor.

While we examine the broad structure of a financing, we also place particular emphasis on certain technical provisions, the absence or modification of which may have a negative impact on a rating. Since our ratings reflect the likelihood of timely payment of debt service, a debt service reserve fund should be established with the trustee to provide a buffer in the event of cash flow difficulties. The debt service reserve fund should be funded on the front end of the financing in an amount equal to either maximum annual debt service or average annual debt service, in those situations where debt service is essentially level. Only 50 percent funding of the debt service reserve fund on the front end will not have a negative impact on the rating if the account will be fully funded by the first principal payment date and the hospital's net revenues available for debt service provided historical coverage of maximum annual debt service on the proposed bonds of at least 1.50 times for the last completed fiscal year or 1.20 times for each of the last two completed fiscal years.

Since third party payers make reimbursements based on the depreciation schedule rather than on a principal repayment schedule, a shortfall between the amount of depreciation expense and the required principal payment will often occur at some point over the life of the bonds. Therefore, to provide adequate protection for the bondholders, it has been our position that a depreciation reserve fund should be established and fully funded to the amount of the shortfall by the year in which the required principal payment exceeds depreciation. The absence of this provision is a negative factor in the rating process unless it can be demonstrated that there is no principal/depreciation shortfall.

Restrictions related to future debt are areas of special rating consideration. In past years, debt covenants in the legal documents were highly restrictive allowing the hospitals little financing flexibility. Recently, there has been a trend toward the loosening of debt restrictions. In our rating process, we have generally favored these trends so that hospitals would have a measure of flexibility to operate more effectively in an increasingly complex financing environment. Our basic approach is to look first to the underlying strength of the institution, the competency of its management and the long-term goals. In addition to the basic additional bonds tests, restraints on alternative indebtedness, interim and short-term debt, and borrowings from the depreciation reserve fund are also reviewed. With the development of multihospital systems recently, a number of them have adopted master indentures, whose convenants cover the entire spectrum of financing alternatives. Again, we look to the basic credit strength of the hospital system in assessing the varied debt clauses.

We expect a hospital to structure its rates and charges in amounts which will produce net revenues at least sufficient to make required debt service payments. In order to provide an early warning signal, if net revenues fall below 1.10 times annual debt service in any fiscal year the hospital would also be expected to call in immediately an independent, nationally recognized consultant to make written recommendations to remedy the situation and to follow such recommendations to the degree possible.

With malpractice litigation having become a major risk to hospitals, we feel that it is warranted that a hospital maintain malpractice insurance at a specified level of at least $300,000 per occurrence and $1,000,000 aggregate per year. The "customarily insured" language is not viewed negatively so long as there is a requirement for an independent consultant's recommendation and annual review. Self-insurance will not negatively affect a rating as long as the program is based on a sound actuarial determination for funding requirements, provides for trustee-held funds, and generally meets federal Medicare reimbursement requirements. Provisions for disposal of assets, mergers and acquisitions, and events of default are also reviewed.

The provisions mentioned above are regarded as providing the minimum level of security necessary for the bondholders. We can rate issues without these provisions, but the absence or modification thereof may have a negative impact on a rating.

INSTITUTIONAL CHARACTERISTICS AND MARKET POSITION

The institutional characteristics (the type and level of the service provided) and the particular aspects of the market, including competition and market share, are important factors in our analysis of a hospital. In considering the type of institution, we tend to view specialty (such as rehab, eye, or psychiatric) hospitals less favorably than general acute care hospitals because of the greater vulnerability of specialty hospitals to changes in technology and medical treatment modes, reimbursement policies, and to demographic shifts. In addition, specialty hospitals possess limited flexibility to alter services in response to a changing market environment. In looking at the level of care provided, greater credit is given to major teaching, research, and regional referral institutions providing tertiary care and to larger medical centers providing essentially primary care. Our feeling is that major institutions are less vulnerable to general economic cycles and to local economic problems because of a lesser reliance on elective procedures which are less serious and may be deferred and because of their broad regional base. The major institutions are also felt to be less vulnerable to shifts to alternative modes of primary care, such as ambulatory, outpatient, and home care or health maintenance organizations.

We also closely examine historical trends in utilization for the preceding five years. The important inpatient statistics are admissions, average length of stay, patient days, number of beds in service, and occupancy. We look at ancillary services, outpatient, and emergency room trends. These trends are considered within the context of the market in which the hospital is situated. We are particularly concerned with the competitive environment, and credit will be given for market dominance or monopoly.

Excess supply resulting from "overbedding" is a major concern, and the hospital's occupancy compared to the average area occupancy is considered. We also analyze service area use rates (admissions and patient days per thousand) to determine whether patients are patronizing local hospitals or leaving the service area in favor of larger hospitals outside the service area.

Conversely, the hospital may be capturing admissions and referrals from outside its immediate service area. In this part of the analysis, our focus is on the hospital's market share and on stability and trends thereof. Reasons for declining market share are examined in close detail and because of their potential impact on market share we also need information regarding any planned hospital expansions within the service area. The economic and demographic characteristics of the service area are also major considerations. Population trends, income levels, unemployment, and major employers in the area are also analyzed in detail to determine the overall impact on the hospital.

The utilization forecasts provided within the feasibility report should be consistent with historical performance. We are particularly concerned with the justification behind forecasts which assume increased market share or increased use rates reflecting greater penetration of the service area. Similarly, the base demographic projections to which use rates are applied should be reasonable and consistent with historical trends.

A more recent phenomenon in the nonprofit hospital industry has been the development of multihospital systems resulting from the consolidation of two or more institutions. The size, economies of scale, and diversification associated with the systems provide strength, and, if supported by other factors, multihospital systems are generally regarded more favorably than individual institutions.

MANAGEMENT FACTORS

The complex environment within which hospitals must function makes it necessary that hospital management be entrusted to trained professionals. Our analysis of management seeks to determine whether the management team exhibits the depth and the experience to provide leadership, to deal effectively with the medical staff, to budget, monitor, and control financial and personnel resources efficiently, and to define the hospital's role and maintain its competitive position.

The analysis begins with the board of trustees. The board is legally responsible for the operations of the institution and for the quality of the medical care provided. The board's composition should be representative of the community and reflect the importance of the institution. If physicians are not represented directly on the board, we look for a mechanism for their participation in the determination of policy. We are also concerned with the structure and activity of board committees with particular consideration given to the board's role in the setting of financial policies.

Our analysis of the administration begins by first reviewing the historical record and noting changes that have occurred over the years. The résumés of the various members are reviewed and the organizational structure is analyzed. We question the management team on budgeting procedures and the involvement of department heads, and the types and frequency of monitoring and variance reports are also discussed. We also evaluate capital budgeting procedures, cash management, and credit policies. The efficiency of the hospital's staffing pattern encompasses certain ratio analyses, such as full-time employee equivalents per occupied bed to industry standards. A final area involves risk management and the hospital's history with malpractice claims and settlements.

While an S&P rating assigned to a major project financing is usually a provisional rating and, therefore, does not address the risk of default during construction we do examine the planning that went into the project as part of our appraisal of management. For example, an architect or construction manager without major hospital experience is cause for concern, as are the absence of maximum price contracts or firm construction bids.

MEDICAL STAFF CHARACTERISTICS

Since the physician is the primary client of the hospital, a detailed analysis of the medical staff is probably the most important single component of our analysis. The base material for our evaluation should consist of the following:

- the number of active and associate staff members and the specialties represented
- the percentage of admissions by age category and the average age of the entire staff
- a list of the top ten admitting physicians, by age, specialty, and percentage of total hospital admissions
- the net additions or deletions to the active staff over the past three years
- the recruitment practices
- the percentage board certified or board eligible
- the number of group practices

- the number and the specialties of physicians located in offices located adjacent to or close to the hospital
- in large hospitals, details concerning the teaching programs and retention of residents

Our analysis seeks to determine the relative strengths and vulnerabilities of the staff relative to the size of the facility, the services offered, the area which it serves, and the availability of physicians in the area. We are particularly concerned with the number of physicians who utilize said hospital as the primary hospital for their admissions and the overlap between staffs of the hospital and competing hospitals. We look for gaps or potential weaknesses in the various specialties, particularly in the case of smaller facilities. Similarly, a medical staff with a high average age or one which is not sufficiently represented in the younger age categories may be indicative of recruiting problems and may forewarn a potentially serious problem. Net additions to the staff in recent years provide an insight into the attractiveness of the hospital to physicians, the compatibility of management and the medical staff, and the acceptance by the staff of new physicians. We are also interested in the reasons physicians may have left the staff. Staff allegiance is particularly important in highly competitive or overbedded areas. Board certification is more relevant in larger institutions. Our concern here is that the staff's credentials are consistent with the role of the institution.

The base of admissions, as reflected by the percentage attributable to the top ten admitters, is particularly important in smaller hospitals. A very small percentage of physicians accounting for a substantial percentage of admissions is regarded as a particular vulnerability in the absence of mitigating factors, as is the presence of several physicians nearing retirement appearing in the list of the top ten admitters. This list also provides insight into areas of weakness, such as a disproportionately high or low percentage of admissions in a particular specialty. The presence of group practices would offer additional comfort.

The location of physician offices is taken into consideration. The location of physicians in offices adjacent to or within close proximity of the hospital reflects the long-term appeal of the institution and is a further indicator of allegiance and commitment. The presence of a physician clinic adjacent to the facility is viewed as a special strength.

We do not take into account the promise of future action, such as the addition of physicians in six months or a year, and while there can be no rigid rule regarding the impact on the rating of the various factors outlined above, in the end the rating is adjusted based on our judgment as to whether the current strengths can be sustained and the deficiencies recognized and corrected.

FINANCIAL FACTORS

This analysis begins with an examination of historical trends for the preceding five fiscal years, plus the current year's interim period, if applicable. In analyzing the income statement we focus on the stability of performance and look for the reasons behind any erratic or negative trends. Profitability, particularly on an operating basis, is of particular concern; and while it is recognized that a substantial excess of revenues over expenses cannot be expected in high cost-based reimbursement environments, persistent overall losses are negatively reflected in the rating. Reliance on nonoperating income to reach a break-even position, depending on the reliability of the source, is also generally viewed negatively.

Historical coverage, defined as the sum of the excess of revenues over expenses plus depreciation and interest, divided by future maximum annual debt service, is computed. While most hospitals will not exhibit 1.00 times or higher coverage on this basis, should the hospital have such historical coverage, it means that timely payment of debt service will not be completely dependent upon the successful and timely completion of the project being financed. Issues of hospitals which do not have such historical coverage receive provisional ratings which indicate that our rating is subject to the successful and timely completion of the project.

In examining the historical balance sheet, we look at liquidity, focusing on cash balances and current ratios. Borrowing for cash flow purposes, decreasing working capital, and high levels of accounts receivable are causes for concern. Generally, accounts receivable which exceed 65 or 70 days, and current ratios (current assets to current liabilities), under 1.5 : 1 are particularly questioned. We also evaluate historical debt to plant and debt to capitalization ratios.

The forecast of financial performance is taken from the feasibility study or, in certain limited circumstances, from internal forecasts. We look for and question things such as revenue growth that is based on assumptions of large volume increases or substantial and disproportionate price increases. Expense estimates should be conservative and well supported. Forecasts should be consistent with historical performance; in particular we question turnaround situations where poor historical performance is forecast to improve.

Our analysis focuses on the first full fiscal year after project completion. At that point, the hospital will have fully booked the new plant and the net revenues available and cash flow will reflect the increased depreciation. Likewise, the hospital will have finished the period of capitalized interest and will be expensing interest. Said fiscal year is regarded as the most crucial, and it is here that the hospital is felt to be most vulnerable.

Coverage of annual as well as maximum debt service is computed, taking into consideration the structure of the debt service schedule. The quality of the coverage is considered as well as the amount of the coverage. Coverage of maximum annual debt service in the first full year in the majority of cases is on the order of two times. We also compute debt burden, measured by maximum annual debt service as a percentage of net operating revenue. Percentages exceeding 10 percent indicate a heavy debt burden: Hospitals generally average in the 6 percent to 8 percent range.

We again compute the liquidity ratios in examining the forecast balance sheet for the first full fiscal year after completion, tracing the cash flow and paying particular attention to the composition of current assets. In considering capitalization, particular emphasis is placed on the ratio of long-term debt to net property, plant, and equipment, since it is this relationship which determines the amount of depreciation which may be retained for future investment and the amount which must be applied to principal payments. This ratio is to a large extent the determinant of future capacity to pay. Generally, the debt to plant ratio is on the order of 80 percent to 90 percent. We also analyze future financing requirements.

The hospital's regulatory and reimbursement environment is also analyzed and the mix of third party payers considered. A high percentage of cost-based payers in itself may not be negatively perceived, but certainly the hospital's response to this environment and its ability to control costs and maximize reimbursement are taken into consideration.

In summary, the financial analysis provides us with an indicator of past performance and a forecast of capacity to pay debt service. The financial analysis is not considered in isolation but is viewed within the overall context of the institution.

Rating Hospital Revenue Bonds*

RATING HOSPITAL REVENUE BONDS

A municipal bond rating is a judgment of the investment quality of a long-term obligation issued by a state or one of its subdivisions. It is based on an analysis that must ask, first, what has the debtor pledged to pay, and second, what is the likelihood that the borrowing unit will be able to keep his or her promises? The rating is the essence of an analysis and is a shorthand statement of the judgment which is reached. It is an evaluative assessment of the protections afforded the bondholder. The rating is a simple, easy-to-understand classification of the credit risks of a municipal bond. It is a judgment which the market finds to be useful in making comparisons and in maintaining liquidity of capital funds.

A rating is assigned each time an issuer comes to market and requests it. Each new sale changes bonded indebtedness and therefore requires a new appraisal. The analytical work on a particular rating is performed by an analyst, under supervision of an officer who is a senior analyst and who has responsibility for a territorial area or a type of municipal bond.

A detailed credit report is written, in which debt factors, legal security, financial matters, service provision, and the area economy are all evaluated. The supervisor then reviews the report and discusses the rating recommendation, which is then presented to the rating committee. The rating committee, in its entirety, consists of senior officers of the municipal research department. Members serve on a rotating basis and consistency is stressed. After a thorough discussion, a consensus is reached and a rating is assigned.

---

* Excerpted from a presentation made by Craig W. Atwater June 22, 1978, at the Executive Program in Health Care Financial Management at Ohio State University, Columbus, Ohio. Updated May 1982. Mr. Atwater is vice president for Moody's Investors Service. Used by permission.

The rating is then communicated to the applicant (either the governmental unit that is issuing the debt, or its financial adviser or underwriter who is assisting the governmental unit). In most cases, the rating is accepted; occasionally it is formally protested. If new information is provided, the rating will be reviewed. This appeal process may or may not lead to a change in rating.

Once a rating is assigned, it is within the public domain and is included in a number of Moody's publications including the weekly *Bond Survey*, the monthly *Bond Record* and in Moody's *Municipal & Government Manual*. The credit report is published and sent to subscribers within a day or two after the assignment of the rating.

All of Moody's ratings are reviewed on a regular basis for as long as the rated debt remains outstanding. Annual financial reports and other information must be supplied on a timely basis. The sale of additional parity bonds will also require a complete rating review.

Since most municipal bonds for acute-care hospitals are revenue rather than tax-supported general obligation bonds, several general comments on revenue bond analysis are appropriate. Revenue bond analysis is in many ways less elusive than analysis of general obligation bonds. Generally, it involves a closed system with a finite number of variables and greater possibilities for quantification. The pledge of security involves an enterprise where the debt is related to an earning asset. The principles of credit analysis are the same, but the analysis shifts from the use of sovereign power of government to extract a tax to the operation of a user enterprise involving benefit analysis. Usually, there is a measurable benefit for which people either are or are not willing to pay. Thus, there are bonds secured by pledges of electric, water, wastewater, toll bridge, college dormitory, off-street parking, toll road, airport, hospital, marine terminal, stadia, and multipurpose civic center/convention revenues.

Among the factors that must be examined are those pertaining to the revenue-producing enterprise, the potential demand, and the legal protections which are safeguards against the unexpected. The physical plant involves engineers' appraisals of the soundness of the system and its ability to produce a service that can be sold at a price consumers are willing to pay. System capability and the ability of management to operate with financial success must also be analyzed. Other factors include the secular, cyclical, and operating characteristics of the industry and the particular system under review.

Legal protections involve detailed examination of the covenants in the trust indenture or bond resolution. Of particular importance is the flow of funds which is established for the enterprise, the additional bonds clause, and the rate covenant. Many difficulties may arise from an improper flow of funds or an additional bond clause that was too liberal in its permissiveness.

And the rate covenant establishes a base by which to measure management and its performance.

The general considerations in the analysis of limited-liability or enterprise revenue bond municipal bonds comprise the following:

1. *Earning assets.* The earning assets, the physical plant or facilities, are carefully studied for their implications, particularly when additions, extensions, or replacements are being undertaken. The additional investment may enhance the earning potential, or it may dilute the preexisting potential. In some instances, expansions have significantly altered the underlying financial or operational characteristics of enterprises, leading to expectations materially different than those formerly obtained. To the extent that the modifications are foreseeable, and in some situations they are inherent, they are relevant considerations in the credit judgment.

2. *Pricing and rate making.* Another set of limits defining credit prospects is the pricing and rate-making policies and procedures. Not only must the policies followed be appropriate to the enterprise, but also the charges must be derived so that they are fair and contribute to the public intent of the project. Additional elements to be considered are the identification of fixed costs against variable costs, the regulation and/or approval process that is required, and charges for capacity and demand.

3. *Technology and secular trends.* Specialized technologies have significant impact on the facilities and operations of most of the enterprises and proprietary-type undertakings. Their effect over time is an important factor in forming analytical judgments. It is generally the cost implications of technological changes that are of analytical interest, though the technical features may of themselves be fascinating to some analysts. In the main, two kinds of changes are involved. One is the gradual improvements in a given technology; the other is a shift to a different process involving equipment or materials significantly different from that previously in use. The effect of the former is usually to increase production at no increase in costs or to increase efficiency and thereby lower costs. The latter shift to a different process may either lower or increase costs. Different constraints obviously pertain to a technology well past its developmental stage than for one in the early stages. This distinction is important in the health care field, especially with the advent of new and improved equipment and processes, such as the CAT scanner. It

is the analyst's function to know, to the extent of an informed layman, the prospects for the technologies important to an issuer. New or radically different technologies pose a more difficult problem. Some innovations are undertaken for purely economic reasons, others due to health or sanitation conditions, or some other kind of necessity. In such an event it is purely fortuitous if costs are affected beneficially. Further, changes of this nature do not necessarily involve invention of a new technology; it may happen that a known technology is at first rarely used, but subsequently must be widely used. It is, therefore, important to know when a routinely and widely used process may have to be supplanted or supplemented by another, and whether that change will be financially advantageous or costly.

4. *Measuring enterprise business.* Most enterprises produce a variety of accurately measurable data on their customers, output, and unit sales. Such data not only facilitate cost comparisons, but also afford a basis for measuring aspects of the business over time that are free of the effects of price changes resulting from inflation/deflation. Moreover, because of standardization within an industry, the performance of an enterprise can be compared with that of the industry generally. Relevant in this analysis are the long-term or secular trends, the short-term or cyclical movements, and the regularly recurring fluctuations resulting from seasonal variation or peaking on an hourly or daily basis.

A number of common risks faced by enterprises emerge:

1. *Failure or impairment of earning assets.* Unless the earning assets are in place and in working order, there can be no earnings. Interruption of the facility's ability to provide the goods or service will interrupt earnings. A major threat to a new enterprise or to a large expansion of an existing system is failure to complete the facilities or to complete them within the time allowed. Two customary protections against such failures are the use of insurance and the issuance of completion bonds. Maintaining a comfortably large working capital is the best protection against interruptions such as labor disputes, weather conditions, and international events.

2. *Inability to borrow.* Bond contracts for limited liabilities invariably contain some kind of restriction or condition controlling the issuance of additional bonds. To facilitate borrowing, interest rate limitations previously in effect have either been raised or eliminated. In addition, various innovative financing mechanisms have been used in

recent years to reduce the perceived risks in entering the long-term market, such as shorter-term bonds or notes, some of which have additional credit support.

3. *Sales or utilization failure.* Disappointing sales or utilization means disappointing revenues, potentially jeopardizing debt service. A serious situation results when the anticipated volume fails to materialize. This can happen because the original anticipations were unrealistic. The credit analyst must seek reassurance of the reliability of projections by considering the experience and reputation of those making the calculations, the information used and the assumptions made, and the actual historical experience of the industry and of the particular enterprise, if established. Another cause of unrealistic volume projection is a perceived need to justify certain annual revenues determined to be necessary to make the project financially feasible. This procedure is putting the cart before the horse, and is a reliable way to ensure a bumpy ride. Miscalculation of demand may also arise from external causes. In this case, the expectations were justifiable when made, but some later development negated the assumptions or invalidated the historical data used.

4. *Failure to control or recoup costs.* The difficulties of cost control, and the hazards of uncontrollable costs, hardly need emphasis after a decade of massive and continuous inflation. Even so, failure to control costs must be included in the specialized risks run by proprietary-type public entities, that is, compared with purely governmental operations, where the power of taxation is at least nominally a protection to the debtor and creditor alike. Failure to recoup costs can be as serious as failure to control them. Defects in price making, whether from defective data inputs or inappropriate pricing schemes, impose a serious handicap on a business, and the risk that there will be such defects is a real one.

Moody's has current ratings on over 500 acute-care hospitals whose capital programs have been financed through nontax-supported municipal bonds. These financings have been for replacement of hospital facilities considered inadequate and nonconforming to present health care standards and for expansion and renovation of ancillary and support facilities for both inpatient and outpatient services. The types of health care facilities include the total range from the modest-sized primary care hospital, to the large regional and specialized health care centers associated with a medical university, to the multisystem health care enterprises. In addition to the financings for the new capital programs, there have also been refundings of debt to achieve a savings in debt charges with the issuance of advance refunding bonds.

Hospital facility financings have been for the nonprofit hospitals via bonds issued either by a health care authority or by a unit of local government. The security arrangements provide that the issuing entity enter into a lease agreement or a mortgage agreement with the hospital under which the hospital as lessee or mortgagor makes payments to provide for debt service on the bonds issued. The source of these payments is a claim on the gross revenues of the hospitals, excluding their restricted gifts and donations. The analysis is concerned with a detailed examination of the covenants contained in the trust indenture or bond resolution of the issuer, as well as for lease-rental or mortgage situations of the relationships between the parties and the particular covenants and promises that the hospital has made. Since the hospitals that have had tax-exempt bonds issued in their behalf are nonprofit undertakings in an industry in which charges and levels of third-party reimbursement are regulated, and since the magnitude of debt being incurred is in many instances substantial relative to that hospital's earnings, the historical net revenues available for debt service are in many cases exceeded by estimated peak annual debt service on the new bonds.

Where historical net revenues are exceeded by estimated peak debt service, projections in a financial feasibility study prepared by independent consultants indicate that the hospital's net revenues following completion of the capital program would be sufficient to service the bonds being offered. These feasibility studies are also prepared in the cases where historical net revenues exceeded estimated peak debt service. These projections are based on various and specified assumptions and conditions and make disclaimers that the occurrence of events or actions not included in the assumptions could affect the projections of usage, earnings, and expenses. To the analyst, it is important that the study contain the narrative, tabular, and assumptions that are comparable and consistent in this field of endeavor, not who prepared the study. In the analysis of hospital enterprises, Moody's employs as an analytical tool medians of certain measures of financial and operating performance from the hospitals that are rated. These are included in our municipal credit reports.

The medians are revised annually. Exhibit 3B-1 depicts the medians calculated for 147 hospital enterprises for the calendar year 1981. They convey various measures of performance and earning capabilities of hospitals which have used tax-exempt bonds for their capital financing program. The medians represent ratios and indices common to revenue-producing enterprises, as well as several unique to the health care enterprises.

The individual hospital's historical financial performance is important, and its operating ratio, net takedown, and peak coverage from historical

Exhibit 3B-1 Current Hospital Enterprise Medians

The following represents the medians calculated on 147 hospital enterprises which have been rated and reviewed by Moody's for the calendar year 1981. The medians convey various measures of performance and earning capabilities of hospitals which have used tax-exempt bonds for their capital financing program. The medians represent ratios and indices common to revenue-producing enterprises, as well as several which are unique to the health care enterprises. The current medians are as follows:

	Median
Operating ratio (%)	90.9
Net take-down (%)	10.9
Peak debt service coverage by historical net revenues	1.18
Peak debt service coverage by estimated net revenues in first full year after project completion	2.20
Debt ratio (%)	43.1
Projected debt ratio (%)	54.4
Bed occupancy (%)	81.4
Number of beds	311
Average length of stay (days)	7.3
Debt svc. safety margin	7.7

DEFINITIONS

Income Statement Definitions and Ratios:

Gross revenue and income:	Operating revenue plus nonoperating revenue.
Operating expenses:	Operating expenses, excluding depreciation, amortization and interest.
Net revenues:	"Gross revenue and income" minus "operating expenses."
Operating ratio (%):	"Operating expenses" divided by total operating revenues.
Net take-down (%):	"Net revenues" divided by "gross revenue and income."
Peak debt service coverage by historical net revenues:	"Net revenues" divided by the estimated maximum annual principal and interest on all outstanding bonds and the bonds to be issued.
Peak debt service coverage by projected net revenues:	Estimated "net revenues" for the hospital during the first full fiscal year following the completion of the capital project financed from the new bonds, divided by the estimated maximum annual principal and interest on all outstanding bonds and the bonds to be issued.
Debt service safety margin:	Net revenues less current debt service divided by gross revenues.

Exhibit 3B-1 continued

Balance Sheet Definitions and Ratios:

Net fixed assets:	Fixed assets minus accumulated depreciation.
Long-term debt:	Gross long-term debt plus the current portion of long-term debt.
Net long-term debt:	"Long-term debt" minus the bond reserve funds/accounts for the payment of bond principal.
Debt Ratio (%):	"Net long-term debt" divided by the sum of "net fixed assets" plus net working capital.
Projected Debt Ratio (%):	Pro forma "Net long-term debt" divided by the sum of "net fixed assets" plus "net working capital" for the first full fiscal year following issuance of the bonds. Figures are derived from feasibility studies.

Utilization Results Definitions and Ratios:

Number of beds:	Represents the average bed complement.
Average daily census:	Total patient days divided by the days in the year (365).
Bed occupancy (%):	Average occupancy of the hospital's patient beds during the year. This ratio is computed by dividing "average daily census" by the hospital's average beds available for that year.
Average length of stay:	Average stay for inpatients, as reported by the hospital for that year. It is computed by taking the total patient days divided by number of admissions or discharges.

Source: Moody's Investors Service.

net, all computed from the last fiscal year, are significant factors in the evaluation and its comparison with the median, or average.

If the trend of historical fiscal performance shows a rise in operating ratio and decline in the net takedown, then there is demonstrated evidence of failure to control or recoup costs, and this is taken into account at the time the bonds are being issued. In some instances, hospitals have recently undertaken, or are in the process of implementing, new or revised procedures to control or recoup costs. The effectiveness of these procedures can be quantified in time through the ratios that are used, but this effectiveness may not be quantifiable at the time the bonds are being sold. In such an instance, there is an element of uncertainty as to whether the procedures will achieve the desired goals.

Debt service coverage is important, and a hospital's ability to cover peak debt service from historical net revenues is taken into account in the evaluation. Above average ratings on hospital revenue bonds are based to a great extent on the coverage levels being significantly above the median. Using ratios in revenue bond analysis is important, but we also recognize one particular enterprise may exhibit characteristics which will contribute to ratios that vary significantly from the median. Our medians include the debt ratio, a balance sheet calculation from the last fiscal year-end, and a pro forma from balance sheets included in the financial feasibility study. High debt ratios will characterize hospitals after issuing their tax-exempt bonds, most notably if most of the project was debt financed. This can be partly minimized through equity contributed by the hospital for the total project, and an indication of historical fiscal performance is the amount of moneys that the hospital is able to contribute to the undertaking. Both historical and pro forma debt ratios are important indices of debt burden.

To keep hospital ratings current and to determine whether the actual financial results are in line with those that had been projected in the feasibility study at the time of the bond offering, Moody's reviews on an ongoing basis the ratings of hospital enterprises following receipt of the latest financial data and other appropriate documentation. Financial data are also received on a summarized basis from certain state-created health facilities. The conditional prefix attached to many of the hospital ratings calls the investors' attention to the need for the issuer to achieve certain conditions, which are predominantly the need for completion of construction and the demonstration of one year's financial seasoning following completion.

The analysis of hospitals requires attention to factors such as the range of facilities and services provided and their historical usage, the educational programs of the hospital, the depth and diversity of the medical staff, and its competitive standing within its area relative to rates, facilities, and utilization. These criteria are important, since hospitals usually are not monopolistic undertakings as are water, sewerage, or electric services. There is competition and an element of choice for the usage of hospital facilities and services by prospective patients. While it is true that a patient goes to hospitals at which his or her physicians have staff privileges, a portion of a hospital's utilization (certainly related to outpatient and emergency-type of activity) may not necessarily be physician-referred. It is important for the analyst to be able to quantify these matters, to determine the distinctive factors of a hospital in its service area. An example is the hospital that is designated as a regional referral center for a specialized procedure or service. While this gives a hospital an advantage over others in its service area, for the analyst it is important to determine the volume of usage of this procedure or service and recognize this specialization requires an investment in the equipment as well as the investment in specially trained personnel. As is the case with other revenue-producing enterprises, an examination of the hospital's financial statements is essential including: the income statement, the balance sheet, and data supplementary or supportive of them.

As with any business with a large number of private customers, the status of accounts receivable is of analytical interest, and the number of days of receivables is an important measure of fiscal performance. The mix of patient revenue sources is important, as well as the historical record of payment by the third-party reimbursers. Evaluation of hospital revenue bonds also takes into account management's ability to obtain full and prompt payment from the third parties.

Hospitals do have vulnerabilities. On two occasions, we have lowered ratings, in stages, to default grade on two general hospitals for which there was no operating history and for which the initial results were well below average. To the extent that a hospital has established itself as a health care facility in an area and has a demonstrable record of acceptance and earnings, the vulnerability to early seasoning is reduced. This factor is also important in the case of a replacement of a hospital within the same service area but at some distance from the existing facility. For start-up hospitals, the availability of money from a source other than hospital revenues (such as appropriations, taxes, or contributions) is a tangible demonstration of support and could be essential in overcoming the start-up problems of sufficient working capital and usage. Consequently, Moody's does not rate hospital revenue bonds for start-up hospitals. We have also made rating reductions for hospitals which have experienced fiscal and administrative problems, and have raised ratings based on a substantial record of sound and improving financial results.

Tax-exempt revenue bond financing for the expansion, replacement, and improvement programs of general hospitals continues. These capital programs will have to demonstrate their need, as approved by the appropriate regional and state health planning agencies. We expect that by the time we are asked to rate hospital revenue bonds the hospital has obtained all its approvals and appropriate certificates of need; we will not rate a hospital for which full approvals have not been obtained as this raises an unnecessary element of uncertainty.

Concern over the costs of health care and a concern for the quality of health care for these costs have spawned frequent articles on these subjects. Hospitals have had to absorb and pass on higher costs for malpractice insurance, energy, supplies, specialized equipment, salaries and benefits for personnel, as well as interest and depreciation expenses. The concern over health care costs has led to the establishment in several states of some form of state agency to monitor and approve rates. Such an arrangement becomes a credit consideration as it affects the hospital's ability to secure rate approval in a timely manner which, in turn, can affect its flows of revenues. An additional concern regarding the proposals for state-created cost control agencies is that these agencies are not a party to the bond contract but they will have an authority over rates; it is important that these state agencies recognize the hospital's promises in their rate covenant and other obligations to the holders of the tax-exempt bonds.

We know that hospital management has studied the implications of federal proposals, including cost containment, cost shifting, competition, and reimbursement limitations. As an analyst, it is important to determine the effects of such pending or proposed legislation on hospitals. Proper questions to be posed to hospital management concern efforts to voluntarily control the growth in costs. What have you done? Can you quantify the effectiveness of your measures? These are proper questions for analysts to ask. Hospital management's ability to control costs and document this gives the investor an indication of its capabilities.

The acute care hospital industry is one that is relatively new to revenue bond financing and will be undergoing the type of seasoning that the toll roads went through in the 1950s, and airports and college housing in the 1960s.

Historically, very few public hospitals financed with general obligations bonds have tried to operate on a self-supporting basis; tax or philanthropic support, or both, was explicit. The third-party payment system has made self-support feasible, but as a basis for revenue bond financing, it is as yet unseasoned. Issuer ingenuity and innovation call for investor and analyst to exercise intelligent skepticism and curiosity.

Many projects represent new or substantially new undertakings, the latter resulting when relatively large additions or other changes significantly outdate historical data. Analysis in these cases requires that significant weight be given to pro forma projections of operating and financial results. The validity of assumptions and the rationale for marked deviations from such past trends require careful evaluation, which must be made in the absence of any longstanding observations; hence, the entire group must be kept under unusually close observation in order that the estimating techniques may be appraised. This will necessarily entail frequent review of new projects, comparing actual experience with projections. The tentative nature of some of the judgments necessary in the developmental stage of a financing device suggest that: (1) uncertainties that might be understood well enough to be tolerated in seasoned industries may be intolerable in these innovative risk situations; and (2) the better quality risks will probably be conceived as those in which there are elements of substantial strength not deriving directly from earnings support.

Popular concern with the level and trend of health facility costs and the record of abuse and ineffectiveness in the Medicaid programs in some jurisdictions suggest that hospital revenue bond financing must receive particularly severe scrutiny within the framework of its medical performance.

It is not within the means or the skill of the credit analyst to determine whether the law is being observed, whether secret corruption exists, or indeed whether medical care and treatment are in accord with the prevailing state of the art. Hence, the experience and reputation of management will assume perhaps significant importance, as will that of consultants.

A final comment on ratings. There is nothing arbitrary, mysterious, or capricious about ratings. It is simply a rationalization and a simplification based on the best analysis the credit analyst can perform. The rating cannot be arrived at through a precisely stated mathematical formula, but involves examining each area of information and their interrelationships, making a judgment modified as necessary by empirical evidence and experience.

Chapter 4

The Financial Feasibility Study

Harvey J. Gitel

The feasibility study has become an important—and often mandatory—document for any public sale of bonds. Its role in the rating process is emphasized by Standard & Poor's Corporation:

> The feasibility study is a necessity in virtually all hospital revenue bond ratings because of the inherent complexities relating to cost accounting, third-party reimbursement, and market position. Only in a very limited number of cases is it possible for us to rate without a feasibility study. These might involve refunding or refinancings or other situations where there is not a major capital project involved, or hospitals we have previously rated. As a guideline, should the hospital show pro forma historical coverage of future maximum annual debt service (i.e., the sum of the excess of revenues over expenditures, depreciation and interest, divided by future maximum annual debt service) of at least 1.25 times for the two consecutive fiscal years immediately preceding issuance, it may be possible for us to rate the issue without a formal feasibility study prepared by an independent firm. Such situations will be evaluated on a case-by-case basis.[1]

The study is usually less essential when debt is privately placed because of the lender's technical and practical ability to conduct its own evaluation based on its specific guidelines. However, any potential lender values a well-prepared study presenting an extensive amount of material in a concise and logical manner whether it is for tax-exempt or taxable debt and whether publicly sold or privately placed.

A health care feasibility study is an independent evaluation of the single most likely future outcome for the plans and programs of the health care facility in question. This study includes the consultants' evaluation of the assumptions used by management and a comprehensive economic and financial forecast. A feasibility study focuses on the cash-generating capacity of the facility and assesses the adequacy of cash flows to meet the hospital's financial needs. While most feasibility studies refer to debt service coverage, which is of interest to bond purchasers, the feasibility study report generally expresses its conclusion in terms of the adequacy of total cash flows and the reasonableness of assumptions upon which the cash flows have been forecast.

The feasibility study normally provides analyses and assumptions of the following:

- the hospital's health care role in the defined service area and the demographic and economic factors affecting future utilization in the service area;
- the potential impact of ongoing or proposed expansion, modernization, and/or program plan changes of other service area hospitals;
- the attitudes toward and support of the hospital's medical staff for the proposed expansion and modernization program;
- the changes in the practice of the medical staff which may affect its future utilization of the facilities;
- the changes in charge rates;
- the impact of contracts, regulations, and third party payer agreements;
- the changes in uncollectible accounts and free services;
- the sources of other operating and nonoperating revenues;
- the hospital's staffing requirements, salary and related fringe benefit costs;
- the hospital's nonwage expenses;
- the timing, cost, and financing assumptions of the program; and
- other anticipated sources and uses of cash during the forecast period, including changes in working capital requirements.

The rating agencies generally require a feasibility study prior to rating the bonds, and bond purchasers use it as a basis for deciding whether to buy a particular bond issue. All parties in the financing program expect the study to be detailed, thorough, and rigorous. Although hospital management is often capable of preparing a feasibility study, the study has evolved as a third-party evaluation of the hospital's financial and operational viability, hence requiring the independence and objectivity of an outside consultant. By working with hospital management, the consultant can help develop reasonable assumptions as the basis for financial statement forecasts.

THE FEASIBILITY STUDY

The health care feasibility study usually contains a financial forecast. It is defined by the American Institute of Certified Public Accountants (AICPA) as follows:

> A financial forecast for an entity is an estimate of the most probable financial position, results of operations, and changes in financial position for one or more future periods. In this context,
>
> - Entity means any unit, existing or to be formed for which financial statements could be prepared in conformity with generally accepted accounting principles or other comprehensive basis of accounting.
> - Most probable means that the assumptions have been evaluated by management and that the forecast is based on management's judgement of the most likely set of conditions and its most likely course of action. "Most probable" is not used in a mathematical or statistical sense.[2]

The AICPA has issued a *Guide for a Review of a Financial Forecast* and plans to publish additional documents on reporting prospective financial information.[3] Although the AICPA guide emphasizes how to review a financial forecast, which is only one part of a feasibility study, it also provides a significant definition of many of the requirements a feasibility study must include.

The forecasts in a hospital feasibility study cover only a limited time frame. The study generally assesses the hospital's ability to meet debt service payments entirely from the hospital's cash flow for a year or two after the construction program is completed. It is generally perceived that the initial years of meeting the increased obligations of the program are the most difficult. The increased uncertainty associated with extended forecasts and the increasing inability of management to decide upon a likely course of action make it necessary to limit the forecast period. However, this factor increases the need to provide appropriate evaluative information to the user of the forecasts.

Because a feasibility study assesses a specific program and course of action, at a specific point in time, it should be completed close to the time at which it will be utilized for marketing a proposed debt issue.

A feasibility study should encompass all aspects of a hospital's operations to provide potential purchasers of the bonds with the complete program. This is important to the hospital, the investment banker, and the feasibility study consultant in avoiding potential future liability to bond purchasers.

The study must involve key hospital administrators to achieve optimum results. One of these persons usually serves as the major liaison for coordinating the feasibility study.

While each consulting firm approaches a hospital feasibility study differently, almost all divide a feasibility study into a series of phases, each having one or more elements. The phases are separately performed but interdependent in overall effect and meaning. Discussed in the following sections are these three phases: (1) demand, market, or facility utilization assessment (the "Demand Analysis"); (2) financial statement forecasting (the "Financial Analysis"); and (3) reporting and review.

Demand Analysis/Facility Utilization Forecasts

This phase of the study establishes the reasonableness of assumptions relating to forecast utilization of the present and proposed health care facilities. Volume forecasts of all major potential revenue sources, as well as the status of third-party contracts and principles of reimbursement, are among the most significant inputs for the financial forecasts.

The scope of the planned expansion project must be defined early in this phase. Care should be taken to identify planned changes in the hospital's operating characteristics and medical programs, as well as changes anticipated in the hospital's physical structure. Defining the project's scope will facilitate the collection of pertinent information and minimize the collection of unnecessary data.

The forecast utilization should be based on assumptions and rationale about the potential supply and demand characteristics of the hospital's primary and secondary service areas as related to the particular facilities, services, and physicians of the hospital. Assumptions and rationale should be developed after investigation of the following factors:

- the potential population growth of the hospital service area obtained from recognized and accepted agencies; analysis of economic and demographic information, obtained through research of published information and supplemented by interviews with appropriate persons;
- the potential need for health care services in the geographic area, based on an evaluation of the population growth and service area health care trends, as well as national trends;

- the ability of the service area's health care delivery system to meet these needs through existing facilities, plus those under construction and planned for construction during the period of the forecast; and
- the indicated patronage of the hospital by patients of the present and prospective medical staff.

Service Area Supply and Demand Analysis

The purpose of these analyses is to evaluate the assumptions about the prospective health care needs of the area the hospital serves, and the indicated capacities of existing or planned facilities and human resources to meet those needs. Steps to be performed should include:

- determination of the boundaries of the primary and secondary geographic service areas which are the hospital's major sources of patients;
- identification of area population levels and special demographic and economic factors in these service areas which explain why the area may be above or below levels of utilization elsewhere;
- determination of the status of third-party contracts, principles of reimbursement, and contract benefits which may affect facility utilization and/or reimbursement;
- collection of information about the services provided by other hospitals in the service area from state and local health planning agencies; and
- collection of data through interviews with other hospitals in or near the service area about the services provided by those hospitals and their plans for changes in service offerings.

Review of the data gathered from these sources results in an estimate of forecast need for services in the area and the hospital's ability to meet these needs. Several techniques are applied to relate expected population trends to various standards of health care needs:

- state health facility planning formulas;
- comprehensive health planning guidelines;
- current and projected use rate (admissions per 1,000 of population) formulas;
- average use rates in the metropolitan area;
- average use rates in comparable communities; and
- market share expectations.

Physician Survey

Except for outpatient services, physicians with admitting privileges are the major source of a hospital's patients.

The size and scope of practice of the hospital's present medical staff significantly affect the extent to which hospital facilities may be utilized. Although need may exist for health care services, the hospital must have the capability to provide such services. If this capability does not exist, then service area demand will not be indicative of the level of services that can be realized at the facilities.

The present medical staff is likely to contribute the major component of facility demand during the forecast period, but other qualified physicians who are presently practicing at other area hospitals and physicians currently entering area practice should also be considered. Details of physician recruitment practices and results are identified to provide an assessment of the long-range potential of the hospital to maintain or increase its utilization. Changes in bed availability, scope of services, management philosophy, or facility appearance may either attract or discourage patronage from physicians having multiple hospital affiliations.

Because a proposed program depends so greatly on support from physicians, their opinions about how the program will modify the facility and how the modified facility or services will influence their patronage are vital. Information may be gathered from a physician survey using written questionnaires, interviews, or both.

In addition to the physicians' attitudes, other factors in evaluating the hospital medical staff's viability and practice characteristics include:

- the ages of physicians;
- the specialties of the physicians;
- the distribution of admissions by age, specialty, and practice type;
- the practice locations of the physicians; and
- the size, recruiting, and retention of the staff.

Forecasting Facility Utilization

Based on the results of the area and hospital statistical analysis and the physician survey and analyses, the hospital's anticipated facility utilization prepared by administration should be evaluated and adjusted, if necessary, to reflect the results of the consultant's analysis and review.

It is likely that the use rates and forecast population factors for the hospital service areas, as well as information from the physician survey, will indicate a range of prospective demand. These factors, together with other relevant data, should be analyzed and compared to historic trends. Using such information, the hospital administrator and other appropriate hospital personnel judge the most probable level of patient utilization for each of the years of the forecast for review by the consultant.

Forecasted utilization of hospital facilities in terms of patient days and other measurements of service, as developed from economic data and from physicians' estimates showing expected utilization, should be classified according to clinical service and revenue-producing departmental categories such as surgical beds, medical beds, obstetrical beds, pediatric beds, nonacute beds, special clinical services, and emergency and outpatient services.

Based on historic trends and information derived from hospital statistics, the physician survey, and industry statistics—for example, the Hospital Administrative Services and the Professional Activity Study—probable utilization of major special service departments such as laboratory, x-ray, and physical therapy can be forecast.

Forecasting use rates for ancillary or special services such as laboratory and radiology represents a difficult but important task. The following procedures are among those that should be considered in this task:

- The contemplated project should be reviewed to determine whether the planned changes will affect the scope of, or demand for, ancillary services to be offered.
- The physician survey and interview process should include questions related to anticipated changes in usage of major ancillary services.
- Historical use rates of ancillary services to inpatients per patient day or admission, and changes in the mode of providing these ancillary services, should be analyzed to determine whether trend adjustments are needed.
- The results of these trend analyses, adjusted for changes in the special services which are expected as a result of the project and for changes indicated in the physician survey, should be applied to forecast admissions or patient days to develop forecast units of inpatient ancillary service per period.
- In circumstances where outpatient activities do not follow an identifiable trend, or in situations where outpatient volumes are changing rapidly, an outpatient/patient origin study to define the specific outpatient service area should be considered. Future service area populations and anticipated outpatient visit rates, adjusted for anticipated service changes and physician utilization changes, can be used to develop forecasts of outpatient volumes.

Final tabulations of expected service levels should provide estimates of prospective use, classified in annual periods, giving consideration to the planned dates for opening new areas of the hospital.

Financial Analysis

The main objective of this phase is to translate the findings of the facility utilization phase into financial statement forecasts. This requires an understanding of the hospital's operating history to develop reasonable forecasting techniques for each account included in the statements. Because of the study's emphasis on cash flow, significant effort is devoted to the statement of revenues and expenses and the balance sheet.

A forecast is made of the cost of operating the hospital at the forecast levels of use. Required staffing, supplies, and other operating costs needed to support forecast service levels are forecast based on the hospital's previous experience, as well as data from governmental and private agencies, adjusted to reflect the specific operating policies and programs of management. In a feasibility study, the following tasks are generally performed.

The future personnel requirements are estimated on the basis of current workload/workforce patterns, with consideration of such factors as:

- existing over or understaffing situations;
- contemplated changes in physical layout;
- contemplated changes in the methods of delivering services; and
- changes in workload volumes.

Dollar forecasts of operating expenses are developed by analyzing wage, salary, and fringe benefit data for personnel, and cost factors for supplies and professional fees. Past costs of supplies and other expenses per unit of services are developed. Average charge data per occasion of service, based upon price trends and probable future charges, are applied to estimated patient utilization to provide estimates of dollar amounts of patient revenues.

Depreciation estimates for the program and normal replacements of equipment are based upon the expected useful lives, firm construction bids, or guaranteed maximum prices, and estimated other costs of the assets. Depreciation estimates are then computed based upon the method expected to be used for both financial reporting and cost reporting purposes. Depreciation estimates for existing assets are based upon existing lives and methods currently used. In addition, annual interest expense based on debt service schedules prepared by the underwriters is analyzed and developed on the basis of appropriate accounting principles.

Income and expense allocations between payers, and contractual arrangements and policies for accumulating charges and rendering billings, are also evaluated so that contractual allowances can be appropriately reflected.

Balance sheet accounts are analyzed for interrelationships and historical patterns as applied to forecast revenue and expense levels and the provisions of the contemplated program. Substantially completed legal documents are reviewed to identify the appropriate flow of funds during and after the construction period. These funds flow requirements are incorporated in the cash flow statements and a test of the adequacy of the financing level is performed.

From such information, a financial forecast of operating income and expenses, cash flow, changes in fund balances, and financial position is prepared. In preparing the financial statement forecast, it is important to incorporate the accounting principles and techniques which management intends to use during the forecast period.

Report Preparation and Reviews

When the financial phase is completed, final forecasts are prepared in customary financial statement form, and presented in a written report which sets forth the principal assumptions, the rationale, and an outline of the purpose of the study, the scope of work performed, the extent of the consultant's responsibility, and the finding regarding the ability of the hospital to meet operational as well as debt service costs.

The consultant must maintain complete objectivity in preparing the feasibility study report. This objectivity should not, however, lessen the style, design, and content of the report for marketing purposes. Bond buyers, and in particular institutional buyers, are utilizing the feasibility study in reaching an economic decision. Consequently, appropriate disclosures of the assumptions behind the financial statement forecasts are necessary, together with information needed to assess the assumptions and draw conclusions concerning other factors which may be material to the long-term viability of the institution.

All parties must recognize that forecasts are subject to uncertainty and that the consultant is not responsible for events occurring after the date of its report. In addition, disclaimers contained in a feasibility study report are necessary to protect all parties from unnecessary legal liabilities.

Feasibility consultants, as part of their work, generally provide for a review by experienced executives who have not been directly involved in the study to ensure the professional quality of the study's conclusions, disclosures, and work program. In addition, the consultant generally requires the right of approval of any reference to the feasibility study or the consulting firm contained in the official statement or prospectus containing the feasibility study.

In addition to submitting the written feasibility study, the consultant generally should accompany representatives of the hospital to the rating agency meetings. During these meetings, the consultant will answer questions pertaining to the study. The consultant should also attend due-diligence meetings. However, participation in preparation and review of the legal documents varies significantly among consultants and depends upon the desires of management.

SELECTING THE CONSULTANT

Health facility feasibility studies are complex jobs requiring:

- knowledge of hospital operations, reimbursement, and methods of health care financing;
- consultant integrity and independence; and
- understanding and ability to apply special health care and Financial Accounting Standards Board reporting procedures and accounting policies.

The feasibility consultant must understand and document the details of the proposed financing and help the financing authority, the health facility, and the underwriters analyze the impact of various alternative financing structures or indenture terms. An experienced health care feasibility consultant can play a significant role in helping underwriters and attorneys structure the proposed financing program. Thus, the importance of selecting an experienced health care feasibility consultant cannot be overstated.

Depth of Health Care Experience

The feasibility consultant must demonstrate extensive health care experience. It is the experience of the consultant that ensures that the feasibility study will reflect the underlying creditworthiness of the proposed financing. Experience can be assessed on the basis of: (1) the capabilities and health care specialization of the firm's staff; (2) the firm's organizational approach to health care services; (3) the firm's commitment to serve the health care industry; (4) the firm's range of comprehensive health care services; and (5) the firm's record of service to health care facilities locally and nationally. Actual experience in performing high-quality health care feasibility studies locally and nationally for a variety of facilities should be valued highly.

Quality of Work

Feasibility studies help to reduce risk by providing information to the issuer, underwriters, rating agencies, and potential investors that is useful in making financing, investment rating, and investment decisions. Consistent, carefully considered common approaches to the study and report on findings must be used to assure decision makers that a comprehensive assessment has been made by the feasibility consultant.

Ultimately, it is people who ensure quality. The project director assigned to the engagement must be an executive with health care experience, qualified in financial forecasting related to public offerings.

Personnel with technical expertise in economics, marketing, and health care planning should be deeply involved in the facility utilization phase of the study. Those with accounting, finance, and reimbursement expertise should be involved in the financial phase.

The project director must assume active, direct supervision of these technical specialists, and take full responsibility for planning and monitoring all significant engagement procedures, including the preparation of the firm's report.

The firm's commitment to ensure quality can also be measured by the independent review process it requires.

National Reputation/Market Acceptance

The feasibility consulting firm must demonstrate the market acceptability of its work. This can be assessed by noting or exploring (1) the number of studies performed by the firm over the last three to five years; (2) the opinions and experiences of other clients, rating agencies, underwriters, financial consultants, and investors; and (3) the firm's ability to be independent and objective.

Experienced hospital feasibility consultants have repeatedly demonstrated their value to hospitals and other members of financing teams in structuring the financing and in other aspects of the financing program. The feasibility study performs an important function in the hospital financing marketplace by providing a detailed and thorough analysis of the hospital's operations. Consequently, the selection of an experienced consultant can yield significant benefits greatly exceeding the cost of professional services.

NOTES

1. Standard & Poor's Corporation, *Municipal and International Bond Ratings—An Overview* (New York: Standard & Poor's Corporation, 1981), pp. 39–40.

2. American Institute of Certified Public Accountants, *Guide for a Review of a Financial Forecast* (New York: The Institute, October 1980), p. 1.

3. *Ibid.*, at Preface.

SUGGESTED READINGS

American Hospital Association. *Budgeting Procedures for Hospitals.* Chicago: AHA, 1971.

American Institute of Certified Public Accountants. *Guide for a Review of a Financial Forecast.* New York: AICPA, 1980.

Berg, Gordon H. "Evaluation of a Hospital as a Long-Term Borrower." *Financial Analysts Journal* 27: 2 (March/April 1971), pp. 23–32.

Chambers, John C.; Mullick, Satinder K.; and Smith, Donald D. "How to Choose the Right Forecasting Techniques." *Harvard Business Review* (July/August 1971), pp. 45–74.

Gitel, Harvey J. "What is a Hospital Feasibility Study and Who Needs It?" *Hospital Financial Management* 11: 9 (September 1981), pp. 47–52.

Griffith, John R. "Measuring Service Areas and Forecasting Demand." In John R. Griffith, Walton M. Hancock, and Fred Munson, eds. *Cost Control in Hospitals.* Ann Arbor, Mich.: Health Administration Press, 1976.

Johns, Lucy; Chapman, Thomas; and Morton, Raphael. *Guide to Financial and Economic Analysis for Health Planning.* San Rafael, Calif.: Lestor Gorsline Associates, 1973.

McLaughlin, Curtis P., and Sheldon, Alan. *Future and Medical Care: A Health Manager's Guide to Forecasting.* Chapel Hill: University of North Carolina, 1974.

Walker, Jerry M. "Feasibility Study Helps Forecast Your Hospital's Financial Future." *Hospital Financial Management* 9: 3 (March 1979), pp. 14–17.

Chapter 5

Corporate Restructuring and Other Planning Considerations

Geoffrey B. Shields

Every long-term financing imposes a variety of constraints on the hospital's freedom to make business decisions during the life of the outstanding bonds. Hospital administrators should bear this fact carefully in mind when drafting the provisions of the debt documents. An ounce of prevention at this stage is worth pounds (and many dollars) of cure after the hospital is committed to restrictive covenants by the financing.

All of the hospital's long-term planning should be reviewed at the time work commences on a bond issue to be certain that everything the hospital wishes to undertake can be achieved under the restrictions imposed by the debt documents. Discussed below are some of the planning considerations that the hospital and its counsel should consider in drafting debt documents. Specific provisions should be broad enough to permit the hospital to achieve its goals in these areas.

CORPORATE RESTRUCTURING

In recent years a large percentage of the nation's hospitals have started to consider, and in many cases implement, plans for corporate restructuring. The goals of such corporate restructurings include (a) maximizing third-party reimbursement, (b) insulating certain functions from rate review, (c) permitting certain expansion without certificate-of-need and Section 1122 approvals, (d) avoiding certain zoning and land use restrictions, (e) improving the quality of management and the hospital's ability to attract additional first-rate administrators, and (f) facilitating the entry into related fields. It appears likely that health care institutions will continue to restructure to achieve these and a variety of other goals.

In drafting debt documents there are conflicting goals of the parties with regard to corporate restructuring provisions. The hospital and its counsel will want the broadest possible authority to give or loan hospital assets and functions to the related organizations created in the restructuring. The underwriters and prospective bond purchasers will be interested in maintaining tight security of the hospital's assets to back the hospital's bonds. Several means of accommodating both interests have been developed. These include:

- *The ability to transfer a limited amount of assets annually.* Some debt documents simply permit the hospital to transfer three to five percent of its assets each year to an affiliated corporation without requiring any payment for this transfer.

- *Annual transfer plus unlimited transfer upon satisfaction of certain conditions.* Recently the Illinois Health Facilities Authority, the Missouri Health and Educational Facilities Authority, and a number of local issuers in other jurisdictions have permitted a certain amount of assets to be transferred upon the satisfaction of certain minimal conditions (including the requirement that the tax-exempt status of the bonds will not be impaired) and will permit unlimited transfers provided that these and certain other conditions, including a guarantee from a transferee to the trustee on the bonds, be entered into at the time of the transfer. An excerpt from an official statement of one such financing explaining this arrangement is attached as Appendix 5-A to this chapter. This type of covenant is designed to permit bona fide transfers of assets and functions while providing that the security interest of the bondholders in these assets and functions will follow the assets and functions.

- *Master indenture provisions.* A related way of dealing with the transfer to affiliates concept is to provide that all or some affiliated corporations of the borrowing hospital corporation enter into and become parties to a "master indenture." The master indenture provides certain limitations on the kind of debt that the affiliated corporations can enter into, while permitting broad latitude for transfer of assets among affiliated corporations. These negative debt covenants for the entire "family" of affiliated corporations assure that as a group their debt remains at an acceptable level. Sometimes this concept is coupled with a mortgage on property of the affiliated corporations or a guaranty for the benefit of the bondholders.

Timing Considerations

The hospital should attempt, where possible, either to complete a restructuring or to have in mind with some degree of certainty the type of corporate reorganization it would like to achieve prior to beginning the processing of its bond issue. This will permit the hospital to be very specific with regard to what corporate structure it wants and what it is willing to pledge as security for the bonds. This will permit the transfer to affiliates language to be tailored specifically to the plans of the hospital and to permit the best type of disclosure to prospective bondholders with regard to such transfers.

The hospital should discuss at some length with prospective underwriters the formulas that those underwriters are willing to adopt to permit restructuring flexibility for hospitals. The hospital should ascertain whether its counsel is competent to advise it with regard to appropriate restructuring language. If it is not, then special counsel should be hired for this purpose.

ISSUANCE OF ADDITIONAL DEBT

The hospital will likely wish to issue additional debt during the life of the outstanding bonds. Traditionally, this need is dealt with in the debt documents by permitting the issuance of additional bonds or parity debt for capital construction and acquisition of equipment and by permitting the hospital to enter into various shorter-term debt arrangements including capitalized leases, working capital loans, and true leases of equipment. In addition, the hospital is generally permitted to borrow money through mortgaging of property not used for health care purposes such as property surrounding the hospital facility that may be used for later expansion of the hospital. The amounts of these types of debt are limited by certain debt tests. In taxable bond issues the debt tests for additional long-term debt are often tied to some ratio of debt to assets. In tax-exempt issues additional debt is usually tied to a ratio of annual debt service to revenues over expenses (fund balances). The hospital should be certain that its debt documents permit it to issue additional parity debt through other issuers and to offer both taxable and tax-exempt parity debt, so long as it meets the additional debt tests. The hospital will want this flexibility in case other issuers should become more attractive for future bond issues. Also, in recent years the U.S. Treasury Department has expressed a desire to abolish tax-exempt hospital bonds. Should this occur, hospitals will wish to be able to issue taxable bonds which rank on a parity with its outstanding tax-exempt bonds.

Other types of additional debt, such as working capital borrowing and capitalized leases, are frequently limited to some percentage of gross revenues or sometimes to a fund balances test. True leases of equipment generally are permitted without restriction. It is important that the hospital insist that its counsel, accountants, and investment bankers carefully review the additional debt covenants to determine that it has flexibility to engage in additional borrowing. Appendix 5-B is an example of additional debt language.

It should be held in mind that the U.S. Department of Health and Human Services and various state agencies have moved to cut back on the revenues of hospitals. This will likely decrease the revenues available for additional debt service in the future and may make it difficult for hospitals to meet the additional debt tests imposed upon them. If they are unable to meet the tests, hospitals will be unable to issue additional long-term debt unless they defease or retire their outstanding debt. Some hospitals have successfully negotiated a provision permitting them to issue additional long-term debt with as low as one-to-one projected debt coverage, provided that low coverage is a result of state or federal action limiting their revenues and so long as they are able to get a consultant's opinion saying that given the rate and reimbursement restrictions imposed upon the hospital it is unable to obtain better debt service coverage. An example of such language is found in Appendix 5-C.

MERGERS AND ACQUISITIONS

Both not-for-profit and for-profit hospitals have been exposed to a merger and acquisition trend of great magnitude over the last decade.[1] It appears that this trend will continue. Economies of scale in both management and product, community disenchantment with supporting community hospitals with tax revenues, the aggressiveness of proprietary chains, reductions in levels of reimbursement, and a variety of other factors are all pushing hospitals and hospital systems to enter into formal merger agreements or into a wide variety of affiliation agreements. Long-term debt documents generally permit mergers and acquisitions so long as certain conditions are met.

A potential acquiring institution should consider several important factors. If a hospital thinks it is possible that it will be acquiring an outstanding hospital facility, it should be sure that it will be able to acquire that facility without having to refinance or defease its own debt. Thus, it will want to provide that it may acquire another hospital facility so long as it meets minimal requirements with regard to debt coverage on a pro forma (combined) basis. It will probably not want to be in a position where the outstanding hospital facility will have to have had positive fund balances in the year or two before acquisition. Attractive to most hospitals is a test that permits the hospital to acquire an outstanding facility so long as the combined pro forma debt of the two facilities will meet either the historical or the future projected debt coverage tests required for the hospital to issue one dollar of additional parity debt.

The institution to be merged into a larger facility should protect its ability to leave outstanding its debt as the nonsurviving entity in a merger. Here again, it should be able to transfer all of its assets to another corporation so long as the surviving corporation will be able, on a pro forma combined basis, to meet certain minimal debt coverage tests. Again, appropriate ratios may be those contained in the additional parity debt test.

Certain other requirements are normally imposed by the underwriters, including the requirement that any outstanding litigation against the other party to a merger not be in excess of certain amounts, that the tax status of not-for-profit hospitals not be affected, that the tax-exempt status of the hospital's tax-exempt bonds not be affected by the merger, and that all state and federal regulatory requirements for such a merger be met.

In summary, the health care institution should be sure that it will have substantial flexibility in corporate reorganization, mergers and acquisitions, and additional borrowing in its debt documents. These concerns should be discussed carefully with the hospital's underwriter prior to commencing the drafting of the hospital's debt documents. The hospital should not assume that its underwriter or bond counsel will offer provisions that are of maximum advantage to the hospital in these areas. Those parties are apt to be equally concerned with tight security for the benefit of bondholders. It will be up to the hospital and the hospital's counsel to negotiate provisions that are of maximum advantage to the hospital without impairing its ability to get a desirable interest rate on its bonds.

NOTE

1. "Multihospital System Survey," *Modern Healthcare*, April 1981, p. 79.

Appendix 5-A

Transactions with Affiliates

Certain transfers of assets to and transactions with Affiliates are permitted under the following conditions:

A. If the Transferred Property is not necessary for the functioning of the Corporation's acute care hospitals, the Corporation may transfer, with or without consideration: (1) 2 percent or less of its properties and assets in any 12-month period; and (2) the following: (a) once only, up to $2 million of cash and securities to a fund-raising foundation of which the Corporation is a substantial designated beneficiary; (b) once only, real property of the Corporation to an Affiliate, if the appraised value of such property does not exceed 3 percent of the assets of the Corporation; (c) the assets and stock (if any) of Health Data Network (a data processing operation of the hospital) to an Affiliate; and (d) in addition, properties and assets (the Transferred Property) in any 12-month period provided such disposition is to an Affiliate; the Affiliate executes an Affiliate Guaranty; and the delivery of certain appraisals, reports, opinions, and similar materials. Such reports should include: (i) a report of an independent certified public accountant (CPA) (which may be the corporation's auditor) that the Net Revenues of the Corporation for the preceding fiscal year are at least 120 percent of the maximum annual debt service on the outstanding Bonds, Additional Bonds, Parity Obligations and other indebtedness of the Corporation; (ii) a report of a nationally recognized hospital consultant chosen by the Corporation that estimates or forecasts Net Income Available for Debt Service for each of the two following fiscal years after disposition of the Transferred Property will be at least 125 percent of the maximum annual debt service on the outstanding Bonds, Additional Bonds, Parity Obligations, and other indebtedness of the Corporation, sufficient revenues and cash flow could be generated to meet the Corporation's operating expenses and debt service on its other long-term debt during such two years, and the Corporation's unrestricted fund balances will not be made negative by reason of such disposition; (iii) an opinion of Counsel to the effect of such disposition on tax exemptions and as to its enforceability and compliance with the Loan Agreement and applicable law; and (iv) an opinion of a nationally recognized Bond Counsel relating to authorization of the transfer under the Act (state authorizing legislation) and the continuing validity of the Bonds and their tax exemption.

B. The requirements for the CPA and consultant reports shall be deemed satisfied if: (1) in the opinion of a nationally recognized hospital consultant applicable laws or regulations have prevented or will prevent the Corporation from generating the debt service coverage required by the reports; (2) the Corporation has generated, and the forecasts or estimates contained in the hospital consultant's report are that it will generate the maximum amount of Net Income Available for Debt Service (in the opinion of such hospital consultant) permitted to be generated by such laws and regulations for such period; and (3) for each of the following two fiscal years, the Net Income Available for Debt Service is forecasted to be at least 100 percent of the maximum annual debt service on the Bonds, Additional Bonds, Parity Obligations, and all other debt of the Corporation.

C. Each Affiliate Guaranty shall: (1) guarantee payment of the Bonds and any Additional Bonds but only to the extent of the fair market value of the Transferred Property at the transfer or at the time of realization upon the Affiliate Guaranty, whichever is higher (the "Fair Market Value"); (2) provide that the obligations under such Affiliate Guaranty may be discharged if the Affiliate pays to the Corporation cash in the amount of the Fair Market Value; provided that, if the Transferred Property so acquired by such Affiliate constitutes a part of the Project or other property financed with bond proceeds, the Affiliate Guaranty may be discharged only if the Affiliate reconveys such Transferred Property to the Corporation or secures the release provided for in the Loan Agreement; (3) provide that the Affiliate may not incur any indebtedness or liabilities except: (a) for unsecured indebtedness for borrowed money of the Affiliate which is subordinated to the Affiliate's obligations under the Affiliate Guaranty and the Bonds, and which shall not exceed 20 percent of the Affiliate's assets; (b) liabilities (other than for borrowed money [except as set forth in clause (a) above] and other than rents payable under lease agreements) incurred in the regular operations of the Affiliate; and (c) liabilities for borrowed money and rents payable under lease agreements, both payable solely to the Corporation or, if payable to other parties then, in aggregate, not in excess of 20 percent of the amount of the Affiliate Guaranty; (4) prohibit mergers by the Affiliate, except with the Corporation or another Affiliate, if the surviving entity assumes the Affiliate Guaranty; (5) prohibit transfers of assets by the Affiliate, except (a) to the Corporation or to another Affiliate if prior to a transfer to another Affiliate certain conditions are satisfied and (b) in the ordinary course of, and as required by, the Affiliate's activities and upon fair and reasonable terms no less favorable to the Affiliate than it would obtain in a comparable arm's length transaction; (6) provide that the Transferred Property will be reconveyed to the Corporation prior to the Affiliate's dissolution; and (7) provide that if the Affiliate fails to pay under the Affiliate Guaranty, the Trustee shall have a right to attach its gross revenues immediately as necessary to make such payments.

D. An affiliate may satisfy and release its Affiliate Guaranty by paying the amount of such Affiliate Guaranty to the Corporation and supplying an opinion of Bond Counsel on the tax status of the Bonds.

E. The provisions described in this Section need not be met if the transfer is otherwise permitted by the Loan Agreement or the Indenture.

F. Except as permitted by the Loan Agreement or required by law, the Corporation will not enter into any transaction with an Affiliate except in the ordinary course of, and as required by, the Corporation's activities and upon fair and reasonable terms no less favorable to the Corporation than it would obtain in a comparable arm's length transaction with a person not an Affiliate.

Appendix 5-B

Permitted Indebtedness

The Corporation covenants and agrees that it will incur no indebtedness or liabilities of any kind with respect to the hospital facilities, other than:

A. Liabilities under the Loan Agreement.

B. Liabilities (other than for borrowed money and other than rents payable under other lease agreements having a remaining term in excess of one year) incurred in the ordinary course of the Corporation's business.

C. Short-term debt, which is defined as debt maturing in one year or less (which is debt other than Funded Debt), limited to a maximum of 20 percent at any time outstanding of the then-preceding year's gross revenues of the Corporation. The amount of this short-term debt must be reduced to zero for a period of 30 consecutive days every calendar year.

D. Funded Debt so long as the Additional Debt test is satisfied. Such Debt may be represented by Parity Obligations in which case the Bond Reserve Fund Requirements do not need to be satisfied.

E. Indebtedness outstanding at any one time not exceeding 10 percent of the Corporation's Fund Balances shown in the most recent annual audited financial statements, consisting of the aggregate of lease or rental payments to be made under the remaining term of leases of real property.

F. Principal indebtedness guaranteed by the Corporation not to exceed, in combination with the principal amount of Permitted Mortgages, 15 percent of total Fund Balances of the Corporation shown in the Corporation's most recent annual audited financial statements.

G. In addition to capitalized leases permitted under (D.), capitalized leases outstanding at any one time the aggregate total minimum scheduled payments on which do not exceed 10 percent of the Corporation's Fund Balances shown in its most recent annual audited financial statements.

H. Assumption of the debt of an acquired, merged, or consolidated entity (in addition to the guaranties permitted by Subsection F above) if: (1) prior to such assumption, the Corporation provides a report by a

Hospital Consultant stating that (after taking account of the proposed acquisition or merger and assumption of debt), the Corporation's Net Income Available for Debt Service, estimated for each of the two full fiscal years immediately following the date of such report, will not be less than 125 percent of the Annual Debt Service for each of such years on the Outstanding Bonds and any other Parity Obligations; (2) the holders of such assumed debt may be entitled to no lien on the assets of the Corporation (other than on the assets securing the assumed debt prior to merger) superior to that of the Bonds or Parity Obligations; or (3) immediately prior to such assumption such debt shall not be in default in accordance with its terms.

I. Notwithstanding the above, the Corporation may also issue on a one-time basis either Parity Obligations or Additional Bonds (1) for completion of the Project in an amount not in excess of $5 million, and (2) for construction, equipping, and payment of expenses related to the proposed new wing of the hospital in an amount not in excess of $9.5 million without regard to any earnings tests so long as the Debt Service Reserve Fund is increased appropriately.

J. Borrowings from the Depreciation Fund.

K. Liabilities of the Corporation as Lessee under true leases for equipment that are not capitalized on the Corporation's balance sheet.

Appendix 5-C

Additional Bonds and Parity Indebtedness

Additional Bonds ranking on a basis of parity and equality with Series 1982 Bonds, or other Parity Debt, may be issued for (i) costs of completion of the Project in an amount not exceeding $5 million, and (ii) costs of construction, equipment, and expenses related to a new wing for the hospital in an amount not exceeding $9.5 million.

In addition, Additional Bonds ranking on a basis of parity and equality with the Series 1982 Bonds (in addition to the Series 1982 Bonds) may be issued from time to time if:

A. Either (1) the Corporation's average annual Net Income Available for Debt Service for the two Fiscal Years immediately preceding the issuance of such Additional Bonds or Parity Obligations, as evidenced by annual audit reports, must have been equal to at least 1.10 times the Maximum Annual Debt Service Requirement on all Funded Debt (including the Additional Bonds or Parity Obligations to be issued and any outstanding Bonds and Parity Obligations issued by the Corporation), or (2) both (a) the Net Income Available for Debt Service for the Corporation's Fiscal Year immediately preceding the issuance of such Additional Bonds or Parity Obligations, as evidenced by annual audits, must have been equal to at least 1.10 times the then current Maximum Annual Debt Service Requirement on all outstanding Funded Debt (including any outstanding Bonds and Parity Obligations), and (b) the Net Income Available for Debt Service, as estimated in writing by a financial consultant, for the average of the two Fiscal Years following completion of the Project will be not less than 1.20 times the Maximum Annual Debt Service Requirement on all Funded Debt, including the requirements on the Additional Bonds or Parity Obligations and any outstanding Bonds and Parity Obligations.

B. However, if a recognized Hospital Consultant delivers a report to the Trustee to the effect that state or federal laws or regulations or other externally imposed reimbursement requirements then in existence do not permit the Corporation to produce the required levels of Net Income Available for Debt Service set forth above, then such levels shall be reduced to the maximum amount then permitted by such laws or regulations or other externally imposed reimbursement requirements, but in no event less than 100 percent.

C. The Corporation shall not be in default and all required payments must be current.

D. The Bond Reserve Fund Requirement corresponding to such Additional Bonds shall be deposited into the Bond Reserve Fund. No such deposit shall be required for issuance of Parity Debt.

E. The balance in the Bond Reserve Fund upon issuance of the Additional bonds shall be not less than the Maximum Annual Debt Service Requirement on all Bonds, including the proposed Additional Bonds. The Bond Reserve Fund shall be pledged for the benefit only of the holders of Bonds (including Additional Bonds) and not for the benefit of the Parity Obligations.

The terms of any such issue of Additional Bonds, their purchase price, and the manner in which the proceeds therefrom are to be disbursed shall be stipulated in writing by the Corporation; and the Corporation and the Issuer shall enter into an amendment to the Loan Agreement to provide for additional loan payments in an amount at least sufficient to pay principal and interest on the Additional Bonds when due, and the Issuer and the Corporation shall otherwise comply with the provisions of Section 207 of the Indenture with respect to the issuance of such Additional Bonds. Any such completion or improvements financed with the proceeds of the Additional Bonds shall become a part of the Hospital Facilities and shall be included under the Loan Agreement to the same extent as if originally included hereunder.

It is acknowledged that the Corporation may incur additional Parity Obligations which constitute Permitted Indebtedness from time to time ranking on a parity with the Bonds, subject to compliance with the terms and conditions of the Loan Agreement.

Chapter 6

Categories of Borrowing

Geoffrey B. Shields

Several threshold decisions must be made when entering into a borrowing. These include decisions on whether the borrowing should be (1) taxable or tax-exempt, (2) a private placement or a public offering, and (3) long-term or short-term.

Each decision will dramatically affect the cost of borrowing and the type of processing of the debt issue.

TAXABLE OR TAX-EXEMPT?

Although the main consideration in the decision whether a hospital should do its financing as a tax-exempt financing or as a taxable financing is one of cost, there are a variety of other factors which the hospital may wish to consider as well.

Cost

The cost savings for a tax-exempt financing are derived from the fact that the holders of tax-exempt bonds do not have to pay federal income taxes on the interest they derive from those bonds. Thus, they are willing to accept lower interest rates than on taxable securities. Historically, this meant the interest rates on tax-exempt hospital bonds of a particular maturity were approximately one-third lower than the interest rates on a taxable bond issue with the same credit quality. However, the interest rate differential between taxable and tax-exempt bond issues occasionally narrows significantly.

For example, in 1975 the impending default of New York City on its bonds resulted for a brief period in tax-exempt hospital bonds issued through the New York Dormitory Authority selling at a higher interest rate than the same quality taxable bonds. Another example occurred in 1981 when tax rates for individuals were substantially decreased and taxes for corporations were cut through a variety of provisions. By late 1981, the differential between taxable and tax-exempt rates had, for the same maturities, dropped to approximately 20 percent and, in some cases, less.

In tax-exempt financings, in addition to a lower interest rate on the bonds, there is an additional potential cost savings through certain "arbitrage earnings" which hospitals can usually derive from the difference between taxable and tax-exempt interest rates. Certain portions of the bond proceeds can be reinvested in taxable securities, yielding a higher interest rate than the interest rate on the bonds. This provides a certain amount of "arbitrage earnings" that lower the effective interest rate to the hospital. The Internal Revenue Code regulations governing the amount of arbitrage earnings permissible on a hospital financing are changed from time to time, and the underwriter and bond counsel should be consulted about ways in which arbitrage earnings can be maximized.

Partially offsetting the lower interest rates and arbitrage earning advantages of tax-exempt bonds are the higher costs associated with issuing tax-exempt bonds. Because (1) bond counsel must be employed, (2) the issuing authority frequently demands a fee, (3) the documents are more complex and longer, in a tax-exempt financing, (4) the structure of a tax-exempt financing is much more complicated, and (5) often a shorter feasibility study or none at all is required in a taxable financing, the cost of preparing a tax-exempt bond issue is higher than that of a taxable bond issue. However, the total cost to the borrowing hospital is almost always less in a tax-exempt bond issue. The underwriter should be consulted about the difference in cost of the two types of issues.

Speed of Issuance

Certain states have detailed requirements for the issuance of tax-exempt bonds which require various filings, hearings, and other time-consuming procedures in order to be able to accomplish a tax-exempt financing. In taxable financings, most of these requirements are not present. The requirements for issuing tax-exempt bonds may include obtaining approval from the local issuer, validation proceedings, and, in certain instances, waiting one's "turn in line" with the issuing entity in order to go to the market.

Flexibility of Financing Terms

Today, financing terms in both taxable and tax-exempt documents are generally fairly flexible and can be structured to meet the needs of the particular hospital. However, in certain cases, state law or the whim of the issuing authority imposes significant limitations on the flexibility of the hospital to structure its bond issue in the form most advantageous to it. For example, some states prohibit loan agreement financings without a mortgage. The structural limitations of a tax-exempt financing should be discussed with the bond counsel, the underwriter, and special counsel to the hospital.

Maximum Term and Structure of Debt Payments

Currently, the public tax-exempt bond market for health facilities bonds will accept bonds with a term of 30 to 35 years to final maturity with level debt service. The public taxable bond market will, except under special circumstances, accept health facilities bonds with a maximum maturity of 20 years or less, and bond issues of less than 10 years are common.

Privately placed tax-exempt bonds can have maturities of 30 to 35 years while taxable private placements are marketable with a maximum of 20 to 25 years.

Annual debt service is held down in many taxable and some tax-exempt financings of ten years or less by requiring only interest to be paid until the final payment on the loan, at which time all principal, plus the final interest payment, are made in one "balloon payment."

Philosophical Considerations

Some hospitals, particularly religiously affiliated hospitals, do not wish to borrow money through a governmental entity. Although the issuer of tax-exempt revenue bonds is generally not liable for payment of principal or interest on the bonds (all of the responsibility for payment rests with the hospital), the bonds must be issued by a governmental entity in order to comply with federal tax provisions (except in 63-20 financings). The philosophical concern with borrowing money through a governmental entity has decreased substantially since the early 1970s so that there are relatively few hospitals and groups of hospitals which today are unwilling to engage in tax-exempt financing.

Some religiously affiliated hospitals have been concerned that the mere existence of their tax-exempt debt and the existence of a governmental issuer for that debt could be used to force them to conduct procedures which violate their religious principles. Such hospitals may wish to insert a provision in their tax-exempt debt documents permitting them to call the bonds should they be required to perform any procedure or do any other act in contradiction of their moral code.

Federal Government Legislative Initiatives

In recent years, both Democrat and Republican administrations have indicated a desire to stop tax-exempt financings by hospitals.

PUBLIC ISSUE OR PRIVATE PLACEMENT

In both taxable and tax-exempt financing the health care institution has a choice between a public issue through an underwriter or a private placement placed with an institutional buyer by a placement agent or underwriter. It is generally difficult to make a private placement at competitive interest rates for an issue over $25 million (unless the issue is AAA) because of the more limited private placement market. For issues under $5 million, a private placement is especially attractive because it permits the hospital to avoid certain substantial front-end costs of a publicly underwritten issue which are less significant when spread over a larger issue.

Interest Rate

Typically the interest rate on the bonds sold in a public issue will be ⅛ percent to ¾ percent lower than in a private placement. The purchaser of a private placement is able to obtain this premium as a trade-off for, among other things, the reduced front-end costs of a private placement.

Use of Funds

Table 6-1 below shows the typical use of funds in a public issue and a private placement, each designed to raise $10,745,000 for a hospital construction project.

As can be seen from Table 6-1, the hospital can raise the same amount for its construction project, $10,745,000, by either a public issue of $15 million or a private placement of $11,750,000.

The size of the private placement, depending on the requirements of the purchaser, might be further reduced by foregoing the feasibility study (at least $50,000) and the rating agency fees (at least $5,000 per rating agency).

The other front-end savings in a private placement come from:

1. reducing capitalized interest by phasing the borrowing to correspond with major construction payouts. This may raise bond counsel fees

Table 6-1 Typical Tax-Exempt Bond Issue—Public Issue or Private Placement

Estimated Uses of Funds	Public Issue		Private Placement	
	Amount ($)	% of Total Borrowing	Amount ($)	% of Total Borrowing
Acquisition, construction, and equipping, including architect's fees	$10,745,000	72.0	$10,745,000	91.4
Net capitalized interest*	1,400,000	9.0	750,000***	6.4
Required funding of debt service reserve fund**	2,250,000	15.0	0	0
Printing	35,000	0.2	0	0
Legal, feasibility study, rating agency, and other fees	120,000	0.8	120,000	1.0
Bond discount or placement fee or bond discount	450,000	3.0	135,000	1.2
Bond issue size	$15,000,000	100.0	$11,750,000	100.0

* Adjusted to reflect capitalized interest on construction fund and debt service reserve fund net of interest earned.

** Equal to one year's maximum principal and interest at interest rate of 14 percent; often not required in a private placement. The principal of the debt service reserve fund is preserved intact to pay off, at the end of the issue's life, the same amount of bonds as originally issued to create the reserve. The cost (or gain) to the institution is the negative (or positive) arbitrage throughout the life of the issue. For a discussion of the Medicare/Medicaid reimbursement considerations to bear in mind when structuring a debt service reserve fund, see Chapter 7.

*** In a private placement, it is often possible to reduce capitalized interest by phasing the borrowing to meet the construction payout schedule.

Source: Gardner, Carton & Douglas.

somewhat since there may have to be a closing with each drawdown from the purchaser;

2. eliminating the printing of an official statement; and
3. the decreased fee to the underwriter required for a private placement.

With these front-end cost savings, why are most health care bond issues public issues? The most important reason is that up-front costs are one-time costs while interest cost differentials last for the life of the financing.

The present value of a ⅛ percent to ¾ percent interest rate differential on a long-term bond issue will displace a very substantial amount of front-end costs. Other reasons include the following:

- Private placement purchasers generally will buy only high-quality issues.
- Public issues often have a longer maturity, allowing a longer spread-out of debt service payments and improved cash flow for the hospital.
- Public issues generally provide the hospital with less restrictive terms.
- Much or all of the "cost" of greater capitalized interest and the debt service reserve fund is made up in interest earnings in the construction fund and the debt service reserve fund. If the debt service reserve fund can qualify as a funded depreciation account for Medicare/Medicaid reimbursement purposes, there can be a very substantial positive earnings impact from having a debt service reserve fund.
- Private placements generally have longer no-call periods and higher call premiums than public issues.

True Cost of Borrowing vs. Interest Rate on the Bonds

Table 6-1 and the discussion following it illustrate that the health care facility should be concerned with obtaining the lowest available cost of borrowing, not the lowest interest rate on the bonds. The following must be considered in determining the true cost of borrowing:

- front-end costs (for example, costs of preparing the bond issue for sale);
- earnings on the construction and debt service reserve funds;
- Medicare/Medicaid and other third-party reimbursement (and offset) treatment of interest expense and interest earned;
- possible costs of early call or advance refunding of the bond issue; and
- administrative costs of hospital personnel in negotiating the loan.

LONG-TERM vs. SHORT-TERM FINANCING

The type of the financing will depend upon the length of time or "term" the hospital wishes to borrow. The chart below depicts the types of financing generally used for different lengths of borrowing. Each may be done on a taxable or tax-exempt basis, except that a publicly issued taxable bond borrowing will generally have a maximum term of no more than 20 years.

Line-of-Credit or Short-Term Note Issue	Letter-of-Credit-Backed Tax-Exempt Short-Term Bond Issue or "Bullet" Taxable Bond Issue	Direct Private Placement with an Institutional Buyer*	Level Debt Service Public Tax-Exempt Bond Issue
1 Year or Less	5 Years	15 Years to 20 Years	30 Years

* Taxable or tax-exempt.

Short-Term Borrowing

Tax-Exempt Commercial Paper

A few hospitals with very high credit ratings (AA) have borrowed through the tax-exempt commercial paper market. This is actually a series of rollovers of tax-exempt note issues, generally each for 15 to 60 days. The various legal requirements for tax-exemption of the debt, including satisfaction of state law requirements, must be met. These notes carry very low interest rates, usually about 50 percent to 60 percent of the interest rates of ten-year tax-exempt bonds of equivalent ratings. The front-end costs are high because a bank line of credit agreement to take out the outstanding notes is required and the processing fees associated with repeated closings are high.

Bank Line of Credit

Conventional lines of credit between a bank and a hospital for a specific sum of money normally provide for payment of interest on a floating basis at prime plus some small premium (½ percent to 2 percent). This loan may be evidenced by an unsecured note or, in some instances, by a lien on accounts receivable requiring a Uniform Commercial Code filing. Generally, the line of credit must be renegotiated or renewed by mutual consent annually. Sometimes the health care facility is restricted in the line of credit agreement from entering into certain other types of borrowing.

A revolving line of credit is a legal commitment to supply credit up to some maximum amount for a longer period, usually one to five years. Table 6-2 lists various types of bank credit agreements.

Table 6-2 Bank Credit Agreements

	Line of Credit	Revolving Credit
Maturity	1 year	1–5 years, sometimes renewable upon certain conditions
Legal status	None	Legal document
Cost*	Bank's prime lending rate plus ½%–2%	Usually bank's prime lending rate plus ½%–2% (a revolving credit agreement may stipulate a provision to convert the loan to a term loan if a percentage of the total is drawn down)
Compensating balances	Usually same as revolving credit agreement, but negotiable	A requirement to maintain demand-deposits balances at the bank in direct proportion to the amount of funds borrowed and/or the amount of the commitment**
Front-end fee	None	Normally a ½% fee due to set up the credit, though this cost may be reflected in the interest rate or compensating balances required
Security Agreements	Promissory note (sometimes loan agreement)	Promissory note Loan agreement

* A hospital should always attempt to negotiate a maximum rate if it expects the loan to remain outstanding for a long period of time.

** A typical provision requires compensating balances of 10 percent of the credit and 10 percent of the used portion of the credit. If a $1 million revolving credit was fully outstanding, $200,000 would be required as compensating balances.

Intermediate Term Credit

"Master (Floating Rate) Note"—Tax-Exempt. A bank may be willing to negotiate a floating rate "master note" with a maturity of three to five years, callable at any time or on a few days' notice, tied to a percentage (usually 65 percent to 70 percent) of the prime rate charged from time to time by the lending bank. Generally no interest has to be paid until the end of the term of the loan.

Three- to Ten-Year Tax-Exempt Bonds with a Letter of Credit. Recently a large number of intermediate term financings have been done for three to ten years backed by bank letters of credit. These may be either private placements or public issues and carry with them substantial letter-of-credit financing costs.

Taxable Five- to Ten-Year Bonds. These may be issued either on a private placement or public issue basis. Generally these are "bullet" loans which require interest to be paid semiannually and payment of all principal upon maturity.

Floating rate notes which are repriced every 7 to 28 days for as long as 10 to 30 years and provide that the holder may "put" the bonds with only a few days' notice are occasionally used in health care financing. They require letter-of-credit backing.

Leases. Equipment lease financing can be used either in a taxable lease or a tax-exempt (sometimes called a "municipal lease") format. Tax-exempt leases must meet the same legal criteria as a tax-exempt bond issue; that is, they must qualify under Section 103 of the Internal Revenue Code for an exemption from federal income tax on the interest portion of the lease and must be permitted under state law. All capitalized leases must be carried as a liability on the hospital's books under Federal Accounting Standards Board Bulletin No. 13. True (noncapitalized) leases are especially useful where first-generation equipment has an undetermined useful life and the lease is directly with the manufacturer.

The hospital should be sure that its long-term debt covenants permit unlimited true lease and capitalized lease financing of equipment.

Long-Term Debt

As discussed above, long-term financing is available through the issuance of either taxable or tax-exempt debt and on either a private placement or a public issue basis.

Variations on terms and original issue discount (including "zero coupon" bonds) provide substantial flexibility in structuring long-term issues.

There are certain credit pooling and third-party credit devices that can be useful, in certain situations, to improve the credit of a health care institution and reduce the interest rate on its bonds. These are discussed in Chapter 17.

What Term for Debt?

There are different reasons for selecting either short- or long-term debt. The shortest-term debts usually have the lowest interest rates. However, use of short-term debt for major capital projects means that the hospital will have to refinance all or most of the principal of the debt, risking significantly higher interest rates later on. Worse yet, when the hospital attempts to refinance, its creditworthiness may have diminished, or the availability of tax-exempt financing may have come to an end. It could then find refinancing so expensive that it will be forced into default.

Also, the Health Care Financing Authority (HCFA) has threatened to treat any balance sheet "gain" from a defeasance of debt as an immediate offset against Medicare reimbursement. If this is done, a hospital will often find it too expensive to defease debt and will have to wait until the end of the term of outstanding debt or until the end of the no-call period to defease.

In addition, administrators often feel it prudent to use depreciation reimbursement to pay all principal on the hospital's debt. This is best accomplished by structuring debt to have level or even diminishing principal payments, depending on the mix of depreciable lives of the financed construction projects and equipment acquisitions. However, the cash flow consequences of this may be unappealing, and the hospital administration may wish to use some of the depreciation reimbursement to fund a depreciation account, with its favorable Medicare reimbursement treatment.

During the last decade most hospitals have chosen to finance their projects with level debt service long-term bonds, which have approximately equal debt service payments each year the debt is outstanding and no balloon payment at the end. This permits a hospital to "lock in" rates available now. It also forces it to pay off principal while it is receiving depreciation reimbursement.

If interest rates fall the hospital can call the bonds (if the no-call period has run) and refinance them with lower cost debt. If the no-call period has not run, then it can defease the outstanding bonds.

In a defeasance, an escrow funded with U.S. government obligations is established for the payment of principal and interest on the refunded bonds. The U.S. government obligations are purchased with the proceeds of the refunding bond issue. The interest rate on the escrowed securities is limited to the interest rate on the refunding bonds by the arbitrage regulations governing advance refundings.

A hospital can capture a substantial part, but not all, of the lower interest rate on a refunding bond. If the interest rate on the bond issue to be refunded is greater than 2 percent above the interest rate on the refunding bonds, it will almost certainly be worthwhile to do a defeasance.

Thus, if the health care facility finances long-term, it can refinance if interest rates drop.

However, because both the Internal Revenue Service and HCFA Medicare reimbursement treatments of defeasance of debt are currently under review, the hospital should consult its reimbursement adviser and its investment banker about the current availability and benefits of defeasance.

Chapter 7

The Medicare Reimbursement Aspects of Tax-Exempt Hospital Bond Financings[*]

Earl L. Metheny

Necessary[1] and proper[2] interest expense arising from both current[3] and capital indebtedness constitutes a cost reimbursable to providers of health care services[4] participating[5] in the Medicare[6] program.[7] Typically, capital indebtedness is that indebtedness incurred from borrowings for financing the acquisition of equipment, the construction or acquisition of new facilities, and the making of capital improvements.[8] The interest expense on such capital indebtedness incurred pursuant to a bond indenture agreement entered into by a provider is an allowable[9] cost of producing health services to the extent that the expense relates to the acquisition or construction of assets related to patient care activities.[10]

The amount of interest expense for which a provider may be reimbursed, however, is reduced by the amount of investment income it may earn.[11] If a provider, for example, should incur $1 million in interest expense pursuant to a borrowing from a nonrelated[12] source for a capital expenditure related to patient care, the $1 million in allowable interest expense will be reduced *pro tanto*[13] by an amount of interest or other income earned pursuant to a provider's investment of its available funds. Investment income accruing from the following sources, however, is sheltered from the offset requirement:[14]

1. income from gifts and grants, whether restricted or unrestricted, and which gifts and grants are held separate and not commingled with other funds;
2. income from a provider's qualified pension funds; and
3. income from funded depreciation.

---

[*] In my wrestle with the financial accounting angel, I have greatly benefited from the coaching of Terrence M. Hiduke of Main, Hurdman, Certified Public Accountants in Indianapolis, Indiana. If it appears on occasion that I have been pinned, such fault is attributable to my own weakness alone.

The funding of depreciation is the practice of setting aside cash, or other liquid assets, in a fund separate from the general funds of the provider to be used for the replacement of the assets depreciated, or for other capital purposes.[15] When a provider funds depreciation, the money in the depreciation fund will normally be invested and will accumulate revenues. To encourage such funding of depreciation, the United States Department of Health and Human Services (HHS) has determined that the income earned by funded depreciation accounts will not reduce the amount of reimbursable interest expense.[16] In formulating the policy of sheltering such investment income from reimbursement offset, the Health Insurance Benefits Advisory Council, established prior to the enactment of the Medicare statute to provide assistance to the Secretary of Health, Education, and Welfare (now HHS) on matters of general policy with respect to health insurance benefits,[17] noted that failure to motivate providers to reserve funds to replace depreciating assets might lead to greater future borrowing by providers and, as a result, greater expenditures under the program to reimburse providers for allowable interest costs.[18] The wise marshalling of hospital resources therefore compels careful consideration of the use of funded depreciation and its sheltered income in planning the financing of new provider facilities. Although income from a provider's qualified pension funds is also sheltered from the interest reimbursement offset, the use of such funds by a provider for its own financing purposes gives rise to significant fiduciary[19] and prohibited transaction[20] problems under the Employee Retirement Income Security Act of 1974 (ERISA)[21] and should be avoided by providers unwilling to subject themselves to the costly, uncertain, and often prolonged process of obtaining an individual exemption for such borrowing from the United States Department of Labor.[22] Income from noncommingled gifts and grants is also sheltered from the allowable interest-offset rules, but in an era of declining philanthropy, the vast majority of providers cannot include such funds in their financial planning.[23] This chapter, therefore, concentrates on the creative use of funded depreciation in the capital financing setting.

The ensuing discussion is divided into four basic parts. First, the characteristics of funded depreciation are examined in light of the regulations promulgated by HHS, the decisions of the Provider Reimbursement Review Board (PRRB), the decisions of the Administrator of the Health Care Financing Administration (HCFA), and HCFA's program instructions. Second, the tests for determining the necessity and propriety of the borrowings, as established by HHS regulations, federal court decisions, PRRB decisions, and HCFA Administrator reviews are set forth. Third, the requirement of capitalization of interest expense during construction is discussed, and methods of mitigating its adverse effect are explored. Finally, the foregoing analysis of funded depreciation is applied to the cash flows into the basic funds established pursuant to a tax-exempt hospital bond indenture with a view to maximizing third-party reimbursement.[24]

THE CHARACTERISTICS OF FUNDED DEPRECIATION

Creation

Voluntary Establishment

In the course of prudent financial planning, a provider may voluntarily establish a funded depreciation account. The account properly should be created pursuant to a resolution of the provider's governing board to segregate cash or other liquid assets to be used for the replacement of depreciable assets and for other capital purposes.[25] While no requirement exists in the regulations or the program instructions that the board vote a formal resolution creating a depreciation fund, the provider nevertheless must create a fund whose characteristics faithfully accord with the essential elements of a depreciation fund authorized under the Medicare regulations or run the risk of a fiscal intermediary's determination that the provider has merely established an asset clearing account for the normal investment of idle cash.[26] It is therefore advisable that the board vote a resolution explicitly authorizing the funding of depreciation to the maximum extent allowable[27] and that a separate account be maintained on the books of the provider and denominated "funded depreciation" to preclude disputes with the fiscal intermediary. Failure to so designate the fund should not prove fatal, however, so long as the other characteristics of funded depreciation are present.[28]

Mandatory Establishment

A provider may be compelled to fund depreciation under the terms of a bond indenture, mortgage, or other lending agreement.[29] The fund thereby established is restricted by the creditors under the terms of the lending agreement, rather than by the governing board in a corporate resolution.

A number of disputes have arisen over whether the interest earned by bond sinking funds and other capital debt reserve funds established pursuant to a bond indenture should be offset against interest expense. In an attempt to quell the controversy, the Dallas Regional Office of HCFA issued Regional Intermediary Letter No. 79-14, which has been generally adhered to by the other Regional Offices. The Letter succinctly summarizes HCFA's prevailing policy in dealing with the question of whether the sinking and other debt reserve funds established pursuant to a bond indenture constitute funded depreciation. When a sinking fund or other debt reserve fund is a requirement of a revenue bond issue, the portion of accrued interest income which is subsequently applied to the payment of interest on the bonds must also be applied to reduce allowable interest expense. The portion of accrued interest income used to retire bond principal, however, does not reduce allowable interest expense insofar as that portion of the bond fund meets the requirements for funded depreciation set forth in Section 226 of the *Provider Reimbursement Manual* and described below.

Liquidity of Fund

The funding of depreciation is described in the program instructions as the practice of setting aside cash or other liquid assets in a separate fund.[30] Liquid assets normally consist of cash in banks and on hand, other cash assets not set aside for specific purposes other than the payment of current liabilities, or a readily marketable investment. In a 1977 Provider Appeal Decision,[31] the Blue Cross Association allowed a provider to invest its funded depreciation in rental property (presumably real property) and to shelter the rental income from reimbursable interest expense offset. The hearing officer permitted this nonliquid investment of the provider's funded depreciation account with the warning that if the provider should in the future borrow to finance a capital project while it has available funded depreciation in any form, including its rental properties, such investment income must offset reimbursable interest expense. The following year, the HCFA Administrator held in *Willis-Knighton Memorial Hospital, Inc. v. Blue Cross Assoc./Blue Cross of Louisiana*[32] that a provider's purchase of a medical office building purportedly to serve as an investment of the assets of a funded depreciation account provided a basis on which to deny the provider's argument that it had funded depreciation. The Administrator held that not only must the assets contributed to a funded depreciation account be liquid, but the investments made with account assets must also be readily available. The Administrator stated:[33]

> Because of the purpose of a funded depreciation account, the availability of these funds to meet all capital outlays which the provider may require or desire is a key element to the establishment, maintenance and use of such funds. Although it is expected that the funds be invested to earn revenue, the accessibility of these funds to meet capital needs is an essential factor in managing the investment of these funds.

The Administrator therefore held that the provider's investment in the construction of a professional office building to attract physicians to the hospital and the subsequent acquisition of long-term notes from the sale of condominiums in the building did not constitute the funding of depreciation within the meaning of 42 C.F.R. § 405.415(e).[34] The Administrator deemed such use of a provider's assets as an investment to fulfill a (presumably health care) need of the provider rather than as an investment to earn revenue for the funded depreciation account.

Amount That May Be Deposited

Because a funded depreciation account provides the means for conserving funds for the replacement of depreciable assets, the amount that may be contributed to such an account is equivalent to the appropriate allowance, as established by the principles enunciated by HHS at 42 C.F.R. § 405.415(a) for the depreciation of buildings and equipment used in the provision of patient care. Allowable depreciation is the total amount of depreciation properly expensed from the date of the acquisition of the buildings and equipment. It consists of either the total accumulated depreciation recorded in the provider's accounting records or the total accumulated depreciation calculated according to the *Provider Reimbursement Manual.*[35] Furthermore, the allowable depreciation expense may be attributable to periods before as well as after a provider's participation in the Medicare program.[36]

Generally, allowable depreciation expense is determined based on the historical cost of the assets prorated over the estimated useful life of the asset using the straight-line method of depreciation.[37] An accelerated method of depreciation, either declining balance or sum-of-the-years digits, may be used only in certain restricted instances.[38] In the event a provider should make extra deposits of funds in excess of its properly accumulated depreciation, any income earned by such excess funds must be applied to reduce allowable interest expense.[39]

Segregation of Funds

Funded depreciation must constitute a fund separate from the general funds of the provider.[40] Funded depreciation must be accounted for separately, and the investment earnings of funded depreciation must accrue to the funded depreciation account or be used for at least one of the purposes described in the next paragraph. The Deputy Administrator of HCFA has held, however, that it is not necessary to segregate a depreciation fund's interest income; only the principal balance need be held and accounted for separately. In the course of planning for the enhancement of a provider's third-party reimbursement, the earnings should be placed either in a separate funded depreciation interest earned account or be allowed to accumulate in the funded depreciation account.[41] Such compounding, of course, increases the amount of a provider's sheltered income.

Permissible Uses

Funded depreciation may not be used for any purpose other than the improvement, replacement, or expansion of facilities or equipment related to patient care.[42] This list of allowable uses of funded depreciation includes the payment of principal on bonds issued for the enumerated capital purposes. The list does not include the use of funded depreciation for the payment of interest due under the bond issue.[43] Partial use of funded depreciation moneys in a bond indenture fund to pay interest due on the bond issue will not, however, entirely destroy their character as moneys constituting funded depreciation. To the extent that expenditures of funded depreciation moneys are applied to the payment of interest, an appropriate adjustment must be made to offset allowable interest expense by the investment income earned by those funded depreciation moneys subsequently used to pay interest.[44] The regulations and program instructions provide generally that if a provider should use deposits in a funded depreciation account for purposes other than the improvement, replacement, or expansion of facilities or equipment related to patient care, the entire account need not be disqualified. In such cases, however, allowable interest expense in the period of withdrawal is reduced to adjust for offsets not made in prior years for earnings attributable to the withdrawn funds.[45]

Source of Funds

The funds deposited in a funded depreciation account must derive from a hospital's operating revenues.[46] The program instructions require that deposits into the fund must accrue from "the cash generated in excess of cash expenses by the noncash expense of depreciation."[47] To allow a provider to fund depreciation using borrowed funds would defeat part of the strategy behind encouraging providers to fund depreciation; that is, to minimize the future borrowing a provider would otherwise be compelled to undertake to replace assets worn out over time and, therefore, to decrease the interest expense reimbursable under the Medicare program. For this reason, if a bond indenture fund is to be accorded the favorable treatment conferred upon funded depreciation accounts, it is vital that the indenture fund not be a warren for bond proceeds.

Furthermore, should a provider borrow money to fund depreciation, the interest paid by the provider on the borrowed money is not an allowable cost. Therefore, if bond proceeds were to be used to fund depreciation, otherwise reimbursable interest expense would become a nonallowable cost.[48] In addition to the disallowance of the interest expense incurred, a provider might be required to offset from allowable interest expense any income accrued by the borrowed funds.

Six-Month Deposit Rule

To qualify as funded depreciation, moneys deposited in the depreciation account, whether voluntarily created or established pursuant to a bond indenture, must remain on deposit at least six months.[49] To prevent the creation of a phantom-funded depreciation account consisting primarily of accounts receivable, cash deposits representing funded depreciation moneys must remain in the account six months or more to constitute a valid funded depreciation account. Moneys representing the funding of depreciation need not be sequestered in a noninterest-bearing account but may, of course, be invested prior to the expiration of the six-month period. If such moneys remain as invested funds attributable to the funded depreciation account beyond the six-month period, the investment income for the entire cost reporting period will be sheltered, and the transactions will be deemed a valid depreciation funding and a valid investment of funded depreciation moneys.[50]

Deposits in the funded depreciation account may consist of a variety of funds or "subaccounts." To assure that the incentives provided under the Medicare program are applied to the promotion of valid funding transactions, the following sequence of withdrawals from a funded depreciation account are recognized under the program. Withdrawals for investment purposes and for the acquisition of additional capital assets, including the payment of mortgage principal, are accounted for on a first-in, first-out (FIFO) basis.[51] On the other hand, withdrawals for general operating purposes or for making loans to any of a provider's general funds are accounted for on a last-in, first-out (LIFO) basis.[52] Therefore, the latest deposit made to the funded depreciation account will be considered the deposit withdrawn for general operating purposes. Insofar as any money loaned from a funded depreciation account to a provider's general operating fund has not been on deposit in the funded depreciation account for at least six months, this rule will preclude a portion, if not all, of the interest payable to the funded depreciation account on a loan to the provider's general operating fund from being deemed an interest expense reimbursable under the Medicare program.

NECESSITY FOR BORROWING

If interest expense incurred on borrowed funds is to be deemed reimbursable, the borrowing must be "necessary." There is no definition of "necessary" or "necessity" in the Medicare Act, but the regulations state:[53]

> Necessary requires that [allowable] interest:
>
> (i) Be incurred on a loan made to satisfy a financial need of the provider. Loans which result in excess funds or investments will not be considered necessary.
> (ii) Be incurred on a loan made for a purpose reasonably related to patient care.

Unfortunately, the program instructions shed no further light on the necessity test; they merely parrot the regulations.[54] To determine whether a borrowing will be deemed "necessary" for reimbursement purposes, inquiries must be made into (a) whether the borrowing will satisfy a financial need and (b) whether such borrowing relates to patient care. There are various reported controversies relating to each of these principal inquiries.

Fiscal Need of the Provider

Fiscal Need Absent

In *Northwest Hospital, Inc. v. Hospital Service Corporation,*[55] the provider borrowed funds to construct a parking lot and professional building, although it had more than $2 million in its unrestricted funded depreciation account. This amount exceeded the cost of the capital improvements. The court held that the provider had adequate working capital from which the construction projects could have been funded. In response to the provider's argument that its governing board was entitled, in its business judgment, to borrow funds rather than deplete its funded depreciation account for the projects in question, the court stated, "Of course it could exercise its business judgment by obtaining a loan instead, but it cannot fairly impose the cost of that discretionary choice on the Medicare program."[56]

In *Peralta Hospital (Oakland, Cal.) v. Blue Cross Assoc./Blue Cross of Northern California,* [57] the provider had approximately $1.6 million in its funded depreciation account when it borrowed the same amount from a bank to finance a land purchase. The land purchase was the first phase of the provider's $20 million expansion program. The provider had decided to use its funded depreciation to acquire other assets in the course of implementing its expansion plans.

The PRRB disallowed the interest expense incurred on the funds borrowed on the ground that the borrowing was unnecessary. The board gave two reasons for its decision: First, the land purchased with the borrowed funds in anticipation of expansion was not considered to be related to patient care; and second, the provider's funded depreciation account had sufficient funds to acquire the land, thereby obviating a need to borrow additional moneys.

In a dispute that came before the PRRB in 1976,[58] a provider's board of directors had adopted a resolution to fund its depreciation account for the specific purpose of replacing assets used in the existing hospital. The resolution clearly restricted the use of those funds for replacement purposes. Subsequently, the provider built a new wing that was not intended to replace any of the existing facilities. Because of the age and condition of the existing facilities, the governing board adhered to the original restriction of using the depreciation fund for replacement purposes only. The provider, therefore, financed construction of the addition through a bond issue, Hill-Burton funds, and borrowings from the depreciation account. The provider argued that the bond issue and borrowings from the funded depreciation account were necessary because they were made to satisfy a financial need of the provider, and because the expenditures were reasonably related to patient care. The fiscal intermediary, on the other hand, in disallowing a portion of the interest charges incurred on the bond issue and removing the capitalized interest charges from the cost of the new facility, contended that the financing and borrowing during construction were unnecessary since the funds in the depreciation account could have been used for these capital expenditures, notwithstanding the restrictions imposed by the governing board. The intermediary supported its argument with citation from Section 222.1 of the *Provider Reimbursement Manual:*

> Unrestricted funds are available for the use of the provider, and the borrowers should use them rather than "borrow" them. The same treatment applies to funds created by the provider's restricting its own funds for particular management purposes.

The PRRB held for the intermediary, stating that the funds in the funded depreciation account are to be available for all capital outlays that may be required, and that the provider may not voluntarily restrict their use:

> Where a provider voluntarily funds depreciation, as opposed to being required to do so by virtue of agreements with creditors, these funds are available for all capital outlays which the provider may require and cannot be voluntarily restricted or earmarked for a specific or future purpose. While the program cannot prevent a provider from self-restricting its funded depreciation for a particular capital purpose, it can disallow as not necessary and proper interest expense incurred on capital borrowing to the extent funded depreciation is available for this purpose.[59]

To hold otherwise, the Board stated, would be to hold contrary to "the reasonable cost concept of the Medicare law."[60]

On occasion, a provider will attempt to "borrow" from its funded depreciation account to finance capital projects. This issue was not fully reviewed in the foregoing case, but it was the central issue in the following case.

In a 1975 PRRB hearing decision,[61] the Board examined a situation in which a provider borrowed $800,000 from its funded depreciation account, which totaled $900,000, to finance construction costing $1.3 million. The PRRB acknowledged that, pursuant to Section 226.1 of the *Provider Reimbursement Manual,* the general fund of a provider may borrow from the provider's funded depreciation and, if the "necessary and proper" test is met, the interest paid by the general fund to the funded depreciation account is an allowable cost. However, the PRRB held that a provider may not "borrow" from its funded depreciation account for capital construction. A provider may restrict general funds to create a funded depreciation account, but the provider may not further restrict the use of funded depreciation for some specific capital purpose and then borrow from that account for other capital purposes. The interest expense incurred by such borrowings will be disallowed.[62]

The full necessity of a bond financing has also been called into question in a case before the Administrator of HCFA in which the provider had lent 20 percent of the proceeds of a bond issue to its benefactor foundation to build a medical office building.[63] The purpose of the bond issue in question was to finance the expansion of the provider. The interest expense on the portion lent to the foundation was held nonreimbursable, for that portion of the bond proceeds was obviously diverted to a use not constituting a financial need of the provider.[64]

Fiscal Need Present

There are two particularly noteworthy cases in which borrowings were apparently unnecessary, either fully or in part, but in which the interest expense thereby incurred was found to be reimbursable.

In *Research Medical Center (Kansas City, Mo.) v. Blue Cross of Kansas City*,[65] a provider had funded depreciation far in excess of the amount borrowed. The provider had borrowed $1,416,000 in 1971 at an interest rate of 4 percent from the United States Department of Housing and Urban Development (HUD) to build a student residence facility. The fiscal intermediary contended that since the provider had more than $6 million in its funded depreciation account, the borrowing did not satisfy a financial need. The PRRB decided in favor of the provider, finding that the loan was "necessary" on the following grounds:

1. By taking advantage of the low interest rate then obtainable on the HUD loan, the provider could reduce future costs of hospital care to the Medicare program.
2. Because the provider had "well-developed" plans at the time of the loan for proper expenditures of its funded depreciation for a definite building program, to have passed up the opportunity to participate in the HUD interest subsidy grant would have led to a depletion of funded depreciation necessitating extra borrowing at a later date for the building program at a higher rate of interest.

Therefore, the Board concluded, the provider's decision to take the loan rather than extract the moneys from the funded depreciation account was a "prudent, cost-conscious management decision." In affirming the board's decision, the HCFA Administrator stated, "Definite planned utilization of the funded [depreciation] account does not, in itself, justify the provider's incurrence of [a] capital loan."[66] Nevertheless, the Administrator held, such definite planned utilization, approved by a state planning agency, and coupled with the provider's ability to obtain a loan at less than one-half the prevailing interest rate is sufficient to defeat a fiscal intermediary's argument that such a loan is unnecessary.[67]

In *Albany Medical Center Hospital (Albany, N.Y.) v. Blue Cross Assoc./ Blue Cross of Northeastern New York, Inc.*,[68] a provider issued bonds in an amount $6.5 million in excess of the cost of construction. In this case, the provider, a nonprofit, general short-term teaching hospital, had contracted with the state dormitory authority to engage in an extensive renovation and construction program. Financing for the program was accomplished through the authority's issuance of $22.5 million in bonds to pay for construction costs of approximately $16 million. To provide security for the bondholders and to assure that the facilities would be properly maintained, the agreement calling for the issuance of the bonds required various reserve funds to be established from the bond proceeds that were to be under a trustee's control and could not be used by the hospital.

The fiscal intermediary concluded that the income earned from the reserve funds prior to the capitalization date of June 30, 1973, had to be offset against the costs of the facilities being constructed, and that the interest earned thereafter by those reserve funds had to be offset against current interest expenses. The intermediary also sought to disallow part of the interest expense on the ground that a portion of the proceeds from the bonds constituted excess borrowing. The PRRB held, however, that because the reserve funds were restricted by the bond indenture agreement and did not constitute working capital and because the borrowing was required as part of a loan made to satisfy a financial need directly related to patient care, the borrowing was necessary and reimbursement of the interest expense should not be disallowed.

Related to Patient Care

In order for a provider to receive reimbursement for its interest expense, the debt in question must also be directly related to current patient care. For this reason, interest due on a bond issue during construction of patient facilities cannot be expensed but must be capitalized. Furthermore, the PRRB in *Peralta Hospital*[69] disallowed any reimbursement for interest expense incurred in the acquisition of land for a hospital facility expansion program on the basis that the land, even though it eventually would be used in the construction of new patient care facilities for the provider, was not "related to patient care."

Denial of reimbursement of interest expense on the ground of insufficient connection with patient care has also arisen in a situation in which a provider borrowed funds to purchase a certificate of need from another hospital to replace its deteriorating facility with a new and larger facility. The PRRB, in a decision affirmed in relevant part by the federal district court, held that the debt did not relate to patient care, that the provider failed to establish that a new facility was the only way to maintain its accreditation, and that the provider failed to establish that the needed upgrading of its existing facility was either impossible or economically infeasible.[70]

The PRRB has also denied interest expense reimbursement on the basis of inadequate relation of the borrowing to patient care in other, more obvious cases. In a 1976 PRRB decision, a provider was denied interest expense reimbursement for the assumption of the debts of a parochial high school and a convent-nursing home pursuant to a corporate reorganization.[71] In a Provider Appeal Decision a year earlier, a provider was denied reimbursement of that portion of interest expense attributable to the construction of a medical office building, which, although owned by the provider, was not used in the care of the provider's patients.[72]

PROPRIETY OF BORROWING

To be reimbursable, interest expense, besides being "necessary," must also be "proper."[73] To be deemed "proper," interest expense must be incurred at a rate not in excess of what a prudent borrower would have had to pay in the money market at the time the loan was made.[74] There has been little dispute over the meaning of this requirement. Furthermore, the interest must be paid to a lender not related through control or ownership or personal relationship to the provider.[75] This second requirement has caused a fair amount of controversy.

The rule that the borrower not be related through control, ownership, or personal relationship to the lending organization is based on the expectation that a provider independent of a lender will be free to exert its maximum economic power to negotiate the lowest interest rate obtainable based on its creditworthiness and financial acumen. The regulatory presumption obtains that if the provider is related to the lender, the absence of self-interested negotiations that typically occur in an arm's length setting will lead to the payment of interest rates higher than those otherwise obtainable and may also lead to unnecessary borrowing.[76] There are two principal exceptions to the unrelatedness requirement. These exceptions apply to loans made prior to July 1, 1966 and to certain loans between a provider and the governing body of its related religious order.[77]

Interest paid to a sole proprietor, partner, stockholder, or related organization on loans made before July 1, 1966 constitutes an allowable cost.[78] Furthermore, interest paid pursuant to loan agreements entered into before July 1, 1966 between the home office and components of a chain operation is also allowable.[79] This exception to the nonrelatedness rule prevails unless the terms and conditions of repayment of such loans are modified in any way after June 30, 1966.[80]

In one interesting case, a not-for-profit hospital issued bonds for the purchase of a related for-profit corporation which had operated the provider. The provider argued that the interest expense on the bonds should be allowed because the terms of the bond indenture were established on June 1, 1966. No proceeds were received, however, until the bonds were actually issued on March 31, 1967. It was held, therefore, that the interest expense was not allowable, for the agreement had to have been effective and the proceeds received prior to July 1, 1966.[81]

The federal regulators have maintained an abiding faith that governing bodies of religious orders will not deal sharply with the Medicare program and with the hospitals they sponsor in the course of lending funds to such providers.[82] Where there is a contractual agreement for the payment of interest on a loan from the governing body of a religious order, and the terms of the loan contemplate repayment, the interest paid by the sectarian provider to its related sponsor is an allowable cost. The loan agreement need not be in writing. The existence of the loan arrangement may be effectively evidenced by appropriate financial statements, provided the arrangement is carried on the records of the provider as a loan to be repaid and it is in fact repaid.[83] Care must be taken by sectarian providers actually to pay the interest expense incurred during a cost reporting period within the succeeding reporting period in order to preserve the reimbursement privilege.[84]

In an unusual case, *Trustees of Indiana University* (*Indiana University Hospitals*) *v. United States*,[85] the Court of Claims refused to enforce the prohibition against the reimbursement of interest expense attributable to loans from a related organization. Although the state of Indiana provides funds to Indiana University, the law of Indiana forbade the use of such funds for the university's affiliated not-for-profit teaching hospitals. Because the hospitals were not legal entities separate from the university, they were unable to borrow funds from outside sources. To compensate for operating losses, the university loaned funds to the hospitals at less than the current rate of interest. Presented with this hard case, the court made questionable law (consistent, however, in its dubiousness with that made not infrequently by tribunals dealing with Medicare issues) and held the interest expense on the loans to the affiliated hospitals to be an allowable cost on the ground that the evil of an unrealistically high interest rate against which the regulation was directed was not present.[86]

Notwithstanding the foregoing, the nonrelated lender requirement does not encompass within its sweep the internally maintained funds of a provider and, consequently, does not render nonreimbursable the interest expense paid on loans from the provider's donor-restricted funds, the funded depreciation account, or the provider's qualified pension fund.[87]

CAPITALIZATION OF INTEREST EXPENSE

Pursuant to Medicare program instructions, interest costs incurred must be capitalized during the construction period as a part of the cost of the facility.[88] Under the principles of Medicare cost reimbursement, the interest costs must be related to health care services rendered.[89] Since services will be rendered only after an asset is put into use, interest expense during construction is capitalized. Those capitalized costs are subsequently amortized over the useful life of the asset constructed or acquired.[90]

The Medicare regulations require that providers follow accounting principles generally accepted in the hospital industry and related fields.[91] The capitalization of interest expense is one area in which the cost reporting requirements of Medicare have historically diverged from generally accepted accounting principles. The degree of such divergence has been a controversial problem, and not easily resolved, for the question of capitalizing interest cost had never been fully addressed in an authoritative pronouncement of a standard-setting body prior to the issuance of Statement of Financial Accounting Standards No. 34 *Capitalization of Interest Cost* (FASB 34) by the Financial Accounting Standards Board (FASB), effective December 15, 1979.

Intermediary Letter No. 51 issued in 1966 informed providers that interest incurred during the construction of an asset may not be expensed but must be capitalized. In addition, Section 206 of the *Provider Reimbursement Manual,* issued in 1968, explicitly requires that interest costs incurred during the period of construction must be capitalized as a part of the cost of the facility. After the construction period, interest on the borrowing is allowable as an operating cost.

When Section 206 was issued, it embodied the position expressed by the American Hospital Association (AHA) *Chart of Accounts for Hospitals,* published in 1966.[92] Ten years later, the AHA published a *Chart of Accounts for Hospitals* more to the liking of many embattled providers, in which it stated, "[I]nterest incurred during construction has traditionally been capitalized as a cost of the related projects; however, it can be charged as a current-period expense."[93] Few program instructions have engendered as much controversy as Section 206, but HCFA and the PRRB have consistently denied challenges to the position that interest expense incurred during the construction period must be capitalized.[94] Intermediary Letter No. 51 and Section 206 of the *Provider Reimbursement Manual* have been unsuccessfully challenged in federal court on the ground that they are inconsistent with the Medicare statute and regulations.[95] The Ninth Circuit Court of Appeals has held that they are exempt from the rulemaking requirements of the Administrative Procedure Act under the benefit exception rule[96] and that the United States Department of Health, Education, and Welfare's interpretation of the statute and regulation was not clearly outside its authority, as determined pursuant to the deferential standard of review accorded to interpretive rules enunciated by the United States Supreme Court in *Skidmore v. Swift & Co.*[97]

In October 1979, FASB issued FASB 34, largely in accordance with a demand from the Securities and Exchange Commission (SEC) that standards be established to curb the increasingly frequent and controversial financial reporting practice of publicly held corporations to capitalize rather than currently expense the interest costs related to the acquisition or construction of certain assets. On November 14, 1974, the SEC issued Accounting Series Release No. 163, imposing a moratorium on adopting or extending a policy of capitalizing interest by registrants (other than public utilities) that had not, as of June 21, 1974, publicly disclosed such a policy.[98] Five years later, on November 6, 1979, the SEC rescinded the moratorium in Accounting Series Release No. 272, on the condition that registrants adopt FASB 34.[99] Although publicly held corporations may have resisted the SEC's position favoring the expensing of interest costs, providers, whether proprietary or not-for-profit, found immediate expensing an attractive cost reporting technique. In rejecting for cost reporting purposes the SEC's position favoring the expensing of interest costs incurred during construction, the PRRB has stated, "[T]he SEC is interested in giving creditors and investors a conservative view of the income of publicly held companies and in restraining the optimism of management."[100] Medicare principles, on the other hand, mandate that costs be related to patient care services rendered; therefore, because such services will be rendered only after the asset under construction is put into use, the interest expense incurred during construction will be reimbursed over its useful life.[101]

The announced objectives of FASB 34 and the Medicare cost reporting rules are essentially the same. The financial accounting purposes of capitalizing interest are to determine an acquisition cost that more nearly reflects an enterprise's total investment in the assets, to create a more nearly accurate matching of expense with related revenues by charging a cost relating to the acquisition cost that more nearly reflects an enterprise's total investment in the assets, and to create a more nearly accurate matching of expense with related revenues by charging a cost relating to the acquisition of a resource that will benefit future periods against the revenues of the periods benefited.[102] FASB 34, however, mandates or, in some instances, permits results different from those mandated by cost reporting requirements. Those different results arise from differences in determining the amount of interest to be capitalized, the capitalization rate, and the capitalization period. It will frequently be necessary, therefore, for providers to keep one set of property and depreciation records for financial reporting purposes and another set for third-party cost reporting purposes.

FASB 34 does not permit the reduction of interest cost based on any amounts that might be earned on unused funds received from a borrowing. In paragraph 49, FASB 34 states, "[D]ue to the fungible nature of cash, it is usually impossible to determine objectively the proportion of the funds expended for a particular purpose that was derived from each source."[103] Furthermore, FASB Technical Bulletin No. 81-5, *Offsetting Interest Cost to Be Capitalized with Interest Income,* explicitly states that FASB 34 does not permit such offsetting. While interest expense is capitalized on a gross basis for financial reporting purposes, the interest expense capitalized must be reduced for cost reporting purposes by any income earned by the borrowed proceeds. If the amount of interest capitalized is materially[104] different for financial statement purposes and cost reimbursement purposes, the difference is recorded as deferred reimbursement or deferred revenue on the balance sheet. Such amount is the difference in depreciable cost basis arising during the construction period at the provider's Medicare utilization rate. The deferred revenue would then be amortized into income as a reduction of contractual allowance expense over the depreciable life of the new facility. For financial reporting purposes, earnings on borrowed funds are usually recognized as nonoperating revenues earned or as "other operating revenues" on the Statement of Revenues and Expenses.

FASB may be on the verge of relinquishing its opposition to the netting of investment income from borrowed proceeds against the capitalized interest on such borrowing. Accountants have argued that in the tax-exempt financing setting, the borrowing is so closely linked with a specific asset to be acquired or constructed as to require a more direct accounting association. Consequently, FASB has been urged that the interest expense associated with the borrowing should be included as a cost of acquiring the asset, but that any interest earned on any related temporary investment of borrowed proceeds should be accounted for as a reduction in the cost of acquiring the asset, and, consequently, as a reduction in the amount of interest cost capitalized. On December 22, 1981, FASB issued a Proposed Statement of Financial Accounting Standards, *Capitalization of Interest Cost in Situations Involving Tax-Exempt Borrowings and Certain Gifts and Grants,* in which it suggested amending paragraph 12 of FASB 34 to require the netting of temporary investment income against the amount of interest expense incurred in a tax-exempt financing, where, typically, the association between the asset financed and the borrowing is direct. Furthermore, the funds flows from the tax-exempt borrowing, temporary investment, and construction expenditures must be closely intertwined and restricted, as is typically the case.[105]

In addition to FASB 34's present lack of a netting of earnings requirement, there is no strict requirement in FASB 34 that a specific rate be used as the capitalization rate. Even if debt is legally associated with the qualifying asset,[106] the enterprise is not obligated to use the rate of the specific borrowing as the capitalization rate once it determines that another rate or combination of rates is more appropriate.[107] In the tax-exempt financing setting, the association between the bond issue and the assets thereby financed is typically so obvious that no capitalization rate may be formulated that will be acceptable for third-party cost-reporting purposes other than one based on the interest rate provided in the bond indenture.

Under FASB 34, the capitalization period ends when the asset is "substantially complete and ready for its intended use."[108] FASB has used this formulation to prevent the continuation of interest capitalization in those situations where completion of an asset is intentionally delayed. Section 206 of the *Provider Reimbursement Manual* provides that for Medicare reimbursement purposes, the period of construction is considered to extend to the date the facility is put into use for patient care. A hospital, expecially a not-for-profit provider with a high cost-reporting utilization rate, would have no rational motivation to continue interest capitalization beyond substantial completion. The sooner the capitalization period is ended and the amortization of costs begins, the earlier the hospital's third-party reimbursement will commence.[109]

The requirement that interest expense be capitalized during construction affects a provider adversely in two ways: First, the provider is reimbursed over a number of years for a cash expense paid in one year; second, the provider is reimbursed with dollars of a lesser value as a result of inflation.[110] One strategy to mitigate these adverse consequences is to put the facility into patient care use in stages as quickly as possible rather than wait until the entire facility is completed.[111]

Furthermore, if a provider's borrowing can be characterized as borrowing for the remodeling of an existing structure, rather than the construction of a new structure, the provider may be permitted currently to expense the interest costs. In *Ravenswood Hospital Medical Center and ECF (Chicago, Ill.) v. Blue Cross Assoc./Health Care Service Corp.*,[112] the PRRB held that the aspect of remodeling warranted the creation of an exception to the general capitalization rule. In that case, the evidence disclosed that patient care, services, and revenues, for instance, were not affected by the remodeling of existing structures. Contrary to the PRRB's typical disposition of the issue, the interest expense incurred during the period of remodeling was held to be related to the current care of patients and therefore could be currently expensed rather than capitalized.

At least one provider has argued before the PRRB that interest costs during construction should be amortized over the term of the bond issue since certain charges connected with a bond issue such as legal expenses in preparing the bond indenture and mortgage, cost of printing certificates, registration costs, and commissions to underwriters are written off over the period of the bond issue and not over the projected useful life of the assets.[113] The PRRB, however, has firmly rejected this position, stating that it can find no basis for relating the interest during construction to the life of the bonds when that interest is part of the cost of acquiring the new facility.[114]

THE BOND INDENTURE

When a provider undertakes a tax-exempt bond financing, upon the issuance of the bonds, the proceeds from the sale are deposited with the trustee designated to serve under the bond indenture. The indenture governs the disposition of the bond proceeds and requires the trustee to apply those proceeds to certain funds established pursuant to its terms. Commonly, the trustee will be required to deposit from the bond proceeds an amount equal to the interest due under the indenture during the construction period into an interest fund; an additional amount equal to the annual debt service requirement (as defined in the indenture) usually must be deposited in the debt service reserve fund; an amount will also be deposited in an expense fund to pay fees and expenses incurred in connection with the issuance and sale of the bonds; and, finally, the balance of the proceeds will be deposited in a construction fund. The program instructions explicitly state that interest payable pursuant to a bond issue is an allowable cost in accordance with the terms of the bond indenture, to the extent that the interest relates to bond proceeds used either to acquire assets for use in patient care activities or to provide funds for operations related to patient care.[115]

In the ensuing analysis of the cash flows into the various standard funds discussed below, the following guiding principles for maximizing third-party reimbursement must be borne in mind: moneys qualifying as funded depreciation should be held as long as possible to accumulate sheltered income in funds whose purpose accords with an allowable use for funded depreciation; and bond proceeds, which cannot qualify as funded depreciation, should be directed to funds whose purposes do not accord with an allowable use for funded depreciation and should be expended prior to operationally derived moneys.

The Construction Fund

The trustee under the indenture is required to apply the balance of the bond proceeds (after certain deposits to other funds for interest and issuance expenses) to a construction fund, whose purpose is to provide a reserve sufficient to pay all costs of construction of the project as they become due. Because borrowed funds can never be a source of funded depreciation, the interest accrued from the proceeds on deposit in the construction fund can never be sheltered from reimbursement offset. In addition to the bond proceeds, however, the provider will typically be required to make additional deposits into the construction fund so that there will be sufficient moneys to pay all costs of construction when due. If any such moneys from the provider might qualify as funded depreciation, those moneys should be separately accounted for, or, if possible, kept physically separate. If they cannot be separately accounted for, the interest earned on them, because they are commingled with bond proceeds, may lose its sheltered attribute and be offset against allowable interest expense in the same manner as interest earned on the bond proceeds.

Surplus moneys remaining in the construction fund after the project has been completed are typically deposited in the bond sinking fund or in the optional redemption fund (if not the same fund as the bond sinking fund) and used to call bonds. Care must be taken to segregate any surplus moneys attributable to bond proceeds flowing into the sinking fund or the optional redemption fund so that the potential or actual funded depreciation character of the other moneys in those funds can be preserved.

The Other Indenture Funds

The following discussion examines the six most common tax-exempt hospital bond indenture funds in addition to the construction fund. There are two basic sources for the moneys that flow into these funds: (1) the bond proceeds and realized interest income thereon; and (2) provider operations and any realized interest on funds set aside from operating income. Care must always be taken to account separately for the different ultimate sources of the moneys that flow into and through the indenture funds. In *Albany Medical Center Hospital*,[116] because of the cascading feature of the flows through the indenture funds, it was not possible after the fact to trace backward to the original source any of the amounts in the indenture funds. The PRRB accordingly held that the total amount of all of the required trusteed funds on the capitalization date (that is, the date of project completion) would be treated for reimbursement purposes as originating from bond proceeds, and directly or indirectly from interest on unexpended bond proceeds. The interest income accrued by those funds, therefore, offset allowable interest expense, thereby reducing the hospital's Medicare reimbursement.

Revenue Fund

The indenture frequently provides for a separate revenue fund into which all payments by the provider on the underlying note, as and when received by the trustee, shall be deposited and held until disbursed to the interest fund and the bond sinking fund. The language in the indenture describing this fund should provide for the segregation of those funds that will be transferred to the interest fund from those funds that will be transferred to the bond sinking fund. Moneys that may qualify as funded depreciation should be channeled to the bond sinking fund. Moneys that do not qualify as funded depreciation should be channeled to the interest fund.

Interest Fund

The uses to which moneys constituting funded depreciation may be put are limited to the improvement, replacement, or expansion of facilities or equipment related to patient care.[117] The payment of principal on bonds issued for the above purposes constitutes an allowable use of funded depreciation; the payment of interest due on such bonds, on the other hand, is not a permissible use of funded depreciation.[118] Moneys constituting funded depreciation should never be placed in the interest fund, for the investment income that had accrued from those moneys and that had previously been sheltered will be used to offset allowable interest expense. Therefore, bond proceeds and provider moneys that fail to qualify as funded depreciation should be placed in the interest fund.

Bond Sinking Fund

Because the payment of principal on bonds issued for the improvement, replacement, or expansion of facilities or equipment related to patient care is an allowable use of funded depreciation, provider moneys that are placed in the bond sinking fund (also called the "principal account") will constitute funded depreciation provided that the other requirements for funded depreciation are met: that is, the fund must be liquid; it may not exceed an amount equal to accumulated depreciation expense; the moneys must be segregated; the moneys must have been on deposit for six months. Income accrued on such moneys while in the bond sinking fund will be sheltered from offset against allowable interest expense.

Debt Service Reserve Fund

The debt service reserve fund is the most congenial habitation for funded depreciation. This fund is typically established to receive an amount sufficient to cause the moneys there on deposit to equal a defined maximum annual debt service requirement on the bonds outstanding. It provides security to the bondholders and promotes the marketability of the bonds. Moneys usually remain in the fund over the term of the bonds and accumulate investment income. If bond proceeds flow into the fund, the interest accrued by the proceeds offsets reimbursable interest expense. If, however, moneys that qualify as funded depreciation are placed in the debt service reserve fund, those moneys will accumulate sheltered investment income. The longer the term of the bonds, the greater the sheltered income earned.

If bond proceeds also flow into this fund, care should be taken to separate those proceeds from the funded depreciation moneys. Language in the bond indenture should provide for the establishment of separate subaccounts to reflect each source of the moneys. Such an approach should preclude a dispute with the provider's fiscal intermediary over the extent of the investment income earned attributable to the moneys constituting funded depreciation. Alternatively, bond proceeds may be flowed out of this fund prior to placing into it moneys that could qualify as funded depreciation.

Usually, the debt service reserve fund is established to compensate for any deficiencies in the interest fund and the bond sinking fund. The fact that the moneys in the debt service reserve fund could potentially flow into the interest fund has not proved sufficient to defeat a provider's claim that the moneys in the fund (when not from bond proceeds) constitute funded depreciation whose investment income is sheltered. In a 1977 PRRB decision, it was held, in relevant part, that:

> [O]nly the portion of the Reserve Fund [that is, the debt service reserve fund] which is used to pay the interest on the bonds does not meet the requirements of Section 226 of the *Provider Reimbursement Manual* [which section sets forth the requirements for funded depreciation]. Therefore, only that portion of these funds is excluded and the rest of the monies are considered to be funded depreciation.[119]

It appears that one can confidently conclude that so long as none of the funded depreciation moneys is in fact used to pay bond interest, the sheltered attribute of the income accruing from those moneys will be maintained. If a subaccount in the fund is maintained for moneys from bond proceeds, the indenture should state that moneys withdrawn to pay bond interest shall derive from that subaccount until exhausted prior to any withdrawal from the funded depreciation subaccount for any interest payments. The greatest reimbursement is achieved by never using operationally derived moneys in the debt service reserve account to meet interest payments; such moneys should flow into the bond sinking fund, or the redemption fund (if separate from the sinking fund), with any excess transferred to the renewal, replacement, and depreciation fund.

Renewal, Replacement, and Depreciation Fund

A renewal, replacement, and depreciation fund can be viewed to some extent as a secondary debt service reserve fund. Moneys in this fund are used to make up any deficiencies in the interest fund, the bond sinking fund, and the debt service reserve fund. This fund may also be used to pay for repairs of the facility built with the proceeds of the debt. So long as no default exists under the indenture or the mortgage, the provider may also withdraw moneys with the trustee's permission for the purchase of capital assets. Inasmuch as the source of the moneys in this fund is provider operating revenue, investment income earned by these moneys is exempt from reimbursement offset, provided that the other requirements for funded depreciation are met. The same concerns discussed above regarding the use of any provider-derived moneys in the fund for bond interest payments also apply here. For this reason, it is advisable to place the interest fund last on the list of priorities for which payments will be made from this fund in the event of any default in the other funds.

Optional Redemption Fund

The optional redemption fund is established to receive funds from the provider, condemnation proceeds or insurance proceeds, or other moneys received by the trustee for the purpose of redeeming bonds. Excess income earned by the debt service reserve fund, and the renewal, replacement, and depreciation fund may also flow into this fund. Moneys on deposit in this fund are typically applied first to make up any deficiencies in the debt service reserve fund and second, to retire bonds prior to their due dates. If the moneys deposited in the fund are derived from the operating revenues of the provider and otherwise have the characteristics of funded depreciation, those characteristics will be maintained, and any income earned will be exempt from offset.

NOTES

1. The term "necessary" in this context is defined at 42 C.F.R. § 405.419(b)(2) (1979) and discussed in detail in the section of this chapter titled "Necessity for Borrowing."

2. The term "proper" in this context is defined at 42 C.F.R. § 405.419(b)(3) (1979) and discussed in detail in the section of this chapter titled "Propriety of Borrowing."

3. Interest on current indebtedness is the cost incurred for funds borrowed for a relatively short term. Such borrowings are for such purposes as supplying working capital for normal operating expenses. *See* 42 C.F.R. § 405.419(b)(1) (1979).

4. The term "provider of services" (or more cursorially, "provider") is one of art under the Medicare regime and is defined in the *Provider Reimbursement Manual* (hereinafter PRM) at § 2402.1 as follows:

> A provider of services means a hospital, skilled nursing facility, home health agency and, for the limited purpose of furnishing outpatient physical therapy or speech pathology services, a clinic, rehabilitation agency or public health agency.

Effective April 1, 1981, the term includes alcohol detoxification facilities; effective July 1, 1981, the term also includes comprehensive outpatient rehabilitation facilities. *See also* 42 U.S.C. § 1395x(u).

5. The term "participating provider" is defined at PRM § 2402.2 as follows:

> A participating provider is an approved provider of service which has entered into an agreement with the Department of Health, Education, and Welfare [now Health and Human Services] (a) to accept payment based on the reasonable cost of the items and services furnished; (b) not to charge the beneficiary or any other person for covered items and services, except deductibles and coinsurance amounts; and (c) to return any money incorrectly collected. In order to participate in the Medicare program, a hospital must meet the Conditions of Participation set forth at 42 C.F.R. § 405.1020–405.1040 (1981) and sign and have accepted by the Health Care Financing Administration (HCFA) a provider agreement (currently Form HCFA-1561).

6. The Medicare program was established pursuant to the Social Security Amendments of 1965, codified as Title XVIII of The Social Security Act, 42 U.S.C. § 1395 *et seq.* (1965).

7. 42 C.F.R. § 405.419 (1979).

8. 42 C.F.R. § 405.419(b) (1979).

9. The term "allowable" is typically used synonymously with the term "reimbursable" throughout this chapter. Nevertheless, it should be noted that a cost may be "allowable" insofar as it is related to patient care and may be entered on a provider's cost report, but such cost will be "reimbursable" only to the extent of a provider's Medicare utilization rate.

10. PRM § 212.

11. 42 C.F.R. § 405.419(b)(2)(iii) (1979).

12. 42 C.F.R. § 405.419(c) (1979). If a provider should borrow from a related organization, the interest expense incurred is allowable only to the extent of the "cost" to the related organization. *See generally* 42 C.F.R. § 405.427 (1966); PRM §§ 1000; 1002–1002.3; 1004–1004.4. There are basically only two situations in which a provider can borrow from a related organization and enter the interest expense as an allowable cost; these situations are discussed in the section of this chapter titled "Propriety of Borrowing."

13. Following such netting, the amount of reimbursement due under Title XVIII attributable to such interest expense is determined through the application of an appropriate cost finding

method. Cost finding is the process of recasting the data derived from the accounts ordinarily kept by a provider to ascertain costs of the various types of services rendered by allocating direct costs and prorating indirect costs. 42 C.F.R. § 405.453(b) (1980). *See generally* 42 C.F.R. § 405.453(d), where the Departmental Method of cost apportionment using the Step-Down Method, the Double-Apportionment Method, the Combination Method, and "more sophisticated methods" are outlined. The objective of cost finding is to determine the Medicare program's share of a provider's total allowable costs. Such share is sometimes referred to as a provider's "Medicare utilization rate" or "cost-reporting utilization rate." The regulations note that the determination of such share or "rate" is "essential for carrying out the statutory directive that the program's payments to providers should be such that the costs of covered services for [Medicare] beneficiaries . . . not be passed on to non-beneficiaries, nor . . . the cost of services for non-beneficiaries be borne by the [Medicare] program." 42 C.F.R. § 405.403(b) (1977).

14. 42 C.F.R. § 405.419(b)(2)(iii). Although not enumerated in the text, interest received as a result of a review by a federal court whereby a decision rendered by the Provider Reimbursement Review Board (PRRB) or a subsequent reversal, affirmance, or modification by the Secretary of the Department of Health and Human Services (HHS) is reversed in favor of a provider (*see* 42 C.F.R. § 405.454(1) (1977)) is also protected from allowable interest expense offset. *Ibid.*

15. PRM § 226.

16. 42 C.F.R. § 405.415(e); PRM § 2262.

17. Social Security Act § 1867, 79 Stat. 286 (1965), 42 U.S.C. § 1395dd (1972).

18. Health Insurance Benefits Advisory Council (HIBAC), Agenda Book, Minutes of Eighth Meeting, April 30–May 1, 1966.

19. The Employee Retirement Income Security Act of 1974 (ERISA) § 404, 29 U.S.C. § 1104 (1975), sets forth the statutory general standards of conduct for ERISA fiduciaries. An ERISA fiduciary, which term includes the sponsor of an employee benefit plan, must discharge its duties with respect to a plan solely in the interest of the participants and beneficiaries and exclusively for the purposes of providing benefits to participants and their beneficiaries and defraying reasonable administrative expenses.

20. ERISA § 406(b), 29 U.S.C. § 1106(b) (1975). The prohibited transactions rules of ERISA forbid an ERISA fiduciary from dealing with the assets of an employee benefit plan in its own interest or for its own account.

21. Pub. L. 93-406, 88 Stat. 832 (1974).

22. ERISA § 408(a), 29 U.S.C. § 1108(a) (1975).

23. The Economic Recovery Tax Act of 1981 (ERTA), Pub. L. 97-34, may engender a further decline in private contributions to not-for-profit hospitals. ERTA § 121 amended §§ 63(b) and (f) and 170 of the Internal Revenue Code of 1954, as amended (the Code), by adding to it §§ 63(i) and 170(i), effective for taxable years beginning after December 31, 1981, for contributions made after that date but not before January 1, 1986. ERTA § 121 introduces the term "direct charitable contribution" into the Code and defines the term at Code § 63(i). Code § 63(b)(1)(C) allows taxpayers to deduct direct charitable contributions from their gross income in arriving at adjusted gross income. Such a favorable deduction is commonly termed an "above the line" deduction. New Code § 170(i) puts strict limits, however, on the amount that can be claimed as a direct charitable deduction and (to avoid duplication) limits direct charitable deductions to those persons who do not itemize their deductions. In 1982 and 1983, nonitemizing taxpayers can take a 25 percent above-the-line deduction for charitable contributions up to a maximum of $100 (resulting in a maximum deduction of $25). In 1984, the above-the-line deduction is still 25 percent of the contributions, but the maximum

limit is $300 (resulting in a maximum deduction of $75). In 1985, the amount of the deduction rises to 50 percent of all charitable contributions, and in 1986 it rises to 100 percent of all charitable contributions. In 1987, however, the direct charitable deduction is extinguished, and taxpayers will not have the benefit of any above-the-line charitable deductions. The chief beneficiaries of the "direct charitable contribution" rules probably will be religious organizations. See Clotfelter and Salamon, *The Federal Government and the Nonprofit Sector: The Impact of the 1981 Tax Act on Individual Charitable Giving* (Washington, D.C.: The Urban Institute, 1981), pp. 22–23 (hereinafter Clotfelter and Salamon). On the other hand, charitable giving to hospitals likely will decline as a result of ERTA. Clotfelter and Salamon, pp. 22–23. The principal basis for this expectation is that the reduction in the marginal tax rates, which most dramatically benefit upper-income taxpayers, who are the principal benefactors of community hospitals, by reducing the highest marginal rate from 70 percent to 50 percent, effective January 1, 1982, will make charitable giving more costly for such individuals. This reduction in the marginal tax rate also extinguishes the former difference in the tax treatment between personal service income and investment income (and thereby repeals the now-vestigal Code § 1348, effective January 1, 1982). ERTA § 101(c)(1).

24. The creative use of funded depreciation for maximizing third-party reimbursement is constricted in its beneficial results with respect to hospitals in those states that have not adopted a system of prospective rate review. *See, e.g.,* Annotated Code of Maryland, Art. 43, § 568 H *et seq.* (1979), and the regulations promulgated thereunder, especially COMAR § 10.37.10.07. It should also be added here, so that any heightened expectations can be immediately deflated, that this chapter contains no discussion of bond discounts and other expenses; bond premiums; the recall of bonds before maturity; defeasance transactions; nor the treatment of debt cancellation costs.

25. PRM § 226.

26. Willis-Knighton Memorial Hospital, Inc. v. Blue Cross Assoc./Blue Cross of Louisiana, HCFA Adm. Dec., *Medicare & Medicaid Guide* [1980 Transfer Binder] (CCH) ¶30,538, *rev'g* PRRB Dec. No. 78-D61, *Medicare & Medicaid Guide* [1979-1 Transfer Binder] (CCH) ¶29,438.

27. *See* the subsection of this chapter, *infra,* titled "Amount That May Be Deposited."

28. Mercy Medical Center of Springfield (Springfield, Ohio) v. Blue Cross Association/Blue Cross of Southwest Ohio, PRRB Hearing Dec. No. 78-D78, *Medicare & Medicaid Guide* [1979-1 Transfer Binder] (CCH) ¶29,561, *aff'd* HCFA Admin. Dec. [1979-1 Transfer Binder] (CCH) ¶29,620; Saint John's Hospital and Health Center (Santa Monica, Ca.) v. Blue Cross Assoc./Blue Cross of Southern California, PRRB Dec. No. 77-D58R, *Medicare & Medicaid Guide* [1979-1 Transfer Binder] (CCH) ¶29,436, *rev'g* PRRB Dec. No. 77-D58, *Medicare & Medicaid Guide* [1977 Transfer Binder] (CCH) ¶28,646. *Compare* PRRB Dec. No. 77-D37, *Medicare & Medicaid Guide* [1977 Transfer Binder] (CCH) ¶28,517.

29. PRM § 226.

30. *Ibid.*

31. Prov. App. Dec. No. 00-76-68 (Blue Cross Association), *Medicare & Medicaid Guide* [1977 Transfer Binder] (CCH) ¶28,395.

32. Willis-Knighton, *supra* note 26.

33. *Ibid.*

34. 42 C.F.R. § 405.415(e) (1979) reads as follows:

Although funding of depreciation is not required, it is strongly recommended that providers use this mechanism as a means of conserving funds for replacement of depreciable assets, and coordinate their planning of capital expenditures with areawide planning activities of community and State agencies. As an incentive for funding, investment income on funded depreciation will not be treated as a reduction of allowable interest expense.

35. PRM § 226.3. In Research Medical Center v. Schweiker (W.D. Mo. 1981), 4 *Medicare & Medicaid Guide* (CCH) ¶31,592, a provider funded depreciation at a level representing the replacement cost of its depreciable assets. In holding that the provider had overfunded its depreciation account, the court stated, "[T]he Medicare regulations do not divorce the meaning of 'depreciation' for the purposes of depreciation expense as an allowable and reimburseable [sic] cost from the definition of 'depreciation' when used in the context of depreciation funding."

36. PRM § 226.3.

37. 42 C.F.R. § 405.415(a)(3)(i) (1979).

38. 42 C.F.R. § 405.415(a)(3) (1979).

39. PRM § 226.3. Research Medical Center v. Schweiker, *supra* note 35.

40. PRM § 226.

41. The Good Samaritan Hospital (Vincennes, Ind.) v. Blue Cross Assoc./Mutual Hospital Insurance, Inc., HCFA Dep. Adm. Dec., *Medicare & Medicaid Guide* [1980 Transfer Binder] (CCH) ¶30,437, *aff'g* PRRB Dec. No. 79-D80, *Medicare & Medicaid Guide* [1980 Transfer Binder] (CCH) ¶30,338.

42. 42 C.F.R. § 405.419(c)(3) (1979).

43. Use of funded depreciation moneys to pay interest expense is not among the enumerated permissible uses of funded depreciation. 42 C.F.R. § 405.419(c)(3) (1979); *See also* PRM § 226.

44. *Ibid.*

45. 42 C.F.R. § 405.419(c)(3); PRM § 226.4.

46. Research Medical Center (Kansas City, Mo.) v. Blue Cross Assoc./Blue Cross of Kansas City, PRRB Dec. No. 78-D57, *Medicare & Medicaid Guide* [1978 Transfer Binder] (CCH) ¶29,230; HCFA Adm. Dec., *Medicare & Medicaid Guide* [1978 Transfer Binder] (CCH) ¶29,242, *aff'g* PRRB Dec. No. 78-D43, *Medicare & Medicaid Guide* [1978 Transfer Binder] (CCH) ¶29,215.

47. PRM § 226.

48. PRM § 226.5; Prov. App. Dec. No. 00-76-9 (Blue Cross Association), *Medicare & Medicaid Guide* [1976 Transfer Binder] (CCH) ¶27,822.

49. PRM § 226.3.

50. *Ibid.*

51. PRM § 226.4.

52. *Ibid.; See* PRRB Hearing Dec. No. 75-D4, *Medicare & Medicaid Guide* [1975 Transfer Binder] (CCH) ¶27,466.

53. 42 C.F.R. § 405.419(b)(2) (1979).

54. See PRM § 202.2.

55. 500 F. Supp. 1294 (N.D. Ill. 1981).

56. *Id.* at 1308. *Accord,* Whitley County Memorial Hospital (Columbia City, Ind.) v. Blue Cross Assoc./Mutual Hospital Insurance, Inc., PRRB Dec. No. 79-D6, *Medicare & Medicaid Guide* [1979-1 Transfer Binder] (CCH) ¶29,652, modified HCFA Adm. Dec., *Medicare & Medicaid Guide* [1979-1 Transfer Binder] (CCH) ¶29,701; *See also* Potomac Valley Hospital (Keyser, W. Va.) v. Blue Cross Assoc./West Virginia Hospital Service, Inc., PRRB

Hearing Dec. No. 80-D79, *Medicare & Medicaid Guide* [1981-1 Transfer Binder] (CCH) ¶30,732, in which the provider chose to borrow for capital construction rather than use cash on hand.

57. PRRB Hearing Dec. No. 78-D67, *Medicare & Medicaid Guide* [1979-1 Transfer Binder] (CCH) ¶29,442.

58. PRRB Hearing Dec., No. 76-D16, *Medicare & Medicaid Guide* [1976 Transfer Binder] (CCH) ¶27,843.

59. *Ibid.*

60. *Ibid.*

61. PRRB Hearing Dec., No. 75-D3, *Medicare & Medicaid Guide* [1975 Transfer Binder] (CCH) ¶27,426.

62. *Ibid.*

63. HCFA Adm. Dec., *Medicare & Medicaid Guide* [1979-1 Transfer Binder] (CCH) ¶29,621, *rev'g* Saint Francis Hospital (Tulsa, Okla.) v. Blue Cross Association/Blue Cross and Blue Shield of Oklahoma, PRRB Dec. No. 78-D79, *Medicare & Medicaid Guide* [1979-1 Transfer Binder] (CCH) ¶29,562. *See* note 64, *infra*.

64. This decision was subsequently reversed in part and remanded, *sub. nom.* Saint Francis Hospital, Inc. v. Harris (N.D. Okla. 1981), 4 *Medicare & Medicaid Guide* (CCH) ¶31,561, on the ground the HCFA Administrator had given no consideration to the foundation's contributions to the provider and had stopped short in his analysis of a complex chain of transactions. The case was therefore remanded for a fuller statement of HCFA's reasoning.

65. Research Medical Center, *supra* note 46, at ¶29,230, is one of a very small group of cases in which the PRRB has held that a provider may borrow at a special, low rate of interest in certain circumstances, rather than use its funded depreciation. *See also* Mercy Hospital (Buffalo, N.Y.) v. Blue Cross Assoc./Blue Cross of Western New York, Inc., PRRB Hearing Dec. No. 79-D56, *Medicare & Medicaid Guide* [1979-2 Transfer Binder] (CCH) ¶30,130, *aff'd* HCFA Adm. Dec., *Medicare & Medicaid Guide* [1980 Transfer Binder] (CCH) ¶30,318.

66. *Ibid.*

67. HCFA Adm. Dec., *Medicare & Medicaid Guide* [1979-1 Transfer Binder] (CCH) ¶29,447, *aff'd sub. nom.* Research Medical Center v. Schweiker, *supra* note 35.

68. PRRB Hearing Dec. No. 78-D43, *Medicare & Medicaid Guide* [1978 Transfer Binder] (CCH) ¶29,215, *aff'd,* HCFA Adm. Dec., *Medicare & Medicaid Guide* [1978 Transfer Binder] (CCH) ¶ 29,242.

69. Peralta Hospital (Oakland, Cal.) v. Blue Cross Assoc./Blue Cross of Northern California, *supra* note 57.

70. Doctors Hospital, Inc. v. Califano (D. D.C. 1978), *Medicare & Medicaid Guide* [1978 Transfer Binder] (CCH) ¶29,233, *aff'g in relevant part, rev'g in part, rem'd in part,* PRRB Hearing Dec. No. 77-D47, *Medicare & Medicaid Guide* [1977 Transfer Binder] (CCH) ¶28,615.

71. PRRB Hearing Dec. No. 76-D59, *Medicare & Medicaid Guide* [1976 Transfer Binder] (CCH) ¶28,112, *modified as to other issues* Soc. Sec. Comm'r Dec., *Medicare & Medicaid Guide* [1976 Transfer Binder] (CCH) ¶28,113.

72. Prov. App. Dec. No. 00-75-06 (Blue Cross Association), *Medicare & Medicaid Guide* [1975 Transfer Binder] (CCH) ¶27,363.

73. 42 C.F.R. § 405.419(b)(3) (1979).

74. 42 C.F.R. § 405.419(b)(3)(i) (1979).

75. 42 C.F.R. § 405.419(b)(3)(ii) (1979).

76. PRM § 218.

77. 42 C.F.R. § 405.419(c)(2) (1979).

78. PRM § 218.2.

79. PRM § 2150.2.

80. *Ibid.*

81. Prov. App. Dec. No. 00-74-28 (Blue Cross Association), *Medicare & Medicaid Guide* [1975 Transfer Binder] (CCH) ¶27,264; *See also* Northwest Hospital, Inc., *supra* note 55, where the court reached the odd result of allowing the portion of interest expense on a loan to a provider from a related organization. With respect to that portion of the loan in excess of ·the seller's depreciated historical cost over the $100,000 paid in cash, the court held that the interest attributable to such portion of the loan was allowable on the unusual (if not irrational) ground that "total disallowance of interest . . . exceeds the statutory mandate that requires the reimbursement of reasonable costs."

82. PRM § 220.

83. All Saints Hospital (Philadelphia, Pa.) v. Blue Cross Assoc./Blue Cross of Greater Philadelphia, PRRB Hearing Dec. No. 79-D63, *Medicare & Medicaid Guide* [1979-2 Transfer Binder] (CCH) ¶30,157.

84. Prov. App. Dec. No. 00-76-59 (Blue Cross Association), *Medicare and Medicaid Guide* [1977 Transfer Binder] (CCH) ¶28,310.

85. (Ct. Cl. 1980), *Medicare & Medicaid Guide* [1980 Transfer Binder] (CCH) ¶30,398, *rev'g.* Prov. App. Dec. No. 00-74-49, *Medicare & Medicaid Guide* [1980 Transfer Binder] (CCH) ¶27,199.

86. For a case to the contrary, on facts highly similar, *see* HCFA Adm. Dec., *Medicare & Medicaid Guide* [1978 Transfer Binder] (CCH) ¶28,913, *aff'g* PRRB Dec. No. 77-D84, *Medicare & Medicaid Guide* [1978 Transfer Binder] (CCH) ¶28,823.

87. 42 C.F.R. § 405.419(b)(3)(ii) (1979).

88. PRM § 206. The parallel in the federal income taxation area is to be found at Code § 189, whose principal purpose is to prohibit deductions with respect to an asset until it is put into use in the trade or business of the taxpayer. See Feder, "Financing Real Estate Construction: The IRS Challenge to Construction Period Deductions," 8 *Journal of Real Estate Taxation* 3 (1981).

89. 42 C.F.R. § 405.451 (1977).

90. PRRB Hearing Dec. No. 77-D40, *Medicare & Medicaid Guide* [1977 Transfer Binder] (CCH) ¶28,520; HCFA Adm. Dec., *Medicare & Medicaid Guide* [1977 Transfer Binder] (CCH) ¶28,600.

91. 42 C.F.R. § 405.406 (1977). The statutory basis for this regulation is to be found at 42 U.S.C. § 1395x(v)(1)(A) (1965).

92. PRRB Hearing Dec. No. 78-D23, *Medicare & Medicaid Guide* [1978 Transfer Binder] (CCH) ¶29,016.

93. *Ibid.*

94. Portland Adventist Hospital (Portland, Ore.) v. Blue Cross. Assoc./Blue Cross of Oregon, PRRB Hearing Dec. No. 81-D68, 4 *Medicare & Medicaid Guide* (CCH) ¶31,474; Portland Adventist Medical Center v. Harris (D. Ore. 1980), 4 *Medicare & Medicaid Guide* (CCH) ¶31,483, *aff'g* PRRB Dec. No. 78-D58, *Medicare & Medicaid Guide* [1978 Transfer Binder] (CCH) ¶29,238; Lexington County Hospital (West Columbia, S.C.) v. Blue Cross Assoc./Blue Cross of South Carolina, HCFA Dep. Adm. Dec., *Medicare & Medicaid Guide*

[1980 Transfer Binder] (CCH) ¶30,428, *aff'g* PRRB Dec. No. 79-D87, *Medicare & Medicaid Guide* [1980 Transfer Binder] (CCH) ¶30,368; John Muir Memorial Hospital (Walnut Creek, Cal.) v. Blue Cross Assoc./Blue Cross of Southern California, HCFA Adm. Dec., *Medicare & Medicaid Guide* [1979-2 Transfer Binder] (CCH) ¶30,053, *aff'g as to this issue*, PRRB Dec. No. 79-D28, *Medicare & Medicaid Guide* [1979-2 Transfer Binder] (CCH) ¶29,960; Alton Memorial Hospital (Alton, Ill.) v. Blue Cross Assn./Health Care Service Corp., PRRB Hearing Dec. No. 79-D26, *Medicare & Medicaid Guide* [1979-2 Transfer Binder] (CCH) ¶29,958; Research Medical Center (Kansas City, Mo.) v. Blue Cross Assoc./Blue Cross of Kansas City, HCFA Adm. Dec., *Medicare & Medicaid Guide* [1979-1 Transfer Binder] (CCH) ¶29,447, *aff'g* PRRB Hearing Dec., No. 78-D57, *Medicare & Medicaid Guide* [1978 Transfer Binder] (CCH) ¶29,230; PRRB Hearing Dec., No. 78-D23, *Medicare & Medicaid Guide* [1978 Transfer Binder] (CCH) ¶29,016; PRRB Hearing Dec., No. 78-D17, *Medicare & Medicaid Guide* [1978 Transfer Binder] (CCH) ¶28,950; HCFA Adm. Dec., *Medicare & Medicaid Guide* [1977 Transfer Binder] (CCH) ¶28,600 *aff'g* PRRB Hearing Dec. No. 77-D40, *Medicare & Medicaid Guide* [1977 Transfer Binder] (CCH) ¶28,520; Good Samaritan Hospital, Corvallis v. Matthews 609 F.2d 949 (9th Cir. 1979), *aff'g* PRRB Dec. No. 76-D14, *Medicare & Medicaid Guide* [1976 Transfer Binder] (CCH) ¶27,823.

95. Good Samaritan Hospital, Corvallis, v. Matthews, *id.* at 609 F.2d 949. It should be noted, however, that one federal district court has held PRM § 206 to be inapplicable in accounting for construction borrowing costs for reimbursement purposes. St. Francis Hospital v. Weinberger, 413 F.Supp. 323 (N.D. Cal. 1975). In that case, however, the construction project in question began prior to the advent of the Medicare program. In his argument before the Ninth Circuit, the Secretary of Health, Education, and Welfare argued that the result in St. Francis Hospital was motivated by the court's desire to avoid an "inequitable retroactivity not present in the instant controversy." The Court of Claims is in accord with the Ninth Circuit. Saint Francis Hospital v. United States, 648 F.2d 1305 (Ct. Cl. 1981). *See also* Research Medical Center v. Schweiker, *supra* note 35.

96. 5 U.S.C. § 553(a)(2) (1966).

97. 323 U.S. 134 (1944).

98. Accounting Series Release No. 163, 6 Fed. Sec. L. Rep. (CCH) ¶72,185.

99. Accounting Series Release No. 272, 6 Fed. Sec. L. Rep. (CCH) ¶72,294.

100. PRRB Hearing Dec. No. 78-D23, *supra* note 92.

101. *Ibid.*

102. ¶7 of FASB 34.

103. ¶50 of FASB 34.

104. The term "material" is not defined in FASB 34; such lack of definition forms one of the bases for dissent for three members of FASB to FASB 34.

105. The following subparagraphs are proposed to be added to the end of paragraph 12 of FASB 34:

    a. Paragraphs 13–15 describe how to determine the amount of interest cost to be capitalized. In situations involving qualifying assets financed with tax-exempt borrowings, the associated agreements include sufficient restrictions to require association of those borrowings with specified qualifying assets. Paragraph 12(b) specifies the accounting for interest cost and interest earned in those special situations. Other than as specified in paragraph 12(b), interest earned shall not be offset against interest cost in determining either capitalization rates or limitations on the amount of interest cost to be capitalized.

b. The amount of interest cost capitalized on the portion of a qualifying asset acquired with proceeds of a tax-exempt borrowing shall be all interest cost of the borrowing less any interest earned on related interest-bearing investments from the date of the borrowing until the asset is ready for its intended use. Interest cost of a tax-exempt borrowing shall be eligible for capitalization on other qualifying assets of the entity when the specified qualifying asset is no longer eligible for interest capitalization (paragraphs 17–19).

106. *See* ¶s 9–11 of FASB 34, which define the term "qualifying asset."

107. *See* ¶s 50–52 of FASB 34.

108. *See* ¶18 of FASB 34.

109. There appears to be a dearth of discussion on the question of when the construction period begins. Compare the relative unimportance of this issue for reimbursement purposes with its significance in federal income taxation, Code § 189. B. L. Cook, "Determining When Construction Period Begins Key to Realty Deductions under 189," 47 *Journal of Taxation* 8 (1977). Note: the volumes of this source cumulate their pagination, so that volume 41, issue no. 2 will begin with, say, page 97.

110. PRRB Hearing Dec. No. 78-D23, *supra* note 92.

111. Lexington County Hospital (West Columbia, S.C.) v. Blue Cross Assoc./Blue Cross of South Carolina, PRRB Hearing Dec. No. 79-D87, *Medicare & Medicaid Guide* [1980 Transfer Binder] (CCH) ¶30,368.

112. PRRB Hearing Dec. No. 79-D58, *Medicare & Medicaid Guide* [1979-2 Transfer Binder] (CCH) ¶30,139.

113. Lexington County Hospital (West Columbia, S.C.) v. Blue Cross Assoc./Blue Cross of South Carolina, *supra* note 111, *aff'd in relevant part,* HCFA Adm. Dec., *Medicare & Medicaid Guide* [1980 Transfer Binder] (CCH) ¶30,437, *aff'd sub. nom.* Lexington County Hospital v. Schweiker (D. S.C. 1981) 4 *Medicare & Medicaid Guide* (CCH) ¶31,516.

114. *Ibid.*

115. PRM § 212.

116. Albany Medical Center Hospital (Albany, N.Y.) v. Blue Cross Assoc./Blue Cross of Northeastern New York, Inc., PRRB Hearing Dec. No. 78-D43, *Medicare & Medicaid Guide* [1978 Transfer Binder] (CCH) ¶29,215, *aff'd* HCFA Adm. Dec., *Medicare & Medicaid Guide* [1978 Transfer Binder] (CCH) ¶29,242.

117. 42 C.F.R. § 405.419(c)(3) (1979).

118. HCFA Deputy Adm. Dec., *Medicare & Medicaid Guide* [1980 Transfer Binder] (CCH) ¶30,437; The Good Samaritan Hospital (Vincennes, Ind.) v. Blue Cross Assoc./Mutual Hospital Insurance, Inc., *supra* note 41, at PRRB Hearing Dec. No. 79-D80; PRRB Hearing Dec., No. 77-D40, *Medicare & Medicaid Guide* [1977 Transfer Binder] (CCH) ¶28,520.

119. PRRB Hearing Dec. No. 77-D40, *supra* note 90.

Chapter 8

The Commercial Bank's Role in Short-Term Financing

Robert G. Donnelley

In November 1980, the University of Chicago issued $65 million in tax-exempt commercial paper through the Illinois Educational Facilities Authority. Used principally to finance the university's medical center and its related hospitals and clinics, the issue marked the first time tax-exempt commercial paper was used to finance a health care institution. The university borrowed short-term because rapidly rising interest rates had effectively precluded it from the long-term bond market.

In the first year of the program, the financing resulted in savings of more than $1.3 million based upon the difference between the original cost of the rejected term bonds and the average cost of the commercial paper program.

Since 1980, the demand for short-term financing for hospitals has exploded. This growth has been fueled most importantly by the unprecedented interest rate levels in the long-term bond markets which have made long-term financing for plant and equipment impossible or confiscatory. However, other factors have included a slowdown in the payments from third-party reimbursers (primarily the government), the impact of inflation on hospital working capital, and the trend toward consolidation within the health care industry.

Unusually high long-term interest rates have forced hospitals to finance long-term construction projects through a panoply of short-term debt instruments created especially to meet this need. Generally, these programs involve commercial bank credit either directly or indirectly in the form of standby lines or letters of credit.

For the future, interest rate volatility is expected to be the norm. Such an environment, coupled with a continued tightening of cost reimbursement, will place an important premium on the knowledge of short-term financing techniques.

SOURCES OF FUNDS

Traditionally, commercial banks have been the primary source of short-term variable rate credit with a maturity of up to eight years. To a limited extent, insurance companies, savings and loans, leasing firms, finance companies, and brokerage houses have also participated in this market. Generally, insurance companies and savings and loans have limited themselves to construction financing; finance and leasing companies to equipment financing; and brokerage houses to situations where the firm handles the institution's investment portfolio and to "bond anticipation notes" issued for one to three years.

The reluctance of commercial banks to make fixed rate loans and the limited capacity of banks to absorb tax-exempt credit have led to the development of private placements and public, short-term note offerings backed by a letter of credit, standby line, or tax-exempt note purchase agreement involving a commercial bank.

TAX-EXEMPT COMMERCIAL PAPER

The most significant of these instruments is commercial paper and its counterpart in the private placement market, the demand master note program. Some major health care organizations, including Kaiser Permanente, have issued taxable commercial paper for some years. The development of the tax-exempt, short-term note program for the University of Chicago and, five months earlier, a similar program for Loyola University, extended these facilities to the tax-exempt market. Both of these programs were issued through the Illinois Educational Facilities Authority—a state agency—which enabled the interest on the paper to be tax-exempt.

Commercial paper consists of short-term, unsecured, fixed rate notes with a maximum maturity of less than one year. Generally, the maturities on such paper are between 15 and 45 days. Initially, commercial paper was issued strictly for working capital and was expected to be paid off from short-term cash flow.

Because of the short maturity, it is required that such paper be backed up by bank lines available in the event such paper cannot be rolled over at maturity.

Buyers of such paper are generally money market funds, bank trust departments, corporations, and similar institutional investors. Paper is generally issued in denominations of $50,000 or more, which limits the demand for such paper from retail buyers. Commercial paper also requires a rating and an offering memorandum. Such borrowing programs are limited only to the best credits—those institutions with ratings of "AA" or better or those that can obtain such ratings with a bank letter of credit. Because of the costs of issuance, the economic size of such programs is $20 million or more.

Tax-exempt commercial paper developed with the growth of tax-exempt money market funds and similar commingled tax-exempt funds established by bank trust departments having a substantial appetite for very short-term, tax-exempt instruments.

COSTS OF COMMERCIAL PAPER

Because of the short maturities, the tax-exempt commercial paper sells at a rate of between 40 percent and 55 percent of prime. The required standby line, note purchase agreement, and/or letter of credit costs an additional ⅜ percent to 1½ percent per annum. The fee charged by the bank increases according to the extent the issue relies upon the underlying bank credit for its creditworthiness.

A separate fee is charged by the sales agent, that is, the investment bank or commercial bank responsible for marketing the commercial paper. These fees are ¼ percent to ½ percent per annum on the average outstanding amount of commercial paper.

DEMAND MASTER NOTES

The tax-exempt demand master note is a variant of tax-exempt commercial paper and is an evolution of taxable demand note programs established by many bank trust departments which purchase the notes for and on behalf of their trust customers. The principal purchasers are bank trust departments and, since 1979, tax-exempt money market funds. Unlike commercial paper, the notes are privately placed. The face maturity is generally for a year or more; the notes, however, are callable on demand with a notice period between 48 hours and 14 days. Generally, such placements do not require an offering memorandum; however, such placements increasingly involve a rating from a recognized rating agency, for example, Moody's and Standard and Poor's.

Master note placements have ranged from $5 million to as much as $65 million. Typically, the rates on such notes are based on commercial bank prime, 90-day or 180-day Treasury bills. Typical rates are 50 percent to 65 percent of prime, 50 percent to 65 percent of 90-day or 180-day Treasury bills, or, occasionally, on a published index for tax-exempt bonds. As in the case of commercial paper, these placements also require support from a commercial bank to provide liquidity in the event a demand for payment is made. The required support can be in the form of a tax-exempt note purchase agreement, a letter of credit, or a taxable or tax-exempt line of credit.

Placement fees for such paper usually range between ½ percent and 1 percent depending on size and difficulty of the credit. This is generally a one-time fee, although some investment banks and commercial banks may charge an additional fee upon renewal of the program. More recently, some places have begun to charge a per annum fee in lieu of a one-time fee. This fee is generally ¼ to ⅝ percent per annum. The cost of the supporting credit is the same as the fees charged for commercial paper— the greater the dependence on the supporting credit, the higher the price charged.

MONEY MARKET FUNDS—A NEW SOURCE OF FINANCING

From their inception in 1979, to the end of 1981, tax-exempt money market funds grew more than $5 billion. As a result, they have become an important indirect source of short-term funds in the form of commercial paper purchases and private placements. These funds are short-term investment vehicles for individuals and trust departments. They solicit funds from the public, and their offering is governed by an official statement. Typically, such funds commit to investing in liquid securities with a maximum maturity of one year. Generally, the portfolio of such funds is restricted to an average life of 120 days. Tax-exempt master notes payable on demand or after a short notice period are desired since their short maturities not only provide important liquidity, but also enable the funds to invest in longer-term, higher-yielding notes.

Because of this new market, the interest rates on commercial paper and demand master notes may be lower than that dictated by the yield curve.

A particular credit may also obtain an additional advantage from a more favorable short-term rating in comparison to the long-term rating. Short-term notes are rated on a different basis than long-term notes. It is easier to qualify for the best rating for short-term notes.

OTHER FINANCING PROGRAMS

The public market has provided yet another source of short-term financing. While the bond market during periods of high interest rates has not been receptive to long-term bonds, hospitals have been able to finance capital projects with three- to five-year notes. Almost always, these notes have required a bank letter of credit or an irrevocable standby line to provide the assurance that the funds to pay the notes will be available at maturity. If not properly structured, such financing has the disadvantage of being inflexible. Moreover, there is no assurance that, upon maturity in three to five years, the time will be favorable for such refinancing. The alternative of advance refunding of the notes in the interim may be cumbersome and costly.

The requirements of such notes are similar to long-term bonds. The costs of such notes, however, are less because such financing carries the lower interest rates of short-term paper. Generally, underwriting fees range between ¾ percent to 2 percent, depending upon the complexity of the issue.

CRITERIA USED BY BANKS IN JUDGING HEALTH CARE CREDIT

The credit analysis used by commercial banks and other institutional lenders is neither mysterious nor complex. Its essential focus is the determination of whether the funds will be available to pay the principal and interest when due.

To support such an analysis, the lender generally will require three to five years of financial statements and for term credit facilities, two to three years of projections. These requirements may be reduced if the cash need is truly a short-term one and the source of repayment is clearly evidenced by the liquidation of receivables or other sources of cash flow.

BALANCE SHEET CHARACTERISTICS

Certain balance sheet items have an important effect on current and term loans. (Current loans are defined as loans of less than one year.) The factor that has an important effect on a financial institution's assessment of creditworthiness is the leverage ratio (total debt as a percent of total assets). Some analysts define "total assets" as total tangible assets or assets net of good will or other intangibles, normally ranging from 40 percent to 85 percent. This ratio measures the health care institution's dependence on debt as a source of capital. Generally, the higher the ratio is, the weaker the credit. In the case of term credits, pro forma debt to equity is also a key ratio.

LEVERAGE RATIO INCREASINGLY IMPORTANT

It used to be fashionable for some management consultants to question the relevancy of leverage in the credit analysis of an acute care hospital, arguing that the system of cost reimbursement, the existence of a limited franchise, and the third party payer system all served to reduce the importance of capital funds.

Moreover, leverage ratio analysis failed to recognize that hospitals may receive a reimbursement for depreciation at a level higher than principal retirement in the early years of a bond issue. Third-party cost-based insurers reimburse on a straight-line basis. If a bond issue is designed to be amortized on the basis of level debt service with larger principal payments due in later years, then reimbursement for depreciation will exceed principal payments in the early years. Most bond issues have weighted the principal payment toward the end of the issue, increasing the differential between depreciation and principal payments.

Recent and dramatic changes in cost reimbursement and the competitive environment, however, have placed an increased emphasis on leverage as a measure of risk. Bank lenders never forsook the measure during the halcyon days of the 1960s and early 1970s. The market apparently has decreased the level of acceptable leverage for health care entities. The maximum acceptable leverage seems to be from 3.5 to 1 to 4 to 1—the range depending upon the overall perception of risk involved with the particular borrower.

WORKING CAPITAL, ACCOUNTS RECEIVABLE

Working capital levels and the makeup of current assets are also important factors. While the account may vary according to the type of organization, a positive working capital level is important.

The age of a firm's accounts receivable is also a key balance sheet factor, as is the trend reflected by the financial statements of prior years. Generally, this factor is measured by the number of days' revenue tied up in patients' accounts. This measurement is calculated by dividing the dollar amount of accounts receivable at the end of the particular accounting period by the average daily revenue for that period. Anything above 70 days' receivable outstanding is above average and requires explanation.

TERM LENDING

Because of the capital-intensive nature of most health care institutions, most short-term lending is in the form of term loans or term loans standby facilities where the period of the loan may be for seven years or longer and repayment is expected either to come from earnings generated by the business or from a refinancing of the debt in the bond market.

While a health care institution differs from a typical business enterprise in its dependence on third-party reimbursement and the existence of a franchise, the financial characteristics of such institutions are similar in that sufficient income must be obtained from operations and other sources to cover current operating expenses and meet principal payments, working capital needs, necessary capital asset expenditures, and contingencies.

PROJECTED DEBT SERVICE COVERAGE

For this reason, the focus on the credit analysis is on the institution's ability to meet these needs. A key analytical tool is projected level of debt service coverage for the period of the financing. This ratio is defined as all principal payments due plus interest plus earnings (after tax if tax is applicable) plus depreciation divided by principal and interest due.

In the case of short-term loans for major capital projects, the principal may be treated as being amortized over a period longer than the term of the loan. In most instances, projected debt service coverage should be no less than 1.2 times during the life of the loan and 1.5 times during the projected amortization period of 20 years.

This ratio is substantially below the medians calculated by Moody's on the 201 hospital enterprises rated and reviewed for calendar year 1980 and reflects the shorter amortization period. The medians reported by Moody's for peak debt service coverage by historical net revenues and peak debt service coverage by estimated net revenues in the first full year after projected completion are 1.59 and 2.20, respectively.

While it is not necessary to project a full payout during the life of a short-term loan financing major capital expenditures, the financial statistics of the health care institution must be strong enough at the maturity of the short-term financing to support a public bond issue or a private placement.

RISK FACTORS

Projected debt service coverage is the principal factor considered. However, the risk factors behind the projections are then reviewed with specific reference to historic and projected sources of revenue and other market characteristics, operating margins, balance sheet characteristics, the management, the medical staff, and the project being financed. Generally, these factors are analyzed in a financial feasibility study. While a formal financial feasibility study may not be necessary, the borrower will have to provide much of the same kind of detailed analysis to support the financing.

REVENUE

A detailed credit analysis includes a thorough review of historic and projected operating revenues and operating margins.

While most lenders value the basic stability of the third-party reimbursement system, they also are beginning to recognize the increasing impact of cost reimbursement cutbacks and the problem of deficits in reimbursement of such programs, particularly in the cases of Medicaid and, to a lesser extent, Medicare.

Patient mix, therefore, has become an increasingly critical factor. A high level of Medicaid, especially in states with recognized financial problems, without offsetting revenue streams, is closely reviewed. Conversely, a substantial proportion of commercially insured and private-pay patients (with a low bad debt experience) is a favorable factor. A Medicaid load of 15 percent to 20 percent without mitigating factors can be considered a problem. A large percentage of cost based business (over 50 percent) can also be a limiting factor without outside revenue sources.

Percentage of bed occupancy to total beds is also a major analytical tool, although the growth of outpatient revenue has lessened the importance of this factor. Generally, an historic percentage of 78.4 percent (based upon current hospital medians published by Moody's Investors Service) and a minimum projected percentage of 80 percent are good benchmarks.

Other revenue sources are also reviewed in detail for their certainty. Such revenues consist of donations and income from rental properties or other operations not directly related to the health care institution. Of particular interest in these days of corporate reorganization is the extent by which such ancillary activities benefit or increase the risk of the obligor. The existence of an organized capital fund development program is especially important in the case of tax-exempt entities.

OPERATING MARGINS

Free competition, cost containment, inflation, and related changes in the health care markets have caused the institutional banker to place an increased emphasis on operating margins. The elimination of regulations and the loss of the exclusive franchise in the airline and trucking industries have led to squeezed margins and losses, and many institutional lenders fear a similar period of adjustment may be imminent in health care. While, in the past, lenders have recognized in the case of tax-exempt organizations that it was not uncommon for such institutions to fix their rates and charges at or close to the break-even level, increasingly, lending institutions are requiring significant surpluses. According to Moody's, hospital enterprise medians for 1980, "net takedown," defined as "net revenue" divided by "gross revenue and income," was 11.3 percent. Gross revenue and income is defined as "operating revenue plus non-operating revenue." Net revenue is defined as gross revenue minus operating expenses, excluding depreciation, amortization, and interest.

A variation from this level generally must be justified by a local regulatory environment that assures an occupancy rate and a level of stable direct and subsidized reimbursement sufficient to minimize the risk of repayment.

A key referent for evaluation of projected debt service coverage is the historical financial statement. However, the following factors must also be assessed: (1) the market; (2) management; (3) medical staff; and, (4) the financial risk unique to the project being financed.

THE MARKET

A detailed analysis of the primary service area is one of the most important factors in the assessment of the creditworthiness of a health care institution. This element of the credit analysis is particularly important if the projections assume increased utilization or an increase in rates and charges. Among the more important elements are:

- *Demographic trends.* Lenders generally are concerned with population growth and changes in per capita income. Obviously, a growing population and a rising per capita income are favorable factors. In the case of hospitals, lenders are also interested in the total number of acute care beds within the service area and whether the ratio of such beds per 1,000 population is increasing or declining.
- *Factors in increased utilization.* If increased utilization is projected and an important factor for repayment, the sources, for example, previously unsatisfied demand, increase in population, and the hiring of additional physicians, will also be analyzed. Changes in the mix of patient revenues will also be reviewed. Comparisons will be made to the regional average of admissions per 1,000 population.

- *Competitive factors.* The borrowing entity's status within the service area will be reviewed, including the ratio of its beds to the total beds of the service area, the fees charged compared to the competition, and its expansion plans compared to those of the competition. In the case of tax-exempt institutions, the fund-raising efforts will be reviewed in relation to those of similar entities.
- *Trend in state regulation.* Because of the importance of regulation in health care, a lender will be very interested in the following issues: Will competition be restricted by certificate-of-need laws? Will reimbursement be further limited? Will regulatory laws increase costs without providing offsetting benefits?

These factors will be assessed for their impact on the trend in patient days and inpatient admissions. An institution's projected occupancy will be evaluated. Occupancy is measured by dividing "average daily census" by the institution's average beds available for that year. In 1980, Moody's ratio showed a bed occupancy of 78.4 percent. The average length of stay was 7.3 days.

Rates charged for services will also be reviewed to determine to what extent they can be raised to generate additional income given the cost reimbursement regulations.

MANAGEMENT

A vital consideration in the credit evaluation of a health care institution is the quality of management and staff personnel. An assessment of work experience and training of key personnel is an important factor. Sometimes a degree in hospital or business administration may be an important indicator. However, good management is generally assessed by the demonstrated evidence of it.

Some of the factors reviewed are:

- Does a dynamic long-range plan exist? Does it properly reflect a corporate strategy suitable to the entity's resources and environment?
- Is the institution accredited by the various agencies and reimbursement programs such as the Joint Commission on Accreditation of Hospitals? Is it certified for participation in Medicare/Medicaid and Blue Cross?
- Does the institution have good personnel policies? Is the supply of nurses sufficient to meet the institution's needs? Are there union problems? Is there management depth?

- Do the financial statements reflect management control? Are the financial ratios better than industry norms?
- Does the institution have effective purchasing policies and good inventory controls? Is it obtaining the most favorable prices for its supplies?
- Is the institution supported by the community? Does it have an involved and knowledgeable board of trustees? Do they appear to be community leaders? Is the board well balanced, with the medical staff represented but not in a position to dominate?

This list is not all-inclusive. An assessment of management is a key consideration.

MEDICAL STAFF

Most financial institutions have recognized the fact that in a very real sense the physician and not the patient is the real customer of the acute care institution. (In the case of a nursing home, this is less true; however, a good medical staff is an essential element.) Physicians normally decide in which hospitals and for how long their patients will be treated.

Among the factors considered are the following:

- How many physicians are on the medical staff? More importantly, what is the number of active admitting physicians measured in terms of total admissions? Ten or fewer accounting for over 50 percent of admissions may be cause for concern.
- What is the number of physicians with their principal practice in the primary service area compared to the number of beds?
- What is the mix of medical specialties, and what are the qualifications of the staff physicians? What percentage are board certified or board eligible? Is there an active recruitment and training program? Does the facility have an internship or residency program? Is there a medical office building near the health care facility?

THE PROJECT

The final item of consideration is the nature of the capital expenditure itself. A financial institution attempts first to insure that there is a demonstrated economic need for the project. In the case of most hospitals, the certificate-of-need procedure is usually sufficient to assure this.

Other considerations include:

- Is the project revenue-generating?
- Are all requirements met for the project, such as certificate of need, planning agency approval, etc.?
- In the case of a construction project, are the architect and contractor experienced? Is the project covered by maximum price contracts? Are there adequate performance and completion bonds? In the case of equipment, is the installer experienced?
- Are the funds adequate to complete the project? Has an adequate contingency fund been provided (usually 15 percent is considered adequate)?

TYPES OF BANK LOANS AND COMMITMENTS—CUSTOMARY TERMS AND COVENANTS

The simplest form of short-term credit is the taxable current bank line. Such a loan is typically self-liquidating and for a period of less than one year. The rate on such financing generally is based upon commercial banks' prime rate. Compensating balances normally charged range between 7½ percent and 15 percent of the outstanding amount of the loan. Sometimes compensating balances are charged on the commitment. Interest is paid quarterly or on maturity, whichever is shorter. Such financing is generally unsecured. The purpose of such loans generally is to meet a short-term seasonal need, such as the carrying of accounts receivable.

Of generally greater importance to health care institutions are term loans. The period during which such loans may be outstanding may be as much as seven years or longer, and repayment is expected to come out of income generated from operations.

Basically, term credits fall into the following types, although a particular credit facility may be a combination of one or more types. These are:

1. *The serial term loan.* This is a credit under which the funds are made immediately available to the borrower and the obligation is made payable serially over the life of the loan on a monthly, quarterly, semiannual, or annual basis. Actual principal payment may vary in amounts, and sometimes a balloon payment is allowed. Such a balloon payment, however, is rarely more than 30 percent of the principal amount of the loan.

2. *Revolving credit.* Under this arrangement, the borrower may avail itself of funds from time to time up to the maximum amount of the commitment with the privilege of repaying and reborrowing during the life of the credit. The borrower has the right to terminate or

reduce the facility at any time upon proper written notice. A revolving credit is a formal commitment of the financial institution to lend the funds according to the term loan agreement regardless of the general availability of funds. For this reason, a commitment fee is charged based upon the unused portion of the credit.

3. *Call or standby credit.* A call or standby credit is an arrangement that grants the borrower a commitment for a period of time under which the borrower can obtain funds from time to time up to the maximum amount available to the expiration date. It differs from the revolving credit in that there exists no right to repay or reborrow funds.

4. *Revolving or standby credit convertible into a serial term loan.* This financing arrangement enables the borrower to convert a revolving or standby credit after a period of time into a serial term loan, payable over a period of years in accordance with the terms of the agreement. This financing program is particularly suited to plant construction. Drawdowns can be scheduled accordingly to meet the progress payment requirements. Upon completion, the borrowing can then be converted so that the earnings generated can service the term obligation. Sometimes, the term loan feature is used to provide a measure of safety in the event permanent financing cannot be arranged on a satisfactory basis.

5. *Standby letter of credit or irrevocable standby line.* Borrowers have increasingly used bank letters of credit and irrevocable standby lines to secure tax-exempt or fixed rate short-term bonds where the creditworthiness of the borrower or term of the financing requires additional security in order to be marketable. A standby letter of credit assures that, upon presentation of certain documents (normally evidence of nonpayment and the bond), the buyer of such notes can collect his or her funds from the issuing bank. Generally, such letters of credit are made out with the trustee on the note issue as beneficiary. In the event funds or payment date are not available from the borrower, the trustee has an automatic call on the issuing bank for the money. The bankruptcy of the borrower is not sufficient to affect the bank's obligation to fund. Letters of credit generally cost between ¾ percent and 1½ percent per annum plus nominal issuance fees. Because of the unconditional nature of the bank's commitment on such letters of credit, the notes backed by such letters usually are rated based upon the creditworthiness of the underlying bank issuing the letter rather than that of the borrower.

Because commercial banks generally have overall limits on the aggregate amount of standby letters of credit issued, banks have begun to issue irrevocable standby lines of credit. Such lines allow drawdowns without condition to make payments when due. Such commitments generally are less secure than letters of credit since the right to draw under the line is that of the borrower, and, in the event of bankruptcy, the treatment of the proceeds from such borrowing may be open to question. Variations on such lines are unconditional rights to sell bonds to a bank in the event of nonpayment or at or up to a fixed period of time. The cost of an irrevocable line of credit is less than a letter of credit. Moreover, with such a backup, a borrower has the opportunity to establish a reputation in the marketplace whereas, under a letter of credit, the buyer all too often merely bases a decision on the credit of the issuing bank.

Standby letters of credit and irrevocable standby lines normally create upon drawdown under them a demand obligation against the borrower. For this reason, a standby term facility covering drawdowns is an important measure of safety. Such a situation is particularly true in the case of tax-exempt borrowing because a repayment of the borrowing by the borrower may extinguish the right to refinance the obligation on a tax-exempt basis.

INTEREST RATES

Term facilities are generally priced at a rate over commercial bank prime based upon the creditworthiness of the borrower and money market conditions. The rate fluctuates as the prime rate changes. Compensating balances of between 5 percent and 20 percent are also normally required. Such balances may be based upon the commitment and/or on the outstanding borrowing.

In the past several years, a number of alternatives have developed to interest rates based upon commercial bank prime rate. These so-called "cost plus" alternatives have included a rate quoted over Eurodollar deposits, commercial bank certificates of deposit, or federal funds, or a variant of these. Generally, such alternatives have been available only for the better credits. Such pricing alternatives as Eurodollar loans and loans fixed over matching certificates of deposit may provide an important advantage of fixing the interest rate for up to six months or more during a period of market volatility.

EURODOLLAR PRICING

Eurodollar pricing is based at a spread (generally ¾ percent to 2 percent) over the Base Eurodollar Rate adjusted for the Federal Reserve requirement. The Base Eurodollar Rate is the rate at which deposits in U.S. dollars are offered to prime American banks in the offshore interbank market at approximately 11:00 A.M. two business days prior to the date of loan takedown or rollover for an amount and period approximately the amount and period of the Eurodollar loans.

Varying Maturities

Maturities for such loans can be fixed for one, two, three, six, twelve months, or longer, as available, with a month defined as a period starting on one business day in a calendar month and ending on the numerically corresponding business day in the next calendar month. Generally, to be eligible, such borrowings must be in amounts of $2.5 million or more.

Notice Requirement

Such borrowings also include a notice requirement: The borrower normally must notify the lender or lenders by 11:00 A.M. two business days prior to takedown or rollover of its intent to utilize the Eurodollar pricing option, with the rate being that in effect on the day of drawdown or rollover. Because such loans are based upon a deposit of fixed maturity, prepayments of Eurodollar pricing-based credits will not be permitted other than at the maturity of the Eurodollar funding deposit.

The applicable reserve requirement is contained in the amendment to Regulation D promulgated by the Federal Reserve in October 1980. This regulation provides for a phased-in reserve requirement reaching 3 percent on February 16, 1984. The calculation for the Effective Eurodollar Rate is: Base Eurodollar Rate (1 − the applicable reserve requirement expressed as a decimal).

CERTIFICATES-OF-DEPOSIT BASED PRICING

A second variant of "cost plus" credit pricing uses certificates of deposit (CD) as the price index. Such pricing may be on a quasi-floating rate basis. For example, the index may be the weekly average rate as reported by CD dealers to and published by the Federal Reserve Bank of New York adjusted for reserves and the Federal Deposit Insurance Corporation's (FDIC) premium costs.

MATCHED FUNDED PRICING

More important, however, is pricing based on matched funded, fixed rate certificates of deposit. A typical fixing is the average of the secondary market bid rates on certificates of deposit of the desired maturity as quoted to the bank lender or lenders at 10:00 A.M. (Eastern Standard

Time) by three CD dealers of recognized standing on the date of loan takedown or rollover. (The "bid rate" is that rate at which buyers offer to purchase a security.)

This base CD rate is then adjusted for the Federal Reserve requirement and net the FDIC's insurance premium costs. The reserve requirement is equal to the sum of the new reserve percentage (3 percent) plus a transition adjustment percentage of the difference between the old reserve percentage (6 percent) and the new reserve percentage (3 percent). The reserve requirement as of February 18, 1982 is 4.5 percent, falling to 3 percent on February 16, 1984. The FDIC insurance premium is generally less than 0.1 percent, but is recalculated on a semiannual basis. The spread or margin on such CD borrowing ranges between ¾ percent and 2½ percent.

The calculation for the effective CD rate is: the Base CD Rate (1 − the reserve requirement) + the FDIC insurance premium. Similar to Eurodollar deposits, maturities on such borrowings can be fixed for 30, 60, 90, and occasionally, for 120 days or longer. All maturities are subject to availability; however, availability is generally not a problem for periods of 90 days or less. The spread on such loans is similar to Eurodollars—¾ percent to 2 percent.

Like Eurodollar borrowings, fixed rate CD borrowings require notification. Generally, the customer must notify the bank or banks two to four days' prior to takedown or rollover of its intention to borrow based upon the CD pricing option, with the rate being in effect on the day of drawdown or rollover.

Minimum borrowings generally range from $2.5 million to $5 million.

Prepayments other than at the maturity of the CD are generally not permitted.

COMMITMENT FEES

On most term credit facilities, a commitment fee is charged to compensate the lender for holding funds available for the future borrowing as agreed. Such a fee applies only to the unused portion of the credit. The rate may vary, but generally is ½ percent per annum. The fee will be adjusted as the commitment is adjusted.

CUSTOMARY CONDITIONS

There is no agreement form that can be used for term loans generally, nor should there be. Each term credit is different from any other, and what may apply to one may not apply to another. The agreement should be custom-fitted to the specific credit situation.

A term loan agreement normally consists of four principal sections: (1) description of the credit and the collateral pledged, if any; (2) representations and warranties; (3) financial covenants; and (4) default provisions. Tax-exempt credits differ in that the parties to the agreement also include the municipal agency through which the funds are borrowed so that the interest is exempt from taxation.

Representations and warranties cover the area of proper authorization and the truth and accuracy of the information provided upon which the loan is based. If either of these is deficient, these provisions allow the lender either to opt not to make the loan or to require immediate repayment.

COLLATERAL

Traditionally, loans of greater than one year to health care institutions have been secured by a mortgage on the plant and/or a lien on equipment. Sometimes, a gross receipts pledge is taken. In the case of an investor-owned concern, the shares in the operating entity may also be pledged. This last has value because the shares usually control the entity that has been granted the franchise or certificate of need.

The mortgage on a hospital has limited value in itself because the facility generally is too specialized to be used for anything other than a hospital. Nevertheless, such security may have value to another health care provider. More importantly, the control over such security may be essential to tap the long-term bond market.

GROSS RECEIPTS PLEDGE

A gross receipts pledge provides that all income accruing from the operation of the health care entity must be used first to satisfy principal and interest payments due on the loan. It is used because certain accounts receivable such as Medicare and Medicaid payments are legally restricted from being used as security.

Since such a pledge is of value only as long as the health care institution continues to operate, the gross receipts pledge may be of limited value in the case of bankruptcy. However, a gross receipts pledge may effectively limit any other borrowing. Some legal authorities believe that such a pledge could force a subsequent lender to give up principal and interest payments made within the statute of limitations.

Sometimes, a health care institution may attempt to collateralize short-term borrowings with liquid investments. While very attractive to the lender, such investments generally cannot be used because of legal restrictions. The Internal Revenue Service regulations governing arbitrage may also limit such pledging in the case of tax-exempt borrowing.

FINANCIAL COVENANTS

The most important, but most misunderstood, aspect of short-term financing is the establishment of financial covenants. Historically (and still today in some foreign countries), such covenants were unnecessary since short-term loans were callable without condition upon demand by the lender (whether the borrower could pay was another matter).

When the lender gave up the right to make demand at will, financial covenants were established to protect the lender. Financial covenants may be many or few depending upon the quality of the credit. In the case of short-term loans, such covenants are usually more comprehensive than those required to support a public bond issue. Unlike a public bond issue, however, a waiver of such restrictions is much easier to accomplish. Such waivers are handled by negotiation with the lender. In the case of a credit agreement involving a number of creditors, usually such agreements may be altered upon the consent of a certain percentage of creditors involved.

Generally, such covenants should be no more restrictive than policies that any conservative management would follow to maintain a good credit standing. They should be designed to prevent any material deterioration in the financial condition of the borrower or credit preferences.

STANDARD REQUIREMENTS

In the case of loans to health care institutions, some of the more important covenants include the following standard requirements:

- Maintenance in good standing of the licenses necessary to operate. In addition to the required operating licenses, such requirements may include the maintenance of accreditation by the Joint Commission on Accreditation of Hospitals, the status of the contracting party in the Blue Cross Plan, and the certification of participation in the Health Insurance for the Aged (Medicare) program. Sometimes, although less frequently, certification for participation in Medicaid may also be required. In the case of tax-exempt health care institutions, maintenance of 501(c)(3) status is also generally required.

- Maintenance of appropriate and adequate insurance, compliance with ERISA obligations, and maintenance in sound and efficient condition of all necessary plant and equipment.
- The payment of all applicable taxes on a timely basis unless contested in good faith.
- Operation of the business in the fields in which it is currently engaged.

Term loan agreements also include financial covenants. The following are generally the principal ones:

- The provision of timely consolidated and consolidating financial statements, normally both on an annual and quarterly basis.
- The maintenance of a minimum level of working capital. The excess of current assets over current liabilities. The purpose is to insure a satisfactory degree of asset liquidity on the part of the borrower.
- A limit on additional indebtedness. This covenant may be a complete prohibition, a dollar limit, or defined as a percentage of net worth or debt service coverage.
- A restriction on liens on assets. In the case of an unsecured loan, this restriction may take the form of a "negative pledge"—an agreement under which the borrower agrees not to grant liens on assets not already encumbered. Purchase money mortgages may be specifically accepted up to a certain dollar amount.
- A limitation on the payment of dividends and/or management fees.
- A restriction on loans or advances to investments in and guaranties of the obligations of other activities. This covenant provides the lender with a measure of control over a borrower's working capital position.
- A prohibition or restriction on mergers or consolidation or restructuring. A term loan is generally based upon a specific business under a particular management with a particular base of assets. A banker should have the right to reconsider lending should the borrower wish to change any of these elements.
- A restriction on the sale of principal assets other than in the ordinary course of business. Such a sale materially affects the business of the borrower.
- A limitation on the sales of notes or accounts receivable, sale and leaseback deals, and lease rentals. All of these transactions are merely alternate forms of long- and short-term borrowing and for this reason, are restricted.

- A restriction on fixed asset expenditures. Such a covenant will be required when there is a need to maintain or increase working capital. The restriction may be expressed as a fixed dollar amount annually as an amount based on annual depreciation on a cumulative or non-cumulative basis.
- A restriction in the voluntary repayment of other term debt. Normally, this covenant requires the payment of bank debt prior to other institutional lenders on the retirement of all term debt on a *pari passu* basis.
- A restriction on maximum indebtedness to invested funds. This covenant may be expressed as total indebtedness to total liabilities and net worth or, in the case of tax-exempt health care institutions, long-term debt divided by the sum of net fixed assets plus working capital.

In addition to these covenants, two others affecting the income stream or cash flow are also generally included. These are a minimum debt service coverage requirement and a related requirement forcing the health care borrower to raise rates and charges to the maximum extent permitted by law in order to maintain the minimum debt service coverage.

While these are the principal covenants, other covenants may be added based upon the particular risks of the borrower or the industry served by the borrower.

DEFAULT PROVISIONS

Default provisions set forth the conditions that will legally allow the lender to accelerate the maturity of the indebtedness or take other action to protect the loan. Such other action may include the appointment of a management consultant to conduct an operational review.

A default may automatically accelerate maturity, but more generally, it is necessary for the lender or lenders to notify the borrower that the entire obligation is due and payable. Depending upon the type of default, the borrower may be granted a period of time after notice to remedy the breach.

Some common default provisions are:

- a materially false representation or warranty by the borrower in connection with the agreement;
- nonpayment of principal or interest when due;
- breach of any covenant;
- bankruptcy of the borrower;

- failure of the borrower to deny and have vacated within a specified time any bankruptcy or reorganization proceedings against it (frequently 30 days);
- appointment of a trustee or receiver or consent by the borrower to the appointment of a trustee for a substantial part of its property in any involuntary bankruptcy proceeding and not vacated within a specified time (frequently 30 days);
- assignment by the borrower for the benefit of creditors or admission in writing of inability to pay debts as they become due;
- failure of the borrower to discharge any judgment against it within a specified time; and
- breach of any other provision of the agreement which is not remedied within a specified period after written notice from the lender.

CLOSING LEGAL OPINION

A legal opinion stating the following is routinely required for any financing:

1. that the borrower is validly organized;
2. that the agreement is validly executed and binding upon it; and
3. that there is no violation of its articles of incorporation, bylaws, or any existing agreement or interest.

Chapter 9

Equipment Financing

Geoffrey B. Shields

During the last few years a wide variety of techniques for financing equipment have been developed. Because of changes in market conditions and tax laws the least expensive method of purchasing equipment will most likely change from time to time. A health care institution should be sure that it has contacted its banker, its investment banker, a leasing company, and the supplier of its equipment for different suggestions on the best way to finance the equipment.

INITIAL CONSIDERATIONS

Several preliminary questions should be considered before undertaking an equipment financing.

Check Outstanding Debt Documents

If the hospital has outstanding debt, the debt documents probably restrict the amount and type of borrowing permitted for equipment purchases. Frequently there are separate permitted indebtedness provisions governing general long-term debt which may be used for equipment purchases, capitalized leases, and noncapitalized leases. The impact of the form of borrowing to finance equipment upon the debt document tests for additional future borrowing should be considered.

Who Bears Risk of Obsolescence?

A lease with the right to cancel at any time without penalty provision places the risk of equipment obsolescence, changes in environmental or health regulations, and changes in use patterns on the lessor. Because of these risks, many hospitals find it desirable to structure their high-technology equipment acquisitions with a provision permitting cancellation at any time with little or no penalty.

Equipment Sharing

Certificate-of-need incentives and the cost savings possible through equipment sharing have resulted in many hospitals turning to sharing of equipment. Sharing can be done in numerous ways, including:

1. ownership of equipment in a shared services facility as is common at large medical centers with several hospitals;
2. each of two or more hospitals providing services (including availability of equipment) not provided by the other hospital(s) in its shared services group; or
3. equipment and services (such as laboratory equipment) provided by an outside vendor and located at the vendor's facility.

Types of Equipment Financing

- Tax-Exempt Bond Issue
  - One-Hospital Issue
  - Pooled Financing
  - Municipal Lease
- Internally Financed
- True Lease
- Capitalized Lease
- Purchase Money Mortgage

TAX-EXEMPT FINANCING OF EQUIPMENT

Equipment can be financed for both not-for-profit hospitals and for-profit hospitals (so long as the $10 million borrowing limitation is observed) through the issuance of tax-exempt bonds. Small bond issues can be privately placed with a local bank, and in some cases large equipment issues have been privately placed or sold publicly by an investment banker. The same rules that apply generally to tax-exempt financing for for-profit and not-for-profit hospitals apply to tax-exempt equipment financing.

Certain questions must be considered for equipment financing, among them the possible need for a feasibility study, the certificate of need, and reimbursement for past capital expenditures.

Need for a Feasibility Study

Equipment financings are rarely large enough to merit the cost of a feasibility study. If the hospital has outstanding rated bonds it is likely that the rating agencies will give the same ratings to a subsequent equipment financing without a feasibility study. If no rating has been received on the hospital's bonds, then it may wish to pursue third-party credit support in the form of either a letter of credit or bond insurance as a means of obtaining a rating without a feasibility study. Alternatively, the most economical format may be to place privately or sell publicly unrated bonds secured by a security interest in the equipment and a guaranty of payment from the hospital to the trustee or bondholder.

Certificate of Need

While a certificate of need (CON) must be obtained prior to purchasing a piece of equipment costing more than the CON threshold amount, in many states CON procedures allow borrowing to be done for future equipment purchases without having a CON in hand. To satisfy the Internal Revenue Code arbitrage regulations the health care facility need simply demonstrate that it anticipates making equipment purchases sufficient to use up the borrowed funds within a three-year period after the borrowing and that the lesser of $100,000 or 2½ percent of the bond issue will be used for equipment purchases within six months of the borrowing.

Reimbursement for Past Capital Expenditures

Depending on the wording of the state enabling legislation, some bond counsel will permit the hospital to reimburse itself from tax-exempt bond proceeds for equipment purchases made in the recent past. This is sometimes an attractive way for a hospital to raise cash.

POOLED EQUIPMENT FINANCING

Some statewide and county health facilities authorities have established equipment financing trusts in which a large bond issue is floated to raise a pool of funds which are then, in turn, loaned to hospitals for equipment purchases. Generally, only hospitals that have outstanding debt rated "A" or better or that have obtained a letter of credit backing their obligations are able to borrow through these pools. Usually money will be available to hospitals for periods ranging up to seven years for the purchase of equipment through such pools. The hospital should contact its health facilities authority and its underwriter about the availability of such an equipment financing pool.

One problem with these financing pools is that generally they permit loans only at a certain specified interest rate, and if interest rates drop after the creation of the pool it may be less expensive for a hospital to finance its equipment through its own bond issue or through one of the other means discussed.

EQUIPMENT FINANCING AS PART OF A LARGER CAPITAL FINANCING

It should be remembered in doing a long-term financing for a major construction project that the hospital may, at the same time, borrow moneys to finance certain equipment acquisitions to be made up to three years after the issuance of the bonds. Such funding for future acquisitions is permitted under the Internal Revenue Code Arbitrage Regulations and is frequently done in bond issues.

LEASES

Tax Considerations

When a 501(c)(3) organization is the lessee, there are restrictions on the investment tax credits available to the lessor (or purchaser of tax credits) which do not apply when the lessee is a for-profit entity. These limitations affect the lease price to a not-for-profit organization. The hospital should be certain that it is not the guarantor or indemnitor of tax-benefits to any other party in a lease transaction.

The Economic Recovery Tax Act of 1981 (ERTA) provides in Internal Revenue Code Section 168 very attractive provisions for leasing that permit sale of investment tax credits and depreciation in a safe-harbor lease transaction when the lessee is a for-profit entity.[1]

MUNICIPAL LEASES

In recent years, certain leasing companies have devised "municipal leases," a tax-exempt financing technique for leasing equipment. These, in essence, are very small sized tax-exempt bond issues for the purchase of equipment with a governmental issuer of debt acting as the financing conduit. The hospital's concern should be that it is given a flat lease rate which cannot be accelerated or increased if the interest portion of the lease is found to be taxable to the individual(s) or corporation(s) financing the lease. This should be of special concern to the hospital in municipal leases because they tend not to be as well documented or as carefully done as full-blown tax-exempt bond issues; and there generally exists a greater risk to the purchaser of a municipal lease that it will be determined that the interest portion of the municipal lease is taxable to the bondholder. The hospital should be sure that the lease provides that it will not be penalized for the inexpert processing of the lease by the leasing company.[2]

LEASE TERMS

There are a variety of factors with which the lessee should be concerned when negotiating any lease, whether a capitalized lease or a true lease. Some of them follow.

Recourse for Product Defects Directly against the Manufacturer

The hospital should be sure that it has a right to legal action for specific performance and damages against the manufacturer as well as against the lessor for redress of damages due to product defects.

Claims and Warranties

The warranties on the equipment that run from the manufacturer to the lessor should be passed through to the lessee in full with a direct right of enforcement by the lessee. The lessee should have the same right of recovery as the original purchaser of the equipment (usually the lessor) with respect to price adjustments, refunds, and other claims arising from the equipment purchase contract between the original purchaser and the manufacturer of the equipment.

Right of Inspection

There should be a full right of inspection of the equipment before the lessee accepts the equipment and this right of inspection should cover some period of time after receipt of the equipment so that there is time to set it up and test it. The lessee should be able to reject the equipment during the inspection period without penalty.

Amending the Lease

The health care institution should negotiate flexibility to amend the lease, and to revise the specifications of the equipment to be delivered. When there are a large number of investors in the lease financing it is helpful if the leasing documents specify that a "lead" investor has authority (within limits) to consent to amendments on behalf of all investors or all investors of the same class.

Subleasing

The lessee should seek the right to sublease the equipment. The sublease provision should permit the lessee to retain any gains from a sublease.

Maintenance

The equipment lease will generally require the lessee to maintain the equipment as a protection for the lessor's residual value interest. The lessee should not consent to provide maintenance in excess of what it would apply to its own equipment or to maintenance standards which impose excessive costs on the lessee.

Recapture of Equipment Purchase Contract

The lessee should have a right to a reassignment from the lessor of the equipment purchase contract in the event that the lease is not consummated.

Representations

The hospital should carefully consider whether any special representations are required of the lessor, including regulatory approvals and qualifications under state and federal law.

Risk of Taxability

In a tax-exempt transaction the lessee should insist that the risk of taxability of the "interest" portion of the lease be borne by the lessor if a subsequent event of taxability is caused by the lessor or if the transaction has failed to meet the original criteria for tax-exemption and the lessor could have taken steps to assure tax-exemption.

Transfer Restrictions

The lessee should consider whether any restrictions should be imposed upon the transfer of the lessor's interest in the lease.

Trustees

The lessee will normally pay the fees of any trustees appointed in connection with an equipment lease financing. Since institutional trust fees vary significantly, the lessee should insist on the right to select the initial trustee and, in nondefault situations, any successor trustee. The hospital should be comfortable that, at the request of the hospital, the trustee will be reasonable in permitting amendments to the lease in cases where it has discretion to permit amendments.

Indemnities

Generally, equipment leases require the lessee to indemnify the other parties to the transaction against various risks and expenses. The lessee should be willing to indemnify the other parties for the risks and expenses that stem from ownership or possession of equipment, including license fees, public liability, and property taxes. However, other indemnities may increase the lessees' exposure to liability beyond what it would have been had the lessee simply purchased the equipment. For example, indemnity against unexpected tax liability commonly includes a "grossing up" provision which requires the indemnitor to make the indemnitee whole, net of taxes on the indemnity payment. Such a provision can cost the lessee more than it benefits the indemnified party. The lessee should carefully consider *each* indemnity it is asked to provide.

Termination Provisions

As discussed above, the lessee may wish to have the lessor bear the risk of obsolescence of equipment, changes in regulations affecting use of equipment, imposition of environmental or other restrictions, and other changes that may make the equipment uneconomical or illegal to use. These and other concerns of the lessee should be specified as exceptions from the typical lease provision which provides that in event of termination the lessee will make a lump-sum termination payment calculated to make the lessor "whole."

Claims against Third Parties

Provisions should be made as to allocation of the beneficial interest in claims against third parties. The lease should authorize the lessee to sue or take other action in the name of the lessor, when necessary, to permit the lessee to assert claims arising from its possession of equipment or other rights under the lease.

"Unwind" Consequences

The lessee may be adversely affected by failure to consummate the lease transaction or by premature termination through the fault of some other party. The lessee should include provisions protecting it against these consequences.

Renewal and Purchase Options

The lessee should pay close attention to the purchase and renewal option provisions. The timing and notice provisions should provide the lessee with adequate time to look elsewhere for replacement equipment should the negotiations prove unsatisfactory.

Modification and Improvement of Equipment

The lessee should negotiate provisions permitting it to modify leased equipment to take advantage of changes in technology or its own changing needs. To the extent the lessee adds significant value to the equipment through these changes it should be able to remove the improvements or, if requested by the lessor, be reimbursed for them by the lessor.

Insurance Covenants

The lessee generally will be required to maintain property damage and liability insurance with respect to the equipment. The lessee should negotiate limits that are within its already outstanding insurance. If the lessee is self-insured to some extent, the insurance covenants of the lease should expressly permit self-insurance.

Surrender of Equipment

At the end of the lease term, if the lessee decides not to exercise its right to purchase (if any), it will be required to tender the equipment to the lessor. Responsibility for the costs of dismantling, shipment (including insurance), and inspections should be specified in the lease.

Expenses

All expenses of the leasing transaction should be clearly specified in the lease documents.

PURCHASE MONEY MORTGAGES ON EQUIPMENT

The hospital can probably obtain financing from its bank with security provided by a purchase money mortgage on the equipment. This will permit the hospital to purchase equipment and to pay back its bank over a period of time, usually approximately coinciding with the normal depreciable life of the equipment. A bank loan can be arranged, where state statutes permit, so that the bank borrowing is on a tax-exempt rather than a taxable basis.

EQUIPMENT PURCHASE CONSIDERATIONS WHEN DRAFTING LONG-TERM DOCUMENTS

Long-term bond documents generally restrict the amount and type of borrowing for equipment that a hospital can do in the future. If this is the case, the hospital should negotiate terms permitting it substantial flexibility as to the types of financing it may employ to purchase equipment. Over time, various factors may influence the hospital to shift from one type of equipment financing to another. Thus, the hospital should be sure that its lawyers are instructed to assure that an unlimited amount of true leasing of equipment can be done and that plenty of latitude is provided to finance leases through (a) tax-exempt bonds secured solely by the financed equipment; (b) parity bonds; (c) capitalized leases; and (d) purchase money mortgages.

NOTES

1. Albert F. Reisman *et al., Equipment Leasing 1981* (New York: Practising Law Institute, 1981) (hereafter Reisman), *especially* Chapter I, Peter K. Nevitt, "Effect of the Economic Recovery Tax Act of 1981 Upon Leasing"; Internal Revenue Code § 168(f) and the regulations issued thereunder.

2. For a detailed discussion of municipal leases *see:* C. Gregory H. Eden *et al.,* "Tax Exempt Municipal Lease Financing: A New Look," *New York Law Journal, Law Journal Seminars—Press* (1980); Reisman, *ibid.,* Chapter 14, Mitchell J. Bragen, "Tax-Exempt Financing and Leasing," p. 463.

SUGGESTED READINGS

Burke, Spencer B. "Bank Counsel's Guide to Equipment Leasing Transactions: Nontax Aspects," *Banking L.J.* 94: 580 (1977).

Coogan, P.; Hogan, W.; and Vagts, D. *Secured Transactions.* Matthew Bender, N.Y. Supp. 1980, esp. Chapter 4A, Coogan, "Leases of Equipment and Some Other Unconventional

Security Devices," Chapter 29A, Mooney, "Treatment by the Courts," Chapter 29B, DeKoven, "Proceedings After Default By The Lessee Under A True Lease Of Equipment."

Eden, C. Gregory H., ed. "Tax Exempt Municipal Lease Financing: A New Look." New York: New York Law Journal, Law Journal Seminars—Press, 1980.

Fogel, Don. "Executory Contracts and Unexpired Leases in the Bankruptcy Code," 64 *Minn.L. Rev.* 64: 341 (1980).

Fritch, Bruce E., and Reisman, Albert F., eds. *Equipment Leasing—Leveraged Leasing* (2d ed.). New York: Practising Law Institute, 1980.

Gutterman, Daniel A. "Equipment Leases as Collateral under the UCC and the New Bankruptcy Code," *U.C.C.L.J.* 12: 344 (1980).

Internal Revenue Code, § 168(f) and the regulations issued thereunder.

Meyers, Philip G. "A Worksheet for Leasing Equipment," *Prac. Law.* 23: 59 (July 15, 1977).

Reisman, Albert F., ed. *Equipment Leasing 1981*. New York: Practising Law Institute, 1981.

Chapter 10

Steps of a Tax-Exempt Financing[*]

Thomas Arthur

Once the decision is made to undertake a long-term, tax-exempt financing, if not before, the health institution will want to form a financing team and decide whether to go public or private. Similarly, reimbursement considerations will be checked, and restructuring and other long-range plans will be noted to assure that the proposed debt instruments and these plans do not conflict. In this chapter it will be assumed that the health institution is a charitable, 501(c)(3) organization (referred to as the "hospital"), and thus able to avail itself of the provisions of the Internal Revenue Code for issuance of tax-exempt debt. It will also be assumed that there will be a public financing.

CHOICE OF FINANCING TEAM

Securities are sold publicly through investment banking firms and, within limits, commercial banks (referred to here as the "underwriter").[1] In public hospital bond financings there is inevitably an "underwriting" where the underwriter purchases the bonds from the issuer in an "at risk," principal transaction.[2] Hospitals are usually free to choose their underwriter, although in some states, if the bonds are to be sold through the state health facilities authority, the selection may be limited or the authority may control the selection. At any rate, it will be assumed in this chapter that an investment banking firm has been chosen to be the underwriter.[3] It will also be assumed that the hospital has selected as the issuing

---

[*] The reader is referred to Chapters 1 through 6, which describe the first steps to be taken when undertaking a tax-exempt financing. Not all of these "first steps" must have been followed or completed in some formal way prior to reaching a decision to go long-term and tax-exempt, but it is necessary for the health institution to have gone through some form of debt capacity analysis.

entity a municipality or other governmental unit of the state (referred to here as the "issuer"), and that the hospital and the issuer have rounded out the team to include the following:

1. hospital[4] and its counsel;
2. issuer and its counsel;
3. underwriter and its counsel;
4. bond counsel;
5. feasibility consultants;[5] and
6. independent accountants.

The stage will thus be set for an underwritten, tax-exempt conduit financing (referred to here as "the closing").

INITIAL REVIEW BY UNDERWRITER

The underwriter is often the first outside party to review the hospital's financing plan fully. This is done informally or in connection with a debt capacity study with the focus on review of proposed uses and sources of funds. The following aspects will be jointly reviewed by the hospital and the underwriter:

1. description and status of the project to be financed (constructing, refunding, reimbursing);
2. sources of funds (equity contributions, other borrowings);
3. impediments to the financing (outstanding debt, enabling laws, hospital governance, other contracts, certificates of need);
4. probable ratings; and
5. selection of any missing team members such as the bond counsel and the feasibility consultant.

INITIAL REVIEW BY ISSUER AND ITS FINANCIAL ADVISER

Statewide authorities are generally more concerned about the quality and terms of a financing than municipalities and local authorities. Depending upon its inclination in this regard, the issuer and its financial adviser (if any) may engage in the same sort of initial review as the underwriter.

PREPARATION OF TERMS LETTER

The underwriter will generally prepare a series of procedural documents which will help trigger the more substantive work to follow. These include the terms letter, a document which can be deceptively short.

It outlines the basic terms so that one of the parties can refer to it later and say, ''Look, that's what we agreed to in the first place.'' This may be in the form of a letter constituting a gentlemen's agreement (an agreement to agree) which is not binding but awkward to ignore. Often there is no letter, just an outline, and the underwriter's promise to underwrite is wholly informal.[6]

The terms letter or outline may include the following:

- the general concept of the project, that is, whether it is a construction financing, a refunding, etc.;
- the approximate principal amount of bonds to be issued and their probable maturities;
- the probable redemption terms;
- the security behind the bonds, that is, whether there will be a real estate mortgage, assignment of gross receipts, etc.;
- the debt service reserve;
- the other funds;
- the limitations on additional and parity[7] debt;
- the permitted encumbrances;
- the rate covenant;[8] and
- the other covenants.[9]

If in the past the issuer or the underwriter has established a pattern of financing terms which tends to fit the proposed financing, the underwriter may simply give the hospital a copy of the official statement used on a recent financing and advise that the terms will be similar except as specified.

OTHER PROCEDURAL DOCUMENTS

The underwriter (or sometimes the issuer if it is a statewide authority) may prepare other useful papers, including a list of parties, a list of documents, and a time schedule.

The *list of parties* gives the names, addresses, and telephone numbers of all persons involved.

The *list of documents* is actually a request for documents to assist in preparing the official statement, to raise issues, and to serve as a commencement of the due diligence process.[10] This lengthy list must include the IRS exemption letters, the certificates of need, all outstanding debt instruments, and the charter and bylaws. Chapter 15 is devoted to due diligence matters and includes a typical document list.

The *time schedule* is the underwriter's (or the issuer's) first estimate of the time requirements. See Appendix 10-A for a time chart. This chart sets forth, in a much more detailed way than would be used in a financing, a series of events leading to the bond closing. It is key that the schedule be realistic vis-a-vis third parties over whom the parties to the financing may have little or no control, including the following:

- notice and meetings of government agencies (including the issuer) whose approvals are required;
- state court validation proceedings;[11]
- certificate-of-need approvals by the state review board;
- rating agency application, review, meeting, and determination;
- receipt of a guaranteed maximum price of any construction project from the hospital's construction contractor;
- notice of redemption of outstanding debt;
- receipt of title reports;
- bond syndication (depending on marketing methods and market conditions); and
- after the sale, printing of the bond certificates.

Thus, the time schedule is drafted around certain assumed critical paths, and the parties to the financing are obliged to accommodate their schedules to meet these limits. Postponements down the line generally result from unexpected delays by these outsiders (rating agencies, validation courts, state review boards, and other public bodies) or from adverse market conditions. Delays can be devastating if the hospital is, for example, faced with an expiring certificate of need or guaranteed maximum price contract or if it is a time of rising interest rates. It is unsatisfactory for the team members with technical roles to play and the capacity to juggle assignments, such as the lawyers, consultants or accountants, to cause the delays.

THE FIRST TEAM MEETING

Customarily, a first meeting is called to bring together all members of the financing team. It is important for the individuals to become acquainted, and there is a good amount of introductory work to be accomplished. It may be the hospital's first opportunity to respond to the terms sheet prepared by the underwriter. Bond counsel and others may have problems with these terms or may not fully understand them.

In this setting, the hospital's representatives are apt to be the least familiar with the steps to a financing, and it is thus appropriate for the proposed time schedule to be reviewed with care for their benefit. The accountants and feasibility consultants may find the schedule too tight, and all parties should take the opportunity, if necessary, to suggest timing changes. The admonishment made earlier in this chapter is worth repeating: It is not satisfactory for the team members to cause delays.

This is the time to review the list of documents with the hospital and its counsel. The person the hospital has selected to be the "strawboss," that is, the person who will be responsible for marshaling all hospital material listed or supplementally requested and submitting it to the other team members, should be introduced at the meeting. This hospital employee must be clearly authorized to set aside the time to do this very necessary work and must have sufficient authority to require others to comply promptly with requests. However, it may not be wise to have the president or the chief financial officer responsible for these details. The efficiency of the financing from the standpoint of the underwriter and other experts is very dependent on the efforts of the strawboss.[12]

The legal printer who is responsible for printing the official statement should be selected no later than this first meeting.[13] Mention should be made of state blue sky filings.[14] Also, the lawyers should determine their various responsibilities. There are set assignment patterns, but with some deviation. The following would be typical:

- *Bond counsel* will draft the indenture and the other bond documents such as the mortgage and security agreement (or lease and guaranty or loan agreement), the bond form, the resolutions, ordinances, and other requirements of the issuer. Bond counsel will review the official statement and draft the sections of it that summarize the bond documents. Bond counsel will preside at the closing and, as the finale, will render the opinion with respect to tax exemption and legality of issuance under state law.

- *Underwriter's counsel* will draft the Bond Purchase Agreement, the agreement among underwriters (if used), and the blue sky survey and legal investment memorandum, and will have a key role in preparation of the official statement and the terms sheet. This counsel's opinion will cover the legality of the issue under securities laws. It may also state that nothing has come to counsel's attention that would lead counsel to believe that the official statement contains any untrue statement of a material fact or omits to state a material fact that would be required to prevent the statements from being misleading.

- *Issuer's counsel* will review all documents and prepare the section of the official statement describing the issuer, and may also undertake other roles such as review of the real estate title documents. This counsel's legal opinion will cover the actions taken by the issuer.
- *Hospital's counsel* will review all documents and handle all real estate aspects—an important role, especially if the bonds are to be secured by a first mortgage. This counsel will often be responsible for obtaining certificate-of-need approvals and other governmental approvals, for handling or at least reviewing litigation matters and describing the litigation in the official statement, and for drafting and reviewing other sections of the official statement applicable to the hospital. This counsel's legal opinion will cover the actions taken by the hospital.

This chapter, indeed this book, frequently uses the word "team" to designate the persons from various firms, companies, and organizations who will combine their skills. The term should not be taken too literally, since there are separate and sometimes conflicting interests among the "players."[15]

FEES AND EXPENSES

The hospital must have a definite understanding with respect to its obligation to pay the fees of the other parties. The hospital pays most fees and costs, including:

- accountants,
- feasibility consultants,
- hospital counsel,
- bond counsel,
- issuer,
- trustee (initial and ongoing fees),
- paying agents (initial and ongoing fees),
- rating agencies,
- printing of the official statement, and
- printing of the bonds.

Customarily, the hospital does not directly pay fees or expenses of the underwriter or the underwriter's counsel, unless there is a default caused by the hospital. These are covered by the underwriter's discount. The hospital does not customarily directly pay the fees of the issuer's financial adviser and counsel in the case of a statewide authority (they are paid by the authority from the fee paid to it by the hospital), but does customarily pay these fees directly in the case of a local authority or municipality which seldom has a prescribed rate schedule to cover its costs and charges as a package.

This may leave certain costs subject to local practice or negotiation, including

- fees and expenses of blue sky filing and printing,
- printing costs of certain underwriting papers, such as the agreement among underwriters, questionnaires, instructions to dealers and notices, and
- fees of issuer's financial adviser and counsel.

These matters should be settled at or before the first meeting. To the extent the hospital asks the underwriter to pick up these costs which could be paid by either party, the underwriter will consider asking for a larger discount.

DRAFTING THE OFFICIAL STATEMENT

One of several parties can take primary responsibility for drafting the official statement, among them a member of the underwriter's staff, the issuer's financial adviser, or underwriter's counsel. The drafters should be trained in preparation of disclosure documents such as prospectuses used in Securities and Exchange Commission filings and blue sky filings. The hospital will be obliged to certify that the official statement does not contain an untrue statement of a material fact or omit to state a material fact that must be included to assure that the statements made therein are not misleading. Counsel for the hospital will be required to give negative assurance with respect to the foregoing as well.[16]

For this reason, counsel should explain the purpose of the official statement to hospital management as an early step. There is no place in the official statement for unsupported opinions and puffery. The account of the hospital and the project should be a balanced presentation which discloses all material negative information. The antifraud provisions of the state and federal securities laws do apply to tax-exempt bond sales, making it clearly in the hospital's best interest to be conservative in writing the official statement. For all of these reasons, it would be a poor decision to select the hospital's development or public relations department to write the first draft of the official statement.[17]

The underwriter will purchase the bonds as a principal, pursuant to the bond purchase agreement; therefore, the hospital is not required to make a selling effort to the public. The interest rate and other terms are determined largely by the bond market on the sales date and by the bond rating. The rating agency examiners are sufficiently experienced to discard salesmanship writing.

The feasibility consultants are charged with preparing a demand analysis which generally describes the hospital, its facilities, administration, services, medical staff, and utilization. This analysis is included in the official statement as an appendix. The consultants' description of the hospital can and should be carefully dovetailed with a similar description in the forepart of the official statement.

THE DRAFTING AND REVIEW PHASE

After the first meeting, the financing team will usually spend a few weeks in a drafting phase. Normally, the bond counsel's and the feasibility consultants' efforts will run ahead of the group drafting the official statement, and it can be assumed that bond counsel, prior to the second meeting, will have drafts of the bond documents. A "shell" form or outline of the official statement and a draft form of the bond purchase agreement may be prepared. Also, the consultants may have prepared drafts of the demand analysis portion of the feasibility study. All of these papers should be reviewed by hospital management.

At the same time, the attorneys should be reviewing the key legal documents pertaining to the hospital to be certain that there are no trouble areas. These are matters of experience and cannot be listed in a definitive way; however, among other matters, early review of the charter and bylaws, tax status, and debt covenants are certainly top priority.

THE SECOND MEETING OF THE TEAM

The second meeting is often devoted primarily to a review of bond counsel's documents (the indenture, mortgage, and security agreement, or lease and guaranty or loan agreement) and perhaps also to a review of the first draft of the official statement. The time schedule will again be reviewed and updated as required.

OTHER MEETINGS OF THE TEAM

Other meetings may follow with the immediate goal being for the team to agree that the status of the various drafts of the bond documents is close enough to final form (with a minimum number of blanks and with typos corrected). The documents can then be submitted to parties who are not part of the team and have not been attending meetings and receiving drafts of documents. In this group would be (a) the rating agencies, (b) the court in any validation hearings,[18] (c) the issuer's governing body and other governmental agencies (as required), and (d) the governing board of the hospital. The number of meetings needed to reach this final proof stage varies; the team simply has to work until the job is done.

DUE DILIGENCE REVIEW

The experts in a public offering may make statements on their own authority or they may make a reasonable investigation with respect to the work of others. To satisfy a part of this burden to investigate, the experts, including the underwriters, go through a "due diligence" review which is a process of making an investigation and leaving tracks to show that the investigation was made.

Therefore, the underwriters and their counsel will hold review sessions usually at the hospital. There are two parts, document review and interviews with key personnel.

Document review should come first. In addition to a review of all documents on the list submitted at the first meeting, counsel will review the corporate records for the last five years or some longer period to enable counsel to see the form of governance as actually practiced, to check on the incumbency of the board and officers, and to search for significant information not yet included in the official statement.

Interviews with key personnel should follow so that the data obtained from the document review can be discussed with the appropriate person. Among those normally questioned are

- the hospital administrator,
- the chief financial officer,
- the hospital attorney,
- the accountants,
- the feasibility consultants,
- representatives of the governing board,
- representatives of the medical staff,
- the architect, and
- the construction contractor.

RATING AGENCY MEETINGS

Rating agency meetings are normally scheduled by the underwriter or the financial adviser to the issuer, if the issuer is a statewide authority. Drafts of the official statement, feasibility study, and financial statements should be sent to the agencies two weeks in advance of these meetings, and another two weeks should be allowed for receipt of the ratings. These times may vary, and the underwriters and the financial adviser will know the current rating agency practice and will advise the other team members in this regard.

Hearings can be held at the hospital or at the offices of the agencies in New York City. The underwriter will supervise this phase and will coach the hospital personnel.

THE PRELIMINARY OFFICIAL STATEMENT

When the official statement is in substantially final form, including the feasibility study and financials, but is still lacking the ratings, name of the trustee, interest rate, maturities, and other related information, it is printed with certain disclaimers written in red vertically along the inner margin of the cover and with the date written in red across the top. This is the preliminary official statement, sometimes called the "red herring."

THE PRICING PERIOD

The underwriters and other dealers use the preliminary official statement to "offer" the bonds. Sales are not final until the offeree accepts and receives a confirmation and the final official statement. The red herring, therefore, has to be in substantially final form. The underwriter's sales effort during a "selling" or "pricing" period may include a "bond syndication" if a group (syndicate) of underwriting firms is formed by the managing underwriter to work jointly on selling the bonds. On smaller public issues, the underwriter will sell all the bonds. The time required for this selling period varies depending on the size, quality and complexity of the financing, but usually runs a week or ten days.

EXECUTION OF BOND PURCHASE AGREEMENT

At the end of the sales period, the underwriter (or underwriters, if a syndicate is formed) will have obtained expressions of interest from offerees, will have an improved feel for the market and will (hopefully) be ready to "commit" to purchase the bonds. The interest rate, maturities, and underwriter's discount are then negotiated with the hospital. There should be no big surprises. When agreement is reached, the issuer, hospital, and underwriters will execute the bond purchase agreement, and the underwriting commitment will have been made.

Just before execution of the bond purchase agreement, it is necessary to hold meetings of the hospital board and the issuer's governing body to authorize the terms, and there may be other filings in validation proceedings and elsewhere at this time. By resolution the hospital board can fix a maximum interest rate and delegate to a board committee or to one hospital officer the authority to commit on the rate, maturities, and discount.

As a condition to execution of the bond purchase agreement, the hospital must cause its independent accountants to submit a "comfort letter"[19] to the underwriter and the issuer. This letter advises that the accountants have carried out certain procedures and made certain inquiries (which are explained to be far less than an audit examination) during the time since the last audit to a recent date and that nothing has come to their attention to lead them to believe that the unaudited statements are not fairly presented.

Often, the trustee is not appointed until this time, and the name of the bank or trust company selected by the parties is then inserted in the final official statement and in the other bond documents. The final official statement is printed, the bond printing is ordered from a banknote company, and the bond documents and other certificates[20] are placed in final form by bond counsel.

THE GAP BETWEEN COMMITMENT AND CLOSING

The traditional reasons for allowing two to four weeks between execution of the bond purchase agreement (the commitment) and the closing are to allow the underwriter time to complete the bond sales, send confirmations and final official statements to the bond purchasers and prepare a list of purchasers, and, finally, to allow the banknote company time to print the bonds. All this happens without much participation by the other team members.

At the same time, however, the team members have certain additional chores. Bond counsel will be submitting the various closing certificates,[21] and these must be reviewed in advance of the closing by the parties who will be obliged to execute them. Awkward situations may develop if the hospital team members are not careful. For example, the hospital normally will be required to execute a "no-arbitrage certificate." This summarizes the use of the proceeds and the various funds and accounts in such a manner as to show bond counsel that there will be no arbitrage of the proceeds that would cause the bonds to lose their tax-exempt status. If substantial construction is involved, bond counsel may ask the architect and the contractor to certify as to the amount necessary to complete the construction, and this figure must dovetail with the information furnished by the hospital in the no-arbitrage certificate.

This sort of activity—asking outside parties such as the architect and contractor to furnish certificates[22]—must be given careful attention by all team members, since at the last minute the completion of the entire financing can rest on a nonteam member who may be relatively unsophisticated in the intricacies of these legal certificates.

Other events that occur during this gap are a review of the bond documents by the newly appointed trustee, the making of final arrangements to refund any outstanding debt as required by the bond purchase agreement, last-minute due diligence, a review by the auditors to support the second comfort letter,[23] and preparation of opinions by the various counsel.

THE CLOSING

Closings are sufficiently technical and complex to be beyond a detailed review. See Appendix 10-A for a sample memorandum of closing documents. Bond counsel supervises the closing process, and it generally takes two days. The first day involves execution of the documents and preparation for last-minute money transfers that occur on the second day. On the evening of the first day, the underwriter will customarily host a dinner for all members of the team.

If construction is involved, bond proceeds will be placed in a construction fund at the closing to be drawn down over the construction period in accordance with the terms of the indenture.

It may be difficult for the uninitiated team member to follow the chain of events at a closing. The secret is that papers delivered in advance are deemed to be delivered in escrow so that everything is considered to take place simultaneously. By honoring this slightly fictitious process, it thus does not matter in what order documents are executed and checks passed.

With the understanding in mind that everything is considered to take place simultaneously, the following are the six major events of the closing depicted in Figure 10-1.

1. Pursuant to the loan agreement (or mortgage and security agreement or lease agreement), the hospital will deliver to the issuer a note (or mortgage note or lease) promising to pay an amount equal

Figure 10-1 Steps of Tax-Exempt Financing

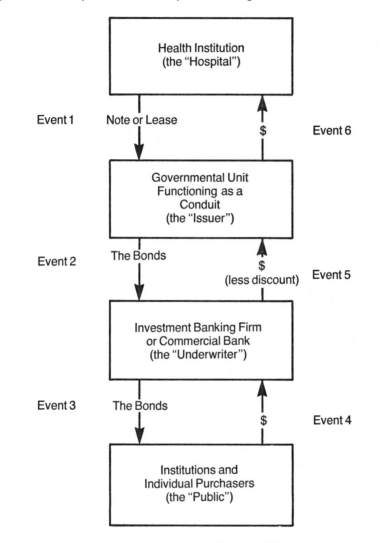

to the bonds in payments which will amortize the bonds (tied to event 6).
2. Pursuant to the indenture, the issuer will execute and the trustee will authenticate the bonds.[24] Pursuant to the bond purchase agreement, delivery of the bonds will be made to the underwriter (tied to event 5).

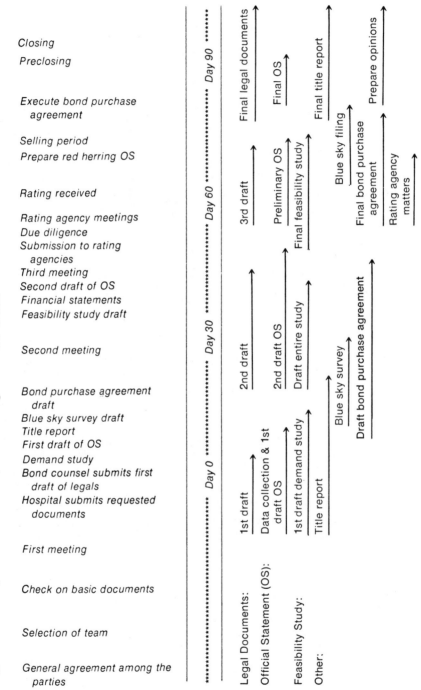

Figure 10-2 Steps to a Tax-Exempt Financing—A Time Chart

3. If the bonds are syndicated, pursuant to an agreement among underwriters, the managing underwriter will allot the bonds to the syndicate members. Then the underwriter (or the underwriting syndicate), by its regular marketing process, will deliver to its (their) customers the bonds, confirmations, and official statements (tied to event 4).
4. Pursuant to the confirmations, the customers will pay the underwriter for the bonds an amount aggregating the public offering price (tied to event 3).
5. Pursuant to the bond purchase agreement and the indenture, the underwriter will pay the issuer for the bonds an amount equal to the public offering price less the bond discount by delivering funds to the trustee (tied to event 2).
6. Pursuant to the loan agreement (or mortgage and security agreement or lease) and the indenture and upon receipt of appropriate requisitions under the indenture, the bond trustee will pay the net proceeds of the public offering to the various bond trust funds[25] and to the hospital (tied to event 1).

Figure 10-2 shows a time line down the middle with the first meeting shown as day zero. Above the time line, the specific events described in this chapter are listed; below, the probable time necessary to complete the key events is shown as lines related to the time line. It must be recognized, however, that every financing is different.

NOTES

1. Since 1933, the National Banking Act (12 U.S.C. § 24), in provisions commonly known as the Glass-Steagle Act, has limited the role of commercial banks in underwritings. The main exception to these limitations has been to permit banks to underwrite general obligation municipal bonds and certain special types of obligations, including issuances for educational purposes which can involve hospitals. The Secretary of the Treasury has indicated that commercial bank underwriting powers should be broadened by permitting them to own investment banking subsidiaries. It is likely, therefore, that the traditional delineation between commercial banks and investment banking firms will be replaced by various polyfinancial organizations and specialty organizations.

2. As opposed to a "best efforts" financing or an agency relationship (as in a private placement). The underwriter will obtain commitments during the selling period, but an underwriter who does not resell all the bonds is still obliged to buy them from the issuer.

3. Investment banking firms are licensed by the Securities and Exchange Commission and by the applicable state commissions and must meet capital requirements to deal in securities. Hospital underwritings are becoming more and more specialized, and investment banking firms usually do not become involved, at least not as managers, unless they are staffed to handle all aspects.

4. Usually the chief financial officer handles matters, although it is also common to have the president take the lead for a hospital.

5. The feasibility consultant submits a report on financial feasibility which is usually attached as an appendix to the official statement. This report analyzes the service area, supply and demand, and projected utilization. Based on stated assumptions, conclusions are reached with respect to a hospital's ability to pay interest and principal on the bonds.

6. This informality is one of the surprising aspects of the underwriting process to the uninitiated. "When will we pin down the underwriter?" the hospital officers may ask. The answer is, only at the last minute when the underwriter has obtained sufficient expressions of purchase interest through its sales force to prompt the underwriter to negotiate and execute the bond purchase agreement. Even after entering into the bond purchase agreement, there are "market outs" to protect the underwriter.

7. "Parity" debt is long-term indebtedness with a right to receive payments of interest and principal equal to (thus on a parity with) the bonds. This equality goes to regular payments and to payments in connection with creditors' remedies as well.

8. The rate covenant is the hospital's undertaking to charge rates sufficient to cover payment of principal and interest.

9. The terms letter or outline will not include the real "punch lines" which are the interest rate and bond discount. These are determined after the pricing period when the bond purchase agreement is executed.

10. The term "due diligence" is used loosely here. It more properly applies to the routine by which the experts involved in a financing registered with the Securities and Exchange Commission make a review and satisfy themselves regarding information furnished to them by the principals to a registered public offering.

11. Some state laws require that a court of equity hear a petition from the issuer and the hospital in support of the financing. There is a public notice, a hearing and an opportunity for other parties to oppose the financing. After a favorable order, there is a period before the order becomes final.

12. This touchy area can strain relationships. If the strawboss is not producing documents and other information required for the team to make progress, underwriter's counsel may ask the hospital's counsel to intercede in the document-gathering process.

13. Therefore, the hospital and the underwriter may have asked printing companies to bid on the work in advance. The underwriter and its counsel should be able to suggest ways of minimizing printing costs.

14. These are actions taken by underwriter's counsel under the state securities laws. It must be remembered that while tax-exempt hospital bonds are normally exempt from registration under the Securities Act of 1933, they are not exempt from all state blue sky laws. The term "blue sky" can be traced to the time when the first of these laws was passed in the early 1900s. It was said that slick dealers were selling securities worth no more than square feet of blue sky.

15. For example, the underwriter or the issuer, if it is a statewide authority, may be interested in serving up a "standard" set of terms while the hospital may have unique needs it wishes to address that deviate from normal terms. Hospital counsel should strive for complete disclosure, perhaps for some special terms and in general for less restrictive covenants. Bond counsel will focus on the tax-exempt aspects and the requirements of state enabling laws. Underwriter's counsel tends to be concerned with challenging the facts and figures submitted by the hospital (part of the due diligence process) and with assisting the underwriter to prepare a total package which will meet the requirements needed in the way of covenants to obtain the anticipated ratings and be most readily acceptable in the market.

16. Much has been written on the liabilities of the various parties to a public offering. If a financing is registered with the Securities and Exchange Commission under the Securities Act of 1933, the drafters follow the appropriate form together with SEC rules and guidelines. In the municipal field these sources do not apply although they may be used as guides. In addition, assistance can be obtained from *Guidelines for Offerings of Securities* (Chicago: Municipal Finance Officers Association of the United States and Canada (MFOA), 1979), available from the MFOA, 180 North Michigan Avenue, Chicago, IL 60601.

17. Chapter 1.

18. Note 11 *supra*.

19. The "comfort letter" is supplied by the hospital's independent certified public accountants. It covers the period after their last audit and, in a negative way, indicates that the accountants made a very limited review and found that nothing came to their attention which caused them to believe that the financial information was not fairly stated. There is usually a comfort letter submitted when the bond purchase agreement is executed and another submitted at the closing.

20. Bond counsel will take the lead in preparing certificates for officers of the hospital and the issuer to execute. These cover various representations and warranties customarily made in any financing, an arbitrage certificate, incumbency certificates, and certificates with respect to the charter, bylaws, and other documents.

21. *Ibid.*

22. Bond counsel may ask for certificates of these parties to support the arbitrage certificates executed by the issuer and the architect. Arbitrage certificates support the concept that the construction project can be completed within a certain time period with the use of a major portion of the moneys furnished from the bond proceeds. They show compliance with the arbitrage regulations (adopted under Section 103(c) of the Internal Revenue Code) which prevent a major portion of the bond proceeds from being invested in securities that will produce a yield higher than the yield on the bonds being sold in the issue.

23. Note 19 *supra*.

24. Bonds are three-party instruments, being executed by the issuer, payable to the bondholder and authenticated by the bond trustee. The authentication simply says that "this is one of the bonds described in the within-mentioned indenture" or words to that effect, and the trustee executes the authentication in a space provided below this language.

25. These are the revenue fund; construction fund (if any); interest fund; special interest fund (if any); redemption fund; repair, replacement, and depreciation fund; and debt service reserve fund. These funds are not always established under the indenture and may not always be funded with the bond proceeds.

Appendix 10-A

Closing Memorandum

<hr>

(Name of Issuer)

<hr>

HOSPITAL REVENUE BONDS
(Name of Hospital)

<hr>

19 ___ SERIES A
CLOSING MEMORANDUM

<hr>

Place
Bond Counsel's Office
Time
Preclosing—Monday, _____, at 2:00 P.M.
Closing—Tuesday, _____, at 9:00 A.M.
Parties
_____, Issuer (I)
_____, Underwriter (U)
_____, Hospital (H)
_____, Trustee (T)
_____, Bond Counsel (BC)
_____, Issuer's Counsel (IC)
_____, Underwriter's Counsel (UC)
_____, Hospital's Counsel (HC)
_____, Hospital's Accountants (A)
_____, Feasibility Consultant (FC)

Preclosing
The parties indicated above will deliver each of the respective documents so indicated below in fifteen (15) copies. The documents will be executed in advance of the Closing by the respective parties thereto and delivered no later than the Preclosing. At that time a Preclosing conference will be held to confirm that all documents and papers are on hand, in

182

proper form and properly executed. All of such deliveries will be deemed to have been made in escrow until the final delivery at the Closing has been made.

Responsibility for preparing or assembling the documents is indicated in parentheticals.

Major Documents

1. Indenture (executed by issuer and trustee) (BC).
2. Loan agreement (executed by issuer and hospital) (BC).
3. Depository agreement (executed by hospital, trustee, and depository bank) (BC).

Documents Relating to the Sale of the Bonds

4. Bond purchase contract with letter of representation (executed by issuer, underwriter, and hospital) (BC).
5. Preliminary official statement (U).
6. Final official statement (executed by issuer and hospital) (U).
7. Rating letters (U).
8. Blue Sky survey/legal investment survey (UC).
9. First comfort letter dated the date of the bond purchase contract (A).
10. Second comfort letter dated the closing date (A).
11. Accountant's letter of consent to use of certified financials (A).
12. Feasibility consultant's letter of consent to use of feasibility study (FC).

Closing Documents Relating to the Issuer

13. Certified copies of resolution of the issuer's authorizing issuance and sale of the bonds (BC).
14. Signature certificate (executed by the officials who sign the bonds) (BC).
15. Certificate of the issuer (executed by issuer's chief executive) (BC).
16. Order of the issuer (executed by issuer's chief executive) (BC).
17. No-arbitrage certificate (executed by issuer's chief executive) (BC).

Closing Documents Relating to the Hospital

18. Certificate as to insurance (BC and HC).
19. Certified articles of incorporation (certified by Secretary of State of hospital's incorporation) (HC).
20. Certified bylaws (HC).
21. Good standing certificate—Secretary of State of hospital's incorporation (HC).
22. Good standing certificate if Hospital is qualified in any other states as a foreign corporation—Secretary of State of applicable state (HC).
23. Resolutions authorizing execution of documents (HC).
24. Certificate of the Hospital (executed by president) (BC).
25. Evidence of compliance with certificate of need law (HC).

26. Evidence that Hospital is an organization described in Section 501(c)(3) of the Internal Revenue Code of 1954, as amended (HC).
27. Supplemental no-arbitrage certificate (executed by president) (BC).
28. UCC-1 financing statement (executed by president) (BC).
Closing Documents Relating to the Trustee
29. Authorization resolution (T).
30. Certificate of the trustee (executed by trustee) (BC).
Closing Documents
31. Receipt for purchase price (executed by trustee) (BC).
32. Receipt for bonds (executed by underwriter) (BC).
33. The Series A Bonds, including specimens (BC).
Legal Opinions
34. Opinion of issuer's counsel (IC).
35. Opinion of hospital's counsel (HC).
36. Opinion of underwriter's counsel (UC).
37. Supplemental opinion of bond counsel (BC).
38. Final opinion of bond counsel (BC).

Closing

At the time of the Closing, each of the parties will receive one signed copy (or executed counterpart) of each of the documents listed above (other than the Series A Bonds), subsequent to the following events:

A. The underwriter will transfer to the trustee an aggregate amount equal to the public offering price less the bond discount less the good faith check previously given to the issuer in immediately available funds, and the issuer will deliver to the trustee an aggregate amount equal to the good faith deposit with interest thereon returned to the underwriter (or included in the check and credited to the underwriter in its transfer).*

B. The trustee will apply the aggregate amount required to the discharge of the existing indebtedness to be discharged (if any, as specified in the order of the issuer).

C. The trustee will release to the underwriter the Series A Bonds in an aggregate principal amount of the bonds sold.

---

* In some cases, interest is not paid to the underwriter on the good faith deposit.

Chapter 11

Forms of Tax-Exempt Financings

Thomas Arthur

The last chapter examined the typical long-term, tax-exempt financing sold publicly with no special features. It was assumed that the health institution was a 501(c)(3) entity. Other tax-exempt forms or variations on the typical theme can be viewed from a number of perspectives:

1. type of institution—charitable or proprietary;
2. single entities or multicorporate or multihospital entities;
3. form of principal and interest payments;
4. form of sale, private or public;
5. form of security; and
6. short-term forms.

Changes in the tax laws and the marketplace make some forms short-lived or subject to considerable change, and new forms are conceived regularly; thus, in the future some of the forms described here may no longer be viable. Any classification is arbitrary, and the classifications overlap.

TYPE OF INSTITUTION—CHARITABLE OR PROPRIETARY

Charitable health institutions qualifying as organizations described in Section 501(c)(3) and exempt from tax under Section 501(a) obviously have an advantage over proprietary institutions when it comes to employing tax-exempt financing. However, the door is not closed completely to the proprietaries.

Proprietary hospitals and business corporations affiliated with proprietary and charitable hospitals may raise capital by issuance of "small issue" industrial development bonds. As previously explained, Section 103 of the

Internal Revenue Code permits municipalities and other local governmental units to issue tax-exempt securities if the user is an exempt person such as a governmental unit or a 501(c)(3) organization.[1] Otherwise, the security is tainted as an industrial development bond, with interest on such bonds not qualifying for the tax exemption unless such bonds are issued to provide funds for certain exempt activities (not relevant to proprietary hospitals) or unless such bonds are issued in certain small issues. These small issues include

- an issue the aggregate amount of which is $1 million or less; and
- an issue the aggregate amount of which is less than $10 million if the aggregate amount of capital expenditures with respect to facilities within the municipality incurred during a six-year period beginning three years before the date of issue and ending three years after such date does not exceed this $10 million amount.[2]

The foregoing is, of course, a simplification of complex tax laws and regulations which are also dependent upon state enabling laws. For purposes of this discussion, however, the important thing to understand is that business corporations such as proprietary hospitals, physicians' office building companies, and other hospital-support organizations can avail themselves of tax-exempt financings in limited amounts. The $1 million exemption is available on a "one shot" basis, regardless of other capital expenditures. The $10 million exemption contains a good many complex twists and is available if total capital expenditures (broadly defined) do not exceed that amount over the six-year period.

For example, a proprietary hospital could participate in a small issue of $1 million, or a group of physicians on the staff of a hospital might arrange for a financing of an office building if all costs are less than $10 million.

The disadvantage that proprietaries suffer with respect to tax-exempt financing is probably compensated for under the Health Care Financing Administration's regulations by recognition that proprietaries are entitled to a reasonable return on equity.[3]

SINGLE ENTITIES OR MULTICORPORATE OR MULTIHOSPITAL ENTITIES

Types of Systems

Multihospital financings present unique challenges. These systems appear in many forms and are classified for purposes of analyzing financing opportunities into basic types as follows:

- *Type 1. Standard multicorporate hospital system under single parent.* These are individual, separately incorporated hospitals owned or controlled by a parent entity (which may be affiliated with a religious organization).

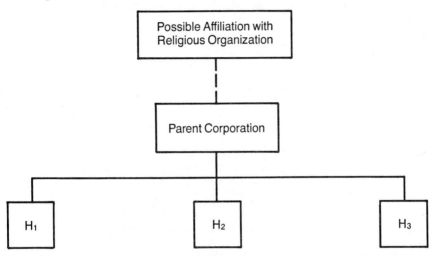

- *Type 2. Single corporation multihospital system.* The individual hospitals are owned outright by one corporation (which may be affiliated).

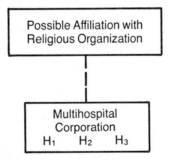

- *Type 3. Multicorporate hospitals under management contracts or other affiliation arrangements.* Independent, separately incorporated hospitals operate under contracts with a management corporation (which will often be the dominant hospital in the group).

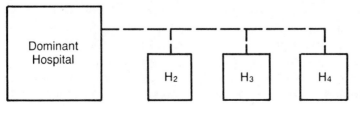

- *Type 4. Independent hospital corporations with security pool.* In this arrangement, independent, separately incorporated hospitals with, perhaps, little common allegiance unite for financing purposes to spread the risks and pool the security and thus increase the credit strength.

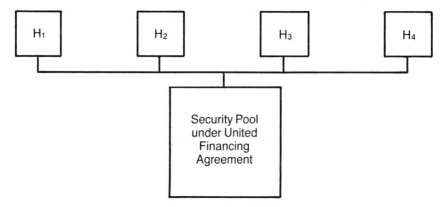

- *Type 5. Combinations of the above.*

Financing Problems

There are several problems inherent in planning any multihospital financing, including dilution of credit strength, a proliferation of the issuers, and limitations on intercorporate guaranties.

Dilution of Credit Strength

If packaged together, it is inevitable that some of the hospitals will be stronger credits than others, and the weaker may dilute the credit strength of the stronger. This may be unsatisfactory to the governing board and creditors of the stronger entity and to rating agencies, state rate-making bodies, and state planning boards as well.

A Proliferation of Issuers

As previously explained, tax-exempt financings flow through local governments or authorities or state authorities. These governmental units can only support hospitals within their jurisdictional limits (with some exceptions), which means that there may be no neat way to bundle a group of hospitals into one united financing package. Instead, there will have to be more than one issuer (1) if, under state enabling laws, a local authority or other local governmental unit must be used as issuer and (2) if the hospitals are located in more than one state, even when there is a statewide authority.

If the parent company is the prime credit, it may be necessary to limit the parent in terms of future liens, mergers, sales of assets, and indebtedness to show the overall strength of the combined group in the eyes of rating agencies and prospective purchasers.

Limitations on Intercorporate Guaranties

Under bankruptcy laws and other laws affecting creditors' rights, it is not always possible for one corporation legally to guaranty the debt of another. State fraudulent conveyances laws may in particular invalidate guaranties among hospital corporations. In a parent subsidiary relationship, there can be three kinds of guaranties:

1. "downstream" guaranties of subsidiary debt by a parent, which do not usually raise problems;
2. "upstream" guaranties of parent debt by one or more subsidiaries, which may be unenforceable; and
3. "cross-stream" guaranties of one subsidiary's debt by one or more other subsidiaries, which also may be unenforceable.

The laws against fraudulent conveyances in effect in all states, either as common law or under the Uniform Fraudulent Conveyances Act, provide that every conveyance made and obligation incurred by a person who is thereby rendered insolvent is fraudulent as to creditors without regard to the person's actual intent if the conveyance is made without fair consideration. In the context of the upstream and cross-stream examples given above, the hospital subsidiary would be the person making the conveyance and incurring the obligation, and the key question would be whether the hospital subsidiary received adequate consideration for its upstream or cross-stream guaranty. The consideration must be measured as of the time of the guaranty, but the enforcement of the guaranty would not be challenged until some later date when the subsidiary would be called upon under the guaranty. By then the original consideration and sound motives for the guaranty might be hard to prove.

There is also the bankruptcy law doctrine of equitable subordination by which the bankruptcy court will subordinate some claims when circumstances warrant. This may occur when a parent corporation has used its control position to its own ends and to the disadvantage of the subsidiary's creditors. Again, the important question is whether the subsidiary benefited from the relationship.

Upstream and cross-stream guaranties can be unenforceable where the subsidiary did not at the time of the guaranty receive fair consideration. Fraudulent intent on the part of the parent (versus the subsidiary's creditors) does not have to be shown.[4] These problems require close consideration by the attorneys and opinions about their applications differ, since there is no case directly on point. One solution is discussed in "The Master Trust" section below.

Partial Solutions

To offset the various financing problems, a number of devices have been tried.

The Parent as Prime Credit

Where the individual hospitals are separate corporations, they can be merged into the parent. The parent can flatly agree not to spin off more than a certain percentage of its assets per year; the parent may agree not to spin off assets unless earning tests are (and will be) met; or the parent and the hospital corporations can agree to reunite by merger if debt service or certain maintenance tests are not met (a kind of shotgun remarriage).

Individual Hospital as the Credit

The "subsidiary" hospital corporation may be the primary credit behind the bonds with a downstream guaranty by the parent or a cross-stream guaranty by a sister hospital. However, cross-stream guaranties in particular raise the problems previously explained relating to bankruptcy and fraudulent conveyances which must be carefully considered.

The Parent as the Credit

Under limited conditions, the parent may be the primary credit with the proceeds going to the "subsidiary" hospital as a capital contribution (with an upstream guaranty) or pursuant to a loan (perhaps with a mortgage assignable as security). Again, bankruptcy and fraudulent conveyances must be considered.

The Master Trust

Hospital chains and individual hospitals with various affiliate entities have availed themselves of a "master trust" arrangement. The parent entity enters into a master trust pursuant to which a series of covenants is adopted to cover all debt of the parent and its "subsidiaries" or affiliates (known as "related obligors"). Any long-term debt of the parent and of the related obligors must be financed through a supplemental indenture and must meet all of these master indenture covenants plus any additional covenants which a future underwriter or other security purchaser may wish to add by placing the additional covenants in the supplemental indenture. This assures each lender that there are certain inviolate terms and yet provides for flexibility in future financing where there can be different obligors, lenders, trustees, and security provisions. One way to deal with these considerations under the master trust arrangement is to limit the amount of each related obligor's guaranty to the amount of benefit (consideration) received by the related obligor by way of asset transfers or by way of being a borrower. For example, if a related obligor financed a $10 million bond issue under the master trust, its reciprocal guaranty cap would be $10 million, and this amount would diminish as the bonds are amortized. State authorities and some lenders may object to the "newness" of this concept and to its broad "open-end" aspects. Moreover, bankruptcy and fraudulent conveyances must be considered.

Debt Service Reserve Trust

It would be possible to create a special debt service reserve to be maintained in a separate trust for the benefit of all hospitals, strong and weak, within a system that is engaged in a series of financings. All participants can be jointly and severally liable for the replenishment of any individual debt service reserve. These reserves would serve as security and could be drawn upon in the event of an insolvency or weakness on the part of one hospital within the group. The stronger members would then be forced to replenish the trust and would have the right to seek reimbursement against the defaulting entity. The amount of the reserve would be severely limited, however, by the arbitrage regulations applicable to various types of bond funds established to secure tax-exempt financing.

CLASSIFICATION BY THE FORM OF PRINCIPAL AND INTEREST PAYMENTS

Theoretically at least, financial planners can conjure unlimited packages of debt securities by varying interest rates and two other factors relating to repayment of the debt principal, namely, duration or term of the security, and method of repayment or amortization.

Duration or term simply refers to the length of time until payment of principal and interest is due. Repayment techniques add complexity. The simplest structure is debt that is all due at once, with no provisions for payments of principal over the life of the debt, sometimes called a "bullet loan." It gives the borrower full use of the principal over the loan life and maximizes the risk that the borrower will not be able to pay all principal at maturity.

The bullet loan can be contrasted with other types calling for systematic repayments.

- *Installment debt* consists of one obligation, made payable periodically in specified partial payments (for example, a ten-year note for $1 million payable in ten annual installments of $100,000 each).
- *Serial debt* consists of a series of separate obligations, made payable at spaced intervals (for example, ten $100,000 notes, payable in each of the next ten years).
- *Sinking fund debt* consists of one obligation with the borrower required to redeem a specified portion at intervals by making sinking fund deposits (for example, a ten-year note for $1 million with the requirement that the borrower must deposit $100,000 each year in a trust account pursuant to which the trustee must redeem from the account $100,000 worth of the notes each year).

Obviously, to the borrower there is little difference in these devices. The average life of the debt is the same in each case. The choice depends on marketing factors.

Short-term debt and debt to be out for only a few years is often issued in bullet loan form, especially if it is a bank loan. There may be an understanding with the bank that the debt will be refinanced prior to maturity. In the early 1980s, as interest rates hit record levels and long-term tax-exempt rates were especially affected, hospitals increasingly turned to this form, not just with banks, but also in public offerings where the obligation is often backed with an irrevocable bank letter of credit.

Longer-term tax-exempt debt that is publicly sold is apt to be a combination of serial debt for the shorter years and sinking fund debt for the longer term. For example, 30-year bonds could be sold as serial bonds for the first 10 years and as sinking fund bonds with a 30-year maturity thereafter. In this example, the sinking fund probably would not start until the eleventh year.

In addition to finding innovative methods of principal repayment, financial planners have also conjured many variations of interest payment.

For example, the interest rate, known in the trade as the "coupon," can be combined with principal discounts and premiums to obtain for the lender a return on investment greater or less than the coupon and to obtain for the borrower an actual cost of money which (including the underwriters' discount) is conversely greater or less than the coupon.

The serial bonds are usually sold at rates which rise with length of maturity and are then followed by the term (sinking fund) bonds which have the highest interest rate.

The serial bonds are usually sold in coupon form and can be bearer bonds or registered bonds. The term bonds are registered. This reflects an investment style: individuals and banks buy the serial bonds, and institutions usually buy the term bonds.

The interaction between serial bonds and the debt service reserve fund is quite interesting. The fund will hold U.S. government securities in amounts sufficient to amortize one year's principal and interest. Thus, as every year goes by and a serial series is paid off, a new series is secured in this almost direct way by U.S. government securities, creating a gilt-edged quality for early maturing serial bonds not fully appreciated in the marketplace.

It is customary to stage the annual principal and interest payments (regardless of the combination of installment, serial, and sinking fund bonds used) to provide for annual level debt service, similar to the familiar practice in home mortgage financing. However, in a hospital financing other factors should be considered, such as:

- In construction financing, an interest account may be separately established to pay interest during construction and funded from bond proceeds with this "capitalized interest."
- Principal may be deferred until after construction.
- Principal may be deferred to dovetail with projected increased cash flow.
- Principal may be balanced with other outstanding debt payments to avoid large payments coming due in certain years and to create an overall level debt service or a smooth curve of debt service.
- Some principal may be amortized, but the bulk may be due at maturity in the form of a "balloon."

Investment advisers and underwriters may feel that uniquely structured payment provisions will affect bond marketability and therefore cost more. For example, as principal is deferred, the average life is extended (a positive factor for the borrower), and the actual cost of money will rise (a negative factor). The hospital's chief financial officer may be willing to pay more for a tailored program. These principal and interest provisions are negotiable.

In addition, and of increasing importance, there may be a floating interest rate. In this form, the interest changes in accordance with some accepted standard, such as the prime rate at a certain bank. The rate can change on the spot when the bank's prime changes, or it can be subject to change at specified intervals. This form became increasingly popular in the early 1980s with high interest costs and the unwillingness of hospitals to commit long-term to high fixed rates. As already suggested, there are many ways to formulate these financings by varying the maturities and interest rates.[5]

Finally, there are "deep discount" and "zero coupon" bonds. These devices first appeared in 1980, and zero coupon bonds were first used by hospitals in 1982.

Deep discount bonds are sold at interest rates below the current market and at sharp discounts. A 30-year, $50 million deep discount issue might sell for a total price of $25 million and, thus, the investor would pay $2,500 for a bond with a face amount of $5,000. The interest coupons are lower than the going rate for ordinary bonds sold at or near par.

The zero coupon bond has been referred to as the "ultimate deep discount issue."[6] It bears no interest and no payments are made until maturity. The chief advantage to the investor is that there is no reinvestment risk. If the investor is bullish (and thinks that interest rates will fall and bond prices will rise), he or she can lock in the yield to maturity and not worry about reinvesting interest income. There can also be certain tax advantages to the investor. On the other hand, because no payment is made until maturity, there is more market risk. (As previously explained, these bullet loans are considered more risky by investors.) Hospital borrowers can benefit from the lower yields and longer life, since there are no sinking fund payments.

Zero coupon bonds issued in the taxable area have had very restricted call privileges, a plus for the investor and a disadvantage to the issuer. Tax-exempt issues, however, provide redemption terms more in line with conventional financing by basing the redemption price on the "compound accreted value," which is determined by compounding the issue price semiannually to the redemption date by the yield to maturity.

CLASSIFICATION AS TO FORM OF SALE

The basic types of sale are the public and private sale, as previously explained. Private sales have certain favorable characteristics, for example:

• They can be negotiated more quickly and at less cost.

- They can be amended much more easily.
- It is generally thought that a sophisticated private investor, such as a bank or insurance company, will be reasonable in bad times and is in a better position to cooperate by waiving defaults or permitting unforeseen changes than is the bond trustee in a public financing.

However, from the negative viewpoint:

- It is generally thought that private placement investors demand higher interest rates.
- The legal documents negotiated in private placements generally include more negative covenants.
- From time to time the institutional market for private placements of tax-exempts can dry up. Some institutions, such as insurance companies, are so structured that tax-exempts are not attractive. Any investor will only want tax-exempt income to the extent the investor is making a profit that makes the lower-yielding tax-exempt bonds attractive (when income taxes are netted against yields on available taxable bonds).

Private financings are placed with money sources that vary from venture capital groups to institutions. These two extremes have completely different capital sources and different investment philosophies. Health care financing, at least of charitable entities, has no appeal to venture capital. However, it is of major interest to banks, pension funds, bond funds, casualty insurance companies, and individuals. Proprietary health institutions may be able to sell equity or combined debt and equity and thus may tap the venture capital market as well as the other types of private investors.

There is a hybrid approach available which combines features of the public and private offerings; it is sometimes called a "limited public offering." A team processes the paperwork in much the manner described in the last chapter, but the bonds are sold to a limited number of investors. The attraction from the hospital's point of view is that the investor is presented with a fully processed set of terms just as the investor would see in a public offering. This is contrasted with the typical private placement where the institution normally imposes its terms at the outset.

In the limited public offering, the hospital hopes to emerge with a better rate and less negative covenants. The hospital must be willing to pay the relatively higher front-end costs.

One reason this arrangement works is that different departments within the casualty companies, funds, and banks may process public deals and private deals, and the idea is to submit the official statement to the department that routinely processes public deals and thus avoid the more formal and hard-fought negotiations encountered on the private side.

The role of the underwriter in the limited public offering can vary. There may be no underwriting whatsoever in the sense that the investment banking firm (either alone or through a syndicate) purchases the bonds as a principal pursuant to a bond purchase agreement and thus is at risk with respect to a public resale. Instead, the investment banking firm may act only as agent for the issuer (and, indirectly, the hospital). The fee or discount paid to the investment banker for arranging the limited public offering would be less than in the full public offering.

The question of transferability of the bonds sold in the limited public offering should be considered. It would seem clear that, in the absence of a covenant not to sell, purchasers can freely transfer the bonds. This may defeat one of the prime reasons to limit an offering, namely to be able to amend more easily and to have better lines of communication with respect to waivers.

CLASSIFICATION BY FORM OF SECURITY

Tax-exempt bonds may be secured or unsecured, and in the latter case should probably be called "notes" or "debentures" rather than "bonds." Generally, there is an effort to provide some security. There are several basic forms of security.

First Mortgage Bonds

In the form of first mortgage bonds, the hospital's real property and fixtures are mortgaged either (1) by transfer of the property to the issuer, which can then mortgage it to the trustee, or (2) by giving a mortgage and security interest to the issuer, which can then pledge it to the trustee. In either form, the hospital may lease the property back or may give a note. The lease rentals or the note payments amortize the bonds. If the property is leased, for bankruptcy law reasons, the hospital will be obliged to guaranty the bonds with the guaranty running directly to the trustee for the benefit of bondholders and not to the issuer.

Lease and Leaseback

Instead of a mortgage, there may be a lease (sometimes called a "ground lease") to the issuer and a leaseback (sometimes called a "sublease") from the issuer to the hospital. The ground lease would be for a longer term than the sublease which would run for the life of the bonds and would amortize them. The extra term of the ground lease would permit the issuer and trustee to negotiate with respect to the property if there were a default; the extra term would simply collapse if the bonds were paid at maturity. The hospital would guaranty the bonds in this case as well. The differences between the mortgage as a security device (with right to foreclose) and the lease (with right of entry and other rights) are subtle and depend on state laws. To the rating agencies and the investing public, the mortgage is considered more secure.

Pledge of Gross Receipts

In most health institution financings, there is a security interest granted to the trustee in all of the institution's gross revenues. This should not be confused with the more traditional and tighter form of accounts receivable financing where all receivables flow through a depository bank and are disbursed to the debtor until there is a default (sometimes called a "lock box arrangement"). Unless there is a default, the hospital would have complete control and freedom to dispose of its revenues as it chooses. It affords the trustee the opportunity to take over on a default and to claim these revenues, but it may not be possible to perfect a security interest in certain important revenues, including gifts, insurance proceeds, and Medicare and Medicaid payments. The pledge is usually part of a security package, which would include the mortgage (or the lease and leaseback) as well.

Debt Service Reserve Fund

This special fund to hold an amount equal to maximum annual principal and interest payment provides significant security and can act as a buffer for a temporarily troubled hospital. The institution's ability to arbitrage the fund minimizes the fact that there is a need to "overborrow" in the first place to create the fund.

Other Collateral

A health institution could pledge as collateral any valuable property, including other real and personal property, land trusts, junior mortgages, paintings, securities (including securities of its subsidiaries), or other assets.

Limits on Security

The institution may very well elect to mortgage only a portion of its facilities. This is negotiable. Naturally one wing or one floor is not very attractive security. It may be that there is more than one campus or that there are natural boundaries making possible a logical separation. On the other hand, there may be after-acquired property clauses which extend the mortgage lien to any property thereafter acquired. A compromise sometimes used is to limit the after-acquired property lien to contiguous property or property within a certain radius or other geographical area.

Third-Party Guaranties

It is possible to include the guaranty of a parent organization or, in limited instances, the guaranty of sister or subsidiary organizations. The problems of fraudulent conveyances and bankruptcy law are encountered on upstream and cross-stream guaranties, as previously explained.

Letters of Credit

With high interest rates it has become more popular to enter into mid-term financings of three to five years. To assure payment (and thus marketability), upon delivery of the bonds the hospital will cause the trustee to receive a "transferable irrevocable standby letter of credit" of a bank with a sufficiently high rating to provide the needed marketability. The hospital will be obligated to reimburse the bank for all payments made under the letter of credit. The terms of this arrangement are embodied in a reimbursement agreement with the bank which may be secured by a mortgage and a pledge to the bank of the hospital's property or by other security.

In this situation, the actual credit behind the bonds on which the rating agencies and investors depend is the bank issuing the letter of credit, not the hospital, and the bonds may be rated as high as AAA. For this reason, the hospital should give any available security to the bank, not to the bond trustee.

The interest rate on these bonds is frequently tied to the prime rate, thus creating what have come to be known as "floating interest rate bonds."

Put Bonds

Instead of an irrevocable letter of credit, the bank may act as a liquidity backup to the bonds in a number of ways. In the case of put bonds, the bank would agree to purchase all bonds tendered back to the hospital at a fixed time by the investors, and the bondholders' "put" would enable the bondholders to treat the bonds as having a maturity encompassed by the duration of the put option.

Standby Agreements

Instead of an irrevocable letter of credit, the bank may act as a liquidity backup by agreeing to make loans in the event the bonds, for various reasons, cannot remain outstanding. Standby terms can be specially written to fit the borrower's needs and the lender's willingness to risk defaults. The bank's standby fees are negotiated based on the likelihood that it might be called on to deliver funds. The standby is substantially similar to a limited letter of credit, and a bank's negotiating posture in this area depends in large measure on how the bank will be required to book these arrangements under generally accepted accounting principles and banking regulations. Standby agreements can provide for taxable and tax-exempt loans, depending on arrangements being made with a governmental unit if tax-exempt treatment is to result. There are generally enough "outs" in the standby agreement to require that the rating agencies look to the hospital as the main credit rather than the bank, so the bonds will not necessarily receive a high rating.

Insured Financings

American Municipal Bond Assurance Corporation and other insurance companies as well have, under certain conditions and pursuant to policy terms, committed to issue policies of insurance that will insure the payment when due of the principal and interest on bonds, including tax-exempt bonds issued by health institutions. If the bond trustee does not receive sufficient funds from the authority (which originally come from the hospital), the trustee is instructed to notify another trustee of the amount needed to make payment. The second trustee then collects from the insurance company and makes the payment.

Again in this situation, the credit behind the bonds on which the rating agencies and investors depend is the insurance company, not the hospital, and the bonds will be rated AAA. The threshold decisions are whether the insurance company will issue a policy and whether the market advantage of the high rating, as opposed to a bond sale with no insurance, more than offsets the cost of the insurance.

Participation Certificates

Official statements for hospital financing may be encountered which refer to the offering of certificates of participation. Such a statement might contain the following language:

Certificates of Participation
Evidencing a Proportionate Interest of the
Holders Thereof in Installment Payments to be Made by the
(NAME OF ISSUER)

Briefly, participation certificates are substantially equivalent to the conventional hospital tax-exempt bonds described in this book. The difference is that, rather than the issuer paying principal and interest directly to bondholders, a new entity is inserted in the form of a bank trust company acting as escrow agent. This agent will issue certificates of participation in a special escrow fund pursuant to agreement with the issuer. The issuer pays the escrow fund an amount that the agent passes along to the certificate holders as principal and interest on the certificates.

Use of certificates of participation is common in the broader area of municipal financing. A city or other governmental unit will enter into an installment sales contract or a lease purchase agreement to acquire needed equipment or other property. Arrangements are often made through a company specializing in municipal financing services (referred to as a "vendor"). The vendor will purchase the equipment and resell (or lease) it to the city and arrange the financing. The vendor's installment sales contract (or lease) will be pledged to the escrow agent as security for the loan. The certificates may be payable only from designated or excess revenues of the city without an obligation to levy a special tax. The entire arrangement is supported by applicable state laws relating to debt of municipalities and other governmental units which are very likely to be independent of the state laws relating to tax-exempt financing of health care institutions.

From this established format in the broader area, it has become acceptable practice in certain states for the municipality to assist hospitals through issuance of participation certificates. The fit is a more natural one for county and municipal hospitals where the project being financed can pertain to the hospital just as it would to the public library or the fire department, but it can be used for other charitable (501(c)(3)) hospitals as well. The vendor or the municipality itself purchases the equipment, facility, or other property, and the hospital is given use of the property through a loan or lease that will provide the dollar flow (through the vendor and municipality) to pay the escrow agent (which pays principal and interest to the certificate holders). The loan or lease will give ownership to the hospital when the certificates are paid.

Hospitals avail themselves of participation certificates when more conventional arrangements are not feasible. This may be because of limitations under applicable state laws, such as usury limits, or perhaps simply because of unclear or insufficient enabling laws to permit conventional financing. Or it may be because the only conventional issuer available to the hospital is an authority who is unable to meet time requirements or who has a policy of imposing unwanted limitations in the form of restrictive terms (which may, of course, be perfectly sound and appropriate) or of imposing unacceptable mandatory rules with respect to the choice of underwriters.

SHORT-TERM TAX-EXEMPT SECURITIES

Tax-Exempt Commercial Paper

In response to the rising public interest in investment funds, particularly in the highly liquid money market funds, tax-exempt investment funds have become an important investment device and capital source. These funds have a special need for short-term tax-exempt securities, known as "tax-exempt commercial paper."

The key aspect of this form is the low interest rate of the commercial paper the tax-exempt investment funds are willing to purchase. However, there are problems involving the newness of this form, the uncertainties of the market, the large amount of paperwork, and the high costs. Also, all parties, including the hospital and its governing board, the rating agencies, and the tax-exempt investment funds, share a common concern with respect to the hospital's continued ability to "roll over" the paper. The main worry is that the federal government will change the tax laws and cut short this device; then large amounts would come due over a short period. The market for this type of paper is limited, and at present it is considered a viable device only for the larger, high credit institutions.

The commercial paper is issued by the appropriate issuer in large amounts for terms of from a few days to 270 days until some agreed limit on principal amount to be outstanding is reached. As the paper comes due, it is "rolled over"; that is, new paper is issued to replace the due paper. There are no provisions for cutting down (amortizing) the principal amount. The paper may be interest-bearing or may sell at an initial discount and be redeemable at par. The interest cost depends on market forces at the time of each rollover. To back up each authority commercial paper note, there must be a compensating hospital note.

To minimize the problems outlined above, especially the threat of a cutoff of the hospital's ability to roll over the paper, the hospital and the authority must enter into a complex series of agreements.

Agent for Sale

A bank or investment banking firm must contract to be agent for the authority in the sale of the paper. This requires experience in selling tax-exempt securities to funds and entails handling frequent transactions for a relatively low fee.

Standby Bank

A bank must act as standby to assure the investors and the authority and hospital that if the paper cannot be rolled over for any reason the bank will provide funds to make the commercial paper payment commitments. The bank arrangement could be an agreement to make a standby loan or it could be by delivery of an irrevocable letter of credit.

The standby arrangements can be two-faceted: an agreement to make a tax-exempt loan through the issuer and an agreement to make a taxable loan directly to the hospital. The reason for this complex dual arrangement is that the hospital would prefer to have the takeout be as a tax-exempt loan at lower rates, but if the tax laws were changed this route might not be possible.

Mechanics of the Transaction

The procedural aspects of rolling over millions of dollars in the ordinary course of business adds significantly to the burden this form puts on all parties.

Put Bonds

The "put bond" developed in an effort to solve the hospital's need to issue long-term debt with advantageous amortization arrangements as well as its need to have reasonable interest rates. On the other hand, it is intended to satisfy the investors' demand for higher rates and their reluctance to go out 25 or 30 years regardless of rate.

Put bonds are issued in the normal way and with customary terms and conditions. They are due and payable over a long term, for example, 30 years.

However, at some intermediate time, the holders have the option of tendering ("putting") to the bond trustee as tender agent all or any part of the put bonds. The time when the tender can be made (the "option date") is some time in the future, for example, in seven years, when the investor feels the need for a chance to get out and also when the hospital feels it will have had time to make other financing arrangements, hopefully in lower interest rate markets, and therefore to refund the put bonds.

Funds to pay for the tendered put bonds are made available by a bank standby agreement. The bank will purchase from the hospital all bonds tendered but will receive a stepped-up interest coupon. Throughout, the bank will be paid a standby fee.

The "put" concept can also be used for short-term notes by having them issued as demand notes payable on three to seven day notice. The notes may also have a fixed long-term maturity, subject to the holder's option to have them redeemed on this short notice. This type of note may be issued on a fixed or on a floating rate basis, the key being that the tax-exempt investment companies are interested in these short-term issues just as they are in commercial paper. When the notes are subject to these very short-term repayments, they are backed by a bank letter of credit or, in the case of stronger credit hospitals, by a bank line of credit. These notes are sold on the basis that the tax-exempt investment companies can treat them as short-term because the holder has the option to demand payment, but the notes are also sold on the understanding that the investment companies probably will not exercise this option. Nevertheless, an investment company may be required to sell to meet its cash needs, especially to pay its withdrawing investors. In such a case, the "put" option would be used and, to protect against this event, a bank backup is required by investors and is just plain prudent on the hospital's part.

The tax-exempt debt can take numerous forms. The health and investment banking industries are charged with devising new ways to raise capital, and local governments and taxing bodies are required to respond. No doubt revisions of the reimbursement system and the tax laws will force further change. It is likely, however, that the different forms outlined here will continue to form the basis of new developments.

NOTES

1. Internal Revenue Code of 1954, as amended (I.R.C.), § 103(b)(3).

2. I.R.C. § 103(b)(6).

3. 42 C.F.R. § 405.429 (1980).

4. For a comprehensive review, *see* Rosenberg, "Intercorporate Guaranties and the Law of Fraudulent Conveyances: Lender Beware," *U. Penn. L. Rev.* 125 (1976): 235.

5. Two complex types, put bonds and tax-exempt commercial paper, are discussed *infra*.

6. Standard & Poor's Corporation, "Rating Deep Discount Bonds," *Standard & Poor's Perspective* (New York: S&P's, 1981), p. 3.

Chapter 12

Key Terms of a Tax-Exempt Financing

Donna S. Wetzler

The legal and business terms of a tax-exempt hospital financing command the attention not only of members of the financing team, but also of rating agencies, prospective purchasers of the bonds, and the financial community. In addition, in a standard hospital bond offering, the hospital may well have to live with these legal and business terms for a period of up to 30 years; future generations will also scrutinize these documents.

Therefore, it is important for all parties to focus carefully on the financing terms, their effect on future hospital operations, and their effect on bond ratings and the marketability of the bonds. It is particularly important that the independent accountants and legal counsel for the hospital evaluate the impact of these terms.

Generally, there is a trade-off between the "liberal" nature of the business terms and the rating the bonds will receive. There are certain "standard" terms the rating agencies are accustomed to seeing; some modifications will be acceptable, but the more the terms vary from the norm, the greater the chance of a lower rating. The underwriter or financial adviser to the issuer generally can give the hospital a good idea of where the rating agency will reach a breaking point.

It is to the hospital's advantage to request from the underwriters a "term sheet" summarizing in a few pages the sorts of key terms discussed below. In that way, basic business terms can be negotiated early and directly between the hospital and the underwriters, without the distractions that arise in large drafting sessions involving all parties to the financing.

The following discussion of key terms primarily will emphasize terms that are regarded as fairly standard in the industry for long-term (generally 30-year) tax-exempt hospital revenue bonds. However, none of these terms is engraved in stone, and substantial leeway always exists.

MATURITY SCHEDULE

Generally, a long-term hospital bond matures in 30 years. Payment of principal usually begins in the year after a construction project is completed, though there is often a delay of an extra year to allow for construction delays.

"Level debt service" is the form of principal and interest repayment most bond offerings take. Basically, "level debt service" is the yearly matching of principal and interest payments so that total debt service remains approximately the same each year. In a level debt service format, principal payments start at a relatively low amount and increase over the term of the bonds, while interest payments start high and decrease. There is, however, considerable flexibility in structuring a hospital's debt service schedule to meet its individual needs. For example, a hospital which forecasts cash flow problems in early years of operations may wish to pack higher principal and interest payments into later years.

OPTIONAL REDEMPTION

Optional redemption provisions provide an "out" for the hospital—that is, the option to prepay the bonds before such prepayment would otherwise be permitted. Optional redemption usually falls into three categories:

1. *Optional redemption.* Usually, long-term hospital bonds may not be redeemed or "called" until ten years after issuance, and then, with a prepayment penalty for a certain number of years. Call periods of less than ten years may present marketing problems, since bondholders generally wish to hold onto their investments as long as possible. Occasionally, five-year call provisions are used; however, in recent financings, three-year and five-year call periods failed to find a receptive market, and the standard ten-year call was instituted. Shorter call periods do work to a hospital's advantage because they permit a hospital to refinance outstanding debt in periods of falling interest rates.

2. *Optional redemption in the event of condemnation or destruction.* If at any time the hospital facility is damaged or condemned and the damage or condemnation exceeds a certain dollar amount (often $250,000) or a stated percentage of value of the property, then the bonds will be subject to redemption from insurance or condemnation proceeds in excess of these amounts.

3. *Extraordinary redemption.* Extraordinary redemption provisions permit a hospital to redeem bonds under certain unique circumstances. One fairly common provision commonly used when religiously affiliated hospitals are involved is a provision permitting redemption at any time without penalty if, by virtue of a court order, the hospital is required because of the financing to operate in a manner contrary to its religious tenets. Generally, such a "religious call" provision also permits redemption at any time with penalty should the hospital believe in good faith that there is a threat that it will be required to operate in a manner contrary to religious teachings.

ADVANCE REFUNDING

Advance refunding provisions, also commonly known as "defeasance" provisions, permit bonds to be paid prior to the normal prepayment date through the deposit with the trustee of moneys sufficient to pay principal and interest to maturity. A defeasance is not the same as a redemption; bondholders continue to hold bonds and to receive principal and interest payments from the moneys deposited with the trustee. However, as in a redemption, the hospital itself is discharged from all of its obligations with respect to the bonds. Basically, then, the advance refunding process is one that allows bond obligations to be erased prior to the date when such bonds could ordinarily be prepaid.

A defeasance can be accomplished on either a "net" or a "full" cash basis; the net cash approach is most favorable to the hospital. In order to effect a full cash defeasance, the deposit with the trustee must be in the actual amount of all principal and interest due on the bonds to maturity. A net cash defeasance, however, requires only that the moneys deposited, together with earning thereon, be sufficient to pay principal and interest on the bonds to maturity.

A hospital should be certain that defeasance provisions are provided in its debt instruments, and that both full cash and net cash options are included. Defeasance language is essential because, in today's market, a drop of 200 basis points (for example, 14 percent to 12 percent) will make it economically worthwhile for a hospital to issue new bonds and use the proceeds to defease the outstanding bonds.

OPEN-END INDENTURE (ADDITIONAL BONDS)

Under an "open-end indenture," later series of bonds can be issued under the same indenture (as supplemented) as earlier series. The later bonds will rank on an equal basis with prior series and, upon default, would have equal rights to the same security.

The original indenture will contain conditions which must be met in order to issue a new series. These conditions generally consist of an either/or ratio test of historical and pro forma debt coverage. Frequently, the historical coverage test requires that net income available for debt service of the hospital for the preceding two years be not less than 110 percent of maximum annual debt service on all long-term debt, including the additional bonds to be issued. If this test cannot be met, a common alternative is a 110 percent historical coverage figure for all long-term debt except the debt to be issued plus a pro forma coverage figure of 120 percent for a certain number of years following such issuance of new bonds.

Frequently, open-end indentures also permit the issuance of "parity obligations." Parity obligations are issued under and are secured by the same open-end indenture, but are issued by a different issuer than the original bonds. The issuer may be either a different governmental entity, in the case of tax-exempt bonds, or may in fact be the hospital or an affiliate of a hospital in the case of taxable bonds. Thus, for example, should no issuing governmental body be available for future bond issues, a hospital may issue taxable "parity" bonds under its old open-end indenture.

PERMITTED INDEBTEDNESS

A critical provision in each hospital financing is that which defines the additional indebtedness the hospital may incur. The "permitted indebtedness" provisions are perhaps those a hospital finds most difficult to live with over the long period that bonds may be outstanding. Therefore, a hospital should carefully evaluate current liabilities and future borrowing needs in order to develop a provision with which it believes it can live comfortably over the changing circumstances of the next 30 years.

"Indebtedness," as it is defined in most debt instruments, means many things; it includes not only additional bonds, but also such liabilities as short-term bank borrowings, rental payments, purchase money mortgages, and capitalized leases.

Permitted indebtedness provisions vary widely, depending on a hospital's financial strength and the views of the underwriter, the issuing entity, and financial advisers who may be involved. Frequently, one sees provisions permitting the incurrence of long-term debt under the same ratio test as used for the issuance of additional bonds. In addition, a catch-all provision allowing additional debt of between 15 percent and 20 percent of adjusted operating revenue is often used.

MERGER

A merger provision should generally allow a hospital to merge with another corporation, provided that (1) the bonds remain tax-exempt after the merger; (2) the surviving corporation remains a tax-exempt entity; and (3) the merger does not impair the surviving corporation's ability to pay the principal and interest on the bonds. In addition, it is common to require the surviving corporation to assume all of the obligations of the hospital with respect to the bonds.

REORGANIZATION

Many hospitals are engaged in realigning their corporate structures to maximize reimbursement and minimize health planning and other governmental constraints. Such restructurings take many forms, but generally involve spinning off into separate affiliated corporations of certain hospital facilities, properties, or operations.

Until very recently, bond documents were not drafted to give a hospital sufficient flexibility to enter into a corporate restructuring. Even now, restructuring language rarely appears in documents without the active prodding of the hospital, its counsel, or an underwriter, since many issuing entities and bond counsel remain philosophically opposed to the concept of restructuring.

Restructuring language generally consists of compromises arrived at by those members of the financing team who are for and against the idea. In general, though, restructuring language provides for the annual spin-off of assets without restriction up to a certain percent (often 5 percent), then the unrestricted spin-off of assets to affiliated corporations, so long as certain conditions are met. These conditions include requirements that (1) the transferred property remain subject to the mortgage or lease, if any, under the indenture; (2) the affiliated corporation execute a lengthy guaranty of the bond obligations and covenants with respect to the bonds; (3) the hospital meet certain debt service coverage tests prior to spinning off assets; and (4) the spin-off will not affect the tax-exempt status of the bonds.

RENEWAL, REPLACEMENT, AND DEPRECIATION FUND

In a standard level debt repayment schedule for a hospital tax-exempt bond, principal payments due in later years may exceed depreciation on the facility. To cover possible cash shortfalls engendered during this "crossover" period, it is traditional to see in bond documents a renewal, replacement, and depreciation fund (the "RR&D fund"), the purpose of which is to fund this shortfall.

However, because hospitals are constantly adding new depreciable plant and equipment, most hospitals never actually need to put money into the RR&D account. Mechanically, this fact is handled by crediting the cost of depreciable property bought by a hospital to the amount the hospital is required to deposit. If moneys are in fact on deposit in the RR&D fund, the indenture generally will permit such funds to be used (1) to purchase depreciable property or (2) to make bond sinking fund or optional redemption fund deposits.

QUALIFIED INVESTMENTS

"Qualified investments" are securities in which a hospital is permitted to invest its trusteed funds, for example, the revenue fund, construction fund, interest fund, sinking fund, debt service reserve fund, RR&D fund, and optional redemption fund. As a general matter, qualified investments are restricted to U.S. government obligations and bank certificates of deposit. In recent years, repurchase agreements and, in some instances, certain grades of commercial paper have also been deemed to be qualified investments in some transactions. Flexibility to invest in instruments such as repurchase agreements, commercial paper, and other money market instruments is advantageous to the hospital, because of the higher interest rates that these instruments usually pay.

EARNINGS ON FUNDS

The trusteed funds under the indenture all earn interest; the indenture directs where that interest will flow. Commonly, in a construction project financing, all income from all funds other than the RR&D fund will be deposited in the construction fund. Following completion of construction, there is really no set pattern as to where moneys must go.

It is often advisable for a hospital to fund the debt service reserve fund from hospital funds rather than from bond proceeds, so that earnings on that fund will not act as a reimbursement offset.

SECURITY

The interests of the bondholders are often secured by property and revenues of the hospital. In some cases of highly rated hospitals, a pledge of hospital gross revenues is sufficient, and no tangible property will be pledged. The pledge of gross receipts should take effect only in bankruptcy; the hospital should fight fiercely against any attempt to institute the old-fashioned "lock-box" approach in which all hospital revenues flow through a bank trustee.

Conflicts often arise between a hospital and the issuing authority as to what real property need be pledged. It is in the hospital's interest to mortgage only the actual hospital facility; other additional properties that are not integral to the operation of a hospital should be excluded in order to facilitate future borrowings and possible corporate restructurings. These sorts of properties include parking garages (often, however, viewed as integral to the hospital and therefore subject to lien), vacant land, professional buildings, income properties, and academic buildings.

Generally, equipment is also pledged whenever a real property lien attaches.

AFTER-ACQUIRED PROPERTY

Today's indentures do not generally require that all property acquired by a hospital after a financing be subject to the lien or mortgage. Rather, the norm is that new property located on the mortgaged land or attached to the mortgaged facility be subject to the lien. Some issuing entities require that any facility, wherever located, that is integral to the operation of the hospital be subject to the after-acquired property clause.

RATE COVENANT

The purpose of a rate covenant is to bind a hospital to agree to maintain rates and charges sufficient to pay debt service and operate and maintain hospital facilities. Generally, the covenant requires that such rates and charges must be at a level that will produce annually net income available for debt service at a fixed percentage (often 110 percent) of maximum annual debt service on all long-term debt outstanding. Generally, the rate covenant provides that if the ratio (or a slightly higher test ratio) is not met, the hospital is required to retain an independent consultant for the purpose of making recommendations with respect to such rates and charges. It is in the hospital's best interest to make sure that a failure to follow such consultant's recommendation will not result in a default. Rather, it is to the hospital's advantage to insist on a covenant in which the hospital agrees to follow such recommendations, so long as the hospital's board of directors deems that that approach is in the best interests of the hospital.

GUARANTIES

In this era of corporate restructuring and diversification in the health care industry, hospitals are increasingly discovering the desirability and necessity of being able to guaranty liabilities of affiliates or of organizations the hospital wishes to acquire. In this regard, it is important that the bond documents give the hospital flexibility to guaranty the debts of others. Frequently, especially in private placement transactions, guaranties are limited to specific dollar ceilings. More leeway may be given the hospital by incorporating the concept of guaranties under the general permitted indebtedness covenants of the documents.

INSURANCE

Bond documents usually require a hospital to maintain specified minimum amounts of insurance with respect to property, general liability, workers' compensation, use and occupancy, boilers, and professional liability. It is particularly important that the documents allow the hospital to self-insure for professional and general liability risks, as well as workers' compensation. Such self-insurance language should be broad enough to encompass insurance pools and captive insurance companies.

Chapter 13

Steps of a Taxable Financing

James R. Wyatt

When a hospital's board of directors authorizes the long-range planning committee to proceed with implementation of a plan to construct new facilities, it is time for administration to review the "first steps" discussed in earlier chapters.

"Would a fund-raising campaign be successful?" "What about our organizational structure?" "How can we improve our financial statements?" These questions should also be addressed quickly.

The planning for a major financing should begin in hospital administration three or four years prior to the actual need for funds. A successful fund-raising campaign not only decreases the ultimate amount of debt but indicates to rating agencies the existence of strong community support. A study of the hospital's existing corporate structure and discussion of alternative corporate alignment are essential before proceeding with a major financing program. In addition, hospital financial officers will want to improve balance sheet and operating statements in anticipation of bond rating agency review and public offering of debt.

ORGANIZATIONAL MEETING

When a decision has been reached to proceed with a taxable bond financing, and when the hospital selection committee has identified the appropriate underwriter for a taxable financing, an organizational meeting should be arranged at an early date. The initial review session, which should include both corporate counsel and underwriter's counsel, will be used to identify various tasks to be performed by members of the financing team, describe the project and its status, discuss sources of funds for the project, and develop an initial time schedule.

An agenda of discussion items at an initial review session should include the following topics.

213

Description of Project

Of primary importance to the investment banker is a thorough description of the construction project to be undertaken. The review should include services to be added or deleted, management estimates of increases or decreases in utilization upon completion of construction and the possible negative impact of the construction program on utilization of existing facilities during the period of construction. The investment banker should be informed of the hospital's long-range plan and whether the proposed project will be followed by a second or third phase of construction in the near future.

Status of Construction Project and Approvals

In order to develop a feeling for the overall time frame of the financing, the investment banker and the banker's counsel should be provided with a chart or table outlining the status of architectural work, the plan for obtaining firm construction contracts or a guaranteed maximum price, the estimated starting date for construction, and the length of the construction or remodeling period.

All parties should also be advised immediately of the status of the application for certificate of need, the state's requirement for 1122 authorization, and any moratorium on construction or approvals in place or threatened to be imposed. The underwriter will use this information in developing a schedule of events.

Estimated Sources and Uses of Funds

Preliminary estimates of construction costs, equipment requirements, architect and construction manager fees, and estimates of interest expense during the construction period should be discussed and evaluated at the organizational meeting. The underwriter and hospital management can then review what hospital resources, such as cash and investments, receipt of building fund contributions, and what income from operations during the construction period could be included in the development of the preliminary sources and uses of funds. It should be recognized that changes in construction estimates, fluctuations in bond interest rates, and assumed investment rates and other variables will necessitate changes and updating of the size of the bond issue necessary to balance the sources and uses of funds calculation.

Public Marketing or Private Placement

After becoming familiar with the proposed construction project, the financial position of the hospital, and the estimated size of the bond issue required, the investment banker will be in a position to discuss the advantages and disadvantages of both public and private sale of the hospital's debt.

The hospital's size, location, reputation, financial position and financing objectives must be carefully analyzed in determining if the investment banker should pursue the arrangement of a private placement of the debt. The investment banker must also evaluate current market conditions and determine the reasonable expectation of finding an institutional lender (most likely an insurance company or pension fund) willing to commit to long-term, fixed-rate, mortgage debt for the hospital.

While certain insurance companies historically have provided funds for hospital construction projects on 25-year fixed rate mortgage bases, in the past few years this type of commitment for conventional, taxable debt has been nearly nonexistent. Continued inflation and related escalation of interest rates have caused many lenders to reduce their percentage of assets in fixed income securities and to seek increased ownership, joint venture, or equity positions in financing opportunities.

Those lenders who continue to provide capital on a taxable basis for hospital expansion projects have required shorter periods of amortization or the option of adjusting interest rates on an indexed basis after each five- or ten-year period.

Taxable bond issues have been reduced in term to 5-, 10-, or 15-year periods in order to gain a more favorable market acceptance. Shorter term issues, while often necessitating a refinancing, offer greater flexibility in security, operating covenants, and prepayment provisions than direct placement financing. Historically, average interest rates on publicly offered debt have been one-quarter to one-half of 1 percent lower than those available from institutional investors.

Preparation of Terms Sheet

Following the initial review session with the underwriter and counsel, the underwriter will begin to prepare an initial draft of a terms sheet which constitutes the conceptual structuring of the bond issue. The initial draft is frequently distributed to members of the financing team for review and comment prior to its use by bond counsel in drafting legal documents. The initial terms sheet will outline the following areas, many of which will continue to be subjects of negotiation throughout the processing of the bond issue.

General Concept

The concept of the taxable bond issue will be dependent, to a degree, on the hospital's objective in the financing. For example, if the hospital is entering into a major construction project it may seek long-term, fully amortized financing. Conversely, if the hospital is financing a smaller project, but anticipates a future major construction program, or lower interest rates in the near future, it may prefer a short-term (five-year) bond issue without scheduled principal payments, and without restrictions on refinancing (generally referred to as a "bullet" loan). On the other hand, the concept will also be affected by general market conditions. As mentioned earlier, in today's volatile bond market, institutional investors are not aggressively seeking long-term, fixed rate investments. The individual investor, with ever-increasing opportunities to invest funds in short-term, liquid securities, is also becoming more reluctant to invest in long-term, fixed rate obligations. Therefore, market conditions have a strong influence on the availability of long-term taxable financing.

Principal Amount, Rates, Maturities

One of the primary advantages of taxable financing is that a corporation may borrow funds for any legal purpose. For example, a hospital may borrow funds for working capital, to acquire facilities that may not be eligible for tax-exempt financing, or to lend to an affiliate corporation. Therefore, the principal amount of a corporate, taxable financing is primarily dependent upon the creditworthiness of the obligor corporation. Interest rates and maturities of a taxable financing today are as volatile as those of tax-exempt financing, and are also determined at the time of marketing of the bond issue. While publicly issued tax-exempt bond issues historically have been marketed to institutional investors, taxable bond issues for health care facilities have been sold primarily to individual investors, or the so-called "retail" market. In today's market, the individual investor is essential to the marketing of both tax-exempt and taxable bond issues.

Again, with such a wide variety of short-term, liquid investment opportunities available to the individual investor, there has been a tendency to shorten the term of the taxable bond issue from 25 years to 15 years and currently, in certain situations, to 5 years. Favorable features of the shorter-term taxable bond issue are elimination of any required principal payments and restrictive prepayment provisions. Consequently, the borrower can quickly assemble a financing for almost any project or purpose and have the flexibility of refinancing the debt at any time.

Selection of Experts

The requirements for selection of experts to work with the hospital and the underwriter in developing the financing differ a great deal in a taxable bond issue compared to a tax-exempt financing. Since no governmental entity (that is, city, county, or state health facility authority) is involved in serving as the conduit issuer of the bonds, fewer experts are involved. Simply stated, the hospital and its counsel are able to negotiate and process the financing directly with the underwriter and underwriter's counsel.

Attorneys

In a typical taxable financing, the hospital will be represented by its corporate counsel, and the underwriter will select its counsel who will draft all documents and assist in preparing the official statement or prospectus. Special, nationally recognized bond counsel is not a requirement of taxable bond financing.

Feasibility Consultants

Financial feasibility reports are not normally required in the taxable bond financing of a health care facility. An underwriter may, however, determine that key elements of a feasibility report (demand analysis for the hospital's services and forecasted debt service coverage) will enhance the rating and marketing of the bond issue, and will suggest that a report be prepared.

A feasibility study may be required to qualify a taxable bond issue for registration with the securities department of certain states if historical financial statements are somewhat marginal.

Feasibility reports for a taxable bond issue are prepared by the same accounting firms and management consultants that prepare reports for tax-exempt financings. A prospective bond issuer should consult with an investment banker to determine if a feasibility report will be required. The feasibility consultant should be selected by the time of the organizational meeting or shortly thereafter.

Selection of Printers

Financial printing firms are available in major cities across the United States. Frequently, taxable bond prospectuses, which are not as complex as tax-exempt official statements, are printed by local printing firms at a substantially reduced fee. The hospital, after consultation with the underwriter, should select the financial printer at the initial financing team meeting, or shortly thereafter, to avoid delays in preparation of the prospectus.

Trustee and Paying Agents

In a taxable bond financing, the hospital has complete flexibility in the selection of a bank to serve as trustee and paying agent. Underwriters will assist the corporation in conducting a survey of area banks to determine if a bank's trust department has experience in administering similar bond issues and if its fees are competitive. The hospital's finance committee or board of directors will review the survey and make a selection. The selection of a trustee is a step that is usually accomplished after preparation of legal documents and prior to completion of marketing of the bond issue.

Bond Ratings

Prior to the rapid growth of municipal financing of hospitals in the mid-1970s, Fitch Investors Service of New York was the only rating agency issuing credit ratings on health care bond financings. Since that time, Moody's Investors Service and Standard & Poor's Corporation have rated the majority of tax-exempt hospital bond issues, while Fitch continues to rate most of the taxable bond issues which are submitted for a rating. Currently, many taxable bond issues are marketed as five- to ten-year term bonds, are sold primarily to individual investors, and are not rated.

Scheduling of Events

The organizational meeting, as discussed earlier in this chapter, will provide a forum for discussion by the hospital and the underwriter of the following items:

1. a description of the project to be financed, the status of the project, and the necessity of any refinancing;
2. available hospital resources, fund raising activities, and other sources of funds for the project;

3. the hospital's general financial position, future projects, and management's objectives in the current financing program; and
4. the remaining experts to be selected to complete the financing term.

After the organizational meeting, the underwriter will be able to prepare a schedule of events and assign responsibilities for various tasks to appropriate team members. The time schedule may have to be revised to accommodate unexpected delays such as the issuance of certificate-of-need or 1122 approvals, receipt of bids or a guaranteed maximum price, or adverse market conditions. In general, delays in the time schedule should not result from a member of the financing team failing to accomplish an assigned task on a timely basis.

A sample schedule of events which outlines each step to be taken in the processing of the financing is included as Exhibit 13-1. A checklist of underwriting steps and required documents is included as Table 13-1.

Exhibit 13-1 Taxable Bond Financing Schedule of Events

Date	Event	Responsible Participant
January	Organizational meeting	Hospital, underwriter's counsel, other selected financing team participants
January	Selection of remaining finance team participants	Hospital administrator and board
January	Preparation of terms sheet, participant distribution list, and preliminary schedule of events	Underwriter
February	Distribution and review of first draft of legal documents, prospectus, and feasibility study	Underwriter's counsel, underwriter, consultants, and hospital
February	Filing of documents of "blue sky" registration of securities in various states	Underwriter and underwriter's counsel
March	Due diligence meeting—to include review of prospectus, financial, feasibility report, corporate minute books, and bond documents	Underwriter, hospital, counsel, and consultants
March	Bond rating agency meeting at hospital and receipt of rating	Financing team participants
March	Public offering of bonds	Underwriter
March	Execution of underwriting agreement, trust indenture, and related legal documents	Corporate officers, counsel, and underwriter
April	Bond closing—to include delivery of legal opinions and distribution of bond proceeds	Underwriter, counsel, trustee, and hospital

Table 13-1 Underwriter's Checklist

		Underwriter	Corporate Trustee	Issuer's File	Issuer's Attorney	Paying Agent				
Name of Corporation										
City and State										
Amount Date										
Type of Security										
2	Financial									
7-20	Legality and Title Opinion, ISSUER									
7a	Legality and Title Opinion, UNDERWRITER									
8	Underwriting Agreement									
9	Prospectus									
10	Specimen Bonds/Notes									
12	Articles of Incorporation									
13, 31, 32	Bylaws, Seal, and Signature									
14	Resolutions—MEMBERS									
14a	Resolutions—BOARD T/D									
15-16	Certificate of Good Standing									
17	Attorney Appointment									
18	Trust Indenture									
18a	Supplemental Indenture									
21	Land Appraisal									
22	Building Appraisal									
26	Survey/Certificate									
28	Architect's Certificate									
30	Source of Funds Certificate									
33	Closing Certificate									
34	Letter of Authentication									

SUBSEQUENT MEETINGS

The schedule of events (or time schedule) will list assignment of tasks, completion dates, and review sessions required to complete the financing program.

The rating agency meeting and due diligence review are particularly important meetings. Hospital administration and the underwriter should prepare detailed agendas, allow adequate time for preparation, and assure appropriate attendance for each meeting.

All participants must develop the confidence through these review sessions that the financing is feasible, the legal documents are appropriate and correctly reflect the transaction, and that the official statement (prospectus) provides complete and accurate disclosure to the investor.

EXECUTION OF THE UNDERWRITING AGREEMENT

When the bond rating has been received and the offering statement is finalized and approved, the underwriter will be prepared to commit to interest rates, maturities, and underwriter's discount. The underwriter and hospital administration will, it is hoped, have held open discussion on these elements of the financing, and there will be no surprises in the underwriting agreement. Upon execution of this document by the hospital and the underwriter, the terms and conditions of the financing have been finalized.

THE CLOSING

The underwriter and underwriter's counsel will work in close coordination with the hospital counsel to assure that legal documents and all related exhibits are available for execution at the closing. The hospital should discuss the appropriate investment of bond proceeds with the trustee bank prior to the closing date and the requirements for disbursement of funds from the construction fund.

Finally, the underwriter will authorize the wire transfer of bond proceeds to complete the financing program.

The purpose of the financing (new construction, refinancing, working capital, or equipment financing) will dictate the structure of the bond issue, required documents, and the schedule of events. While each financing will be tailored to meet the issuer's requirements, it is hoped that this discussion of taxable bond financing will be of assistance to the reader.

Chapter 14

Forms and Key Terms of a Taxable Financing

William D. Gehl

Hospitals, both nonprofit and for-profit, may publicly offer debt securities to raise needed capital for construction, modernization, and rehabilitation of their facilities. Funds may also be obtained to refinance existing debt. Taxable financing involves the issuance of bonds or notes, the interest on which is not exempt from federal income tax. Taxable debt financing is an important and versatile alternative to tax-exempt financing. In some cases it may be the only available means of financing because of the lack of a tax-exempt vehicle to issue tax-exempt securities. Taxable financing does not limit the hospital in its use of proceeds, as may be the case in tax-exempt financing; the underwriting process generally is swifter than the time period needed to arrange tax-exempt financing, and the hospital may avoid entanglement with yet another governmental agency. Costs of issuance of the debt may also be significantly less than the tax-exempt route.

This chapter will describe various forms of taxable financing, as well as some of the basic terminology a hospital will encounter along the road to publicly offering an issue of debt securities. The types of financing and the terms discussed herein relate to long-term issues, which may be anywhere from 10 to 15 to 20 years. Primarily the marketplace determines the length of a public debt issue. During certain economic climates, such as during periods of rapid interest rate escalation, investors simply will not buy (at a reasonable price) securities having too long a term. They choose to remain more flexible and, therefore, seek investments with shorter maturities.

TYPES OF SECURITY

There are various methods of collateralizing debt securities issued by hospitals, but the basic concept entails pledging some form of property to secure repayment of a loan. The property may be real estate, buildings, equipment, fixtures, securities, or even revenues generated by the borrowing institution. In certain instances, the loan may also be guaranteed by some related party, such as a holding company's guaranty of the debt of one of its subsidiaries. In other cases, the security may be in the form of an agreement not to further encumber the property of the borrower. Debt obligations collateralized by specific property are commonly referred to as bonds. Unsecured debt obligations typically are called notes.

Mortgage

The most common type of security used by hospitals to secure debt is the real estate mortgage. In this transaction a hospital conveys an interest in its real property to a third party for the benefit of the lender. The property conveyed must be described accurately in the conveyance document, which is called a trust indenture. The third party who receives the interest in the real property, called the trustee, is usually a bank or trust company. If personal property also is to be pledged to secure the loan, it must be fully described in the indenture, and financing statements must be prepared and recorded in addition to the indenture itself.

The mortgage lien may be a first mortgage, in which case it takes priority over any other pledge of the mortgaged real estate by the hospital. If the first mortgage lien permits, the borrower may give other lenders a lien on the same property, either on a parity basis or subordinate to the first lien, that is, a second mortgage, and so on for each subsequent pledge. In some cases, the indenture will provide for the issuance of subsequent series of bonds secured on a parity with the first mortgage bonds. These subsequent series bonds will also be first mortgage bonds, and they will share equally and ratably in the property pledged as security for the first issue of bonds.

Leasehold Mortgage

If the hospital leases the ground on which its facilities are built, rather than owning the real estate, it may be able to provide security for a bond issue by pledging its interest in the long-term lease to the trustee.

If the trustee were to foreclose, it would obtain title to the leasehold interest and would have to continue to make rent payments in order to maintain possession of the facilities. The trustee, in turn, may choose to realize on the security by selling, assigning, or subleasing the leasehold interest; however, the trustee would have to abide by the terms of the lease concerning assignments and subleases. Pursuant to the mortgage, the leasehold mortgagee may be able to take possession and cure defaults if, for example, the facilities were to fall into disrepair. This would permit immediate action to prevent further dissipation of the collateral rather than the lengthy time period foreclosure would require.

A leasehold mortgage is subordinate to the landowner's right to receive rent payments from the borrower. In certain cases, it may be possible to have the owner of the real estate subordinate the right to receive rent to the lender's interest in the leasehold mortgage. If so, the lender will have a mortgage on the real estate itself.

Since a default in payment of rent by the hospital to the landlord would result in a termination of the lease and the subsequent loss of the leasehold mortgagee's security, the leasehold mortgagee will want full protection against such an occurrence. The leasehold mortgagee will require receipt of notice of any default and that notice be sent to the tenant as well. The mortgagee will also require the right to cure any default by the tenant.

Loan Agreement with a Negative Pledge

The use of the negative pledge as a form of security occurs most often when a hospital issues debt securities not secured by a mortgage or some other type of collateral. In essence the hospital issues direct obligation notes that are not secured by land, buildings, equipment, or furnishings of the hospital. In the event of default, the noteholders will have the status of unsecured creditors and will, therefore, be subordinate to the security position of any mortgage bonds previously issued by the hospital. The noteholders cannot foreclose on the properties of the hospital.

Therefore, in order to offer some protection to the noteholders, the indenture under which notes are issued will often contain a negative pledge agreement whereby the hospital agrees not to create any new debt secured by the real or personal property of the hospital unless the new debt is subordinate to the notes. The negative pledge may be an absolute prohibition of any new secured debt, or it may limit the amount of secured debt that can be created in the future. In this way the noteholders are able to maintain their priority.

Unsecured

In those instances in which a hospital has previously encumbered its property with outstanding mortgages it may be either impractical, because of a favorably low interest rate, or impossible, because of prepayment restrictions, to refinance its outstanding long-term secured debt. The hospital may, however, continue to borrow funds for construction or other purposes on an unsecured basis if the hospital has sufficient net worth and cash flow to service additional debt. The creditworthiness of the hospital is the primary factor in determining whether the hospital has the ability to market its unsecured notes to the public.

In the event of a default, the holders of unsecured notes will have the status of general unsecured creditors. All property of the borrower that is pledged to secure other debt generally will be unavailable to repay the unsecured notes in the event the hospital files for bankruptcy.

BASIC TERMS

The basic terminology of debt financing is common to both bond and note issues. Individual circumstances will tailor these common terms and conditions to the specific needs of the hospital undertaking the proposed financing. Items such as full or partial amortization, for example, must be considered in respect to the term of the proposed securities, the hospital's cash flow, and, of course, market conditions.

Term

The period of time the hospital has to repay its debt obligations is referred to as the term of the debt. Each issue of bonds or notes has a stated term or period over which such loan must be repaid. In cases of short-term debt, such as five-year bonds or notes, the hospital may be required to pay interest only (not principal) during the term. At the end of five years it must repay or refinance the total principal amount borrowed. Longer-term debt issues of ten to fifteen years generally amortize ("pay back") the principal partially or fully over the term of the loan.

Serial

Bonds or notes issued as serials have various interest rates and stated maturities. The entire term of the issue may be 15 years, for example. However, each serial within that term will have a stated maturity and a stated interest rate. Partial amortization of the bond or note issue is obtained through the use of serials. This type of financing offers the advantage of lower interest rates in the early years with slightly higher rates reserved for the longer maturities.

Sinking Fund

Bonds or notes requiring the periodic payment of funds to the trustee for use in redeeming the bonds or notes prior to maturity are called sinking fund bonds or notes. The trustee maintains a separate sinking fund account for the hospital and the hospital agrees to deposit sufficient funds to redeem a certain percentage of the bonds or notes each year.

Permitted Encumbrances

In the case of first mortgage bonds, the indenture securing the bonds usually provides for other encumbrances in addition to the lien of the indenture. These kinds of "permitted encumbrances" typically include:

- the lien of taxes and assessments not delinquent;
- easements, rights of way, zoning ordinances, licenses, reservations, or restrictions; and
- rights of lessors to, or purchase-money liens or charges upon, fixtures, equipment or other personal property leased or purchased under conditional sales, lease-purchase, or other security agreements.

Open-Ended Indenture

This kind of indenture allows a hospital to issue from time to time one or more series of bonds under the same indenture in addition to the initial series of bonds. Limitations and conditions for issuance of additional bonds are imposed on the hospital. The proceeds are often restricted to payment of the cost of construction or other acquisition of additions or improvements to the property of the hospital already subject to the lien of the indenture. Proceeds of such additional bonds may also be used for retiring existing indebtedness of the borrower.

An additional debt test imposes a restriction on the amount of additional bonds which may be issued by the borrower under the existing indenture. The aggregate principal amount of the additional bonds, together with the principal amount of all bonds outstanding after issuance of the additional bonds, is limited to a percentage of the fair value of all of the hospital's land, buildings, and equipment that is subject to the lien of the indenture. It is to the advantage of the hospital not to be too restricted; however, total mortgage debt amounting to 65 percent to 75 percent of fair value is not at all uncommon.

When the subsequent series of bonds is offered, a supplemental indenture, containing the particulars of such additional bonds, including the date of issuance, maturities, interest rates, payment dates, and redemption prices is executed by the hospital.

Other Debt Outstanding

In addition to the debt financed through the issuance of bonds, a hospital may have other debt outstanding, either at the time of issuance of the original bonds or at dates subsequent thereto. Other debt may be short-term, incurred in the ordinary course of business for the current operation, maintenance, and repair of the hospital's facilities, including advances from third party payers and obligations under reasonably necessary employment contracts. The hospital may also incur funded debt in addition to the bonds issued pursuant to the indenture. Funded debt is usually defined in the indenture, and it generally means all of the hospital's debt for borrowed money, or debt which has been incurred in connection with the acquisition of assets plus the capitalized value of the debt of the hospital under any lease of real or personal property which is capitalized in accordance with generally accepted accounting principles on the balance sheet of the hospital and which has a maturity of one year or more.

Funded debt is limited by a debt test, just as the amount of additional bonds that may be issued pursuant to an open-ended indenture is limited to a percentage of the fair value of the hospital's property subject to the lien of the indenture. Before additional funded debt can be incurred, the debt test may require that after giving effect to the issuance of funded debt, the ratio of funded debt to net worth is not more than 4.0 to 1.0.

Alternatively, the test may require that net income available for funded debt service in the last two fiscal years was not less than 125 percent, for example, of the hospital's maximum annual funded debt service requirement in respect to all funded debt outstanding after giving effect to the issuance of the additional funded debt.

In other cases, a hospital may be permitted to incur additional funded debt on the basis of a feasibility report which shows that the hospital's estimated average annual net income available for funded debt service during the three fiscal years following the issuance of the additional funded debt will not be less than 125 percent, for example, of the maximum annual funded debt service requirement of the hospital in respect to all funded debt outstanding after the issuance of the additional funded debt.

Call Provisions

The hospital may be limited in its ability to refinance its outstanding bonds due to specific prohibitions against redemption of those bonds during the early years of their term. These prohibitions may be complete in that no bonds may be redeemed for a period of one to five years from date of issue, or the prohibition may simply ban the use of borrowed funds to effect redemptions during the early years. In the latter case, the hospital may be further restricted to a specific amount of bonds which can be redeemed each year with its own funds. If the hospital exceeds the permitted amount, it must then pay a premium of usually 1 to 2 percent of the principal amount of the bonds redeemed in excess of the permitted amount.

The length of the call period varies; however, bond issues having maturities of 10 to 15 years will typically offer the investor call protection during the first 2 to 5 years. The length of the call period is primarily a marketing decision because investors want to lock in their rate of return for a specified period of time.

Merger or Acquisition

For-profit hospitals generally are prohibited during the term of the financed debt from acquiring other companies into themselves unless, after giving effect to such acquisition or merger, the hospital is in full compliance with the terms and conditions contained in the existing trust indenture. The typical debt tests, net worth requirements and dividend restrictions, would determine whether a merger or an acquisition could take place.

Nonprofit hospitals are not permitted to merge into any other corporation or convey substantially all of their hospital facilities or their properties and assets to any other corporation unless the surviving corporation is nonprofit and it assumes the outstanding debt of the hospital.

Property Included in Mortgage

A trust indenture securing repayment of first mortgage bonds contains a description of all of the hospital's property pledged to the trustee as collateral for the bond issue. Since the indenture is a recorded document, the public is put on notice of the trustee's interest in the hospital's property during the duration of the bond issue. Other lenders will be aware of the bondholder's prior interests and may not lend funds to the hospital unless they too obtain adequate security.

The pledged property may consist of real estate, all buildings and improvements on the real estate, and all fixtures, equipment, apparatus, and machinery located in or upon such land or buildings. Equipment subject to leases generally is not included in the lien of the indenture.

While each financing situation must be analyzed in light of the particular hospital's financial condition, there may be situations where, because the size of the contemplated debt is relatively small compared to the hospital's fair market value, the hospital is not required to pledge all of its real estate to the trustee. Furthermore, there may be situations where the hospital has pledged some of its property to secure other financings, and it still has property of sufficient value available to adequately secure additional borrowing.

After-Acquired Property

The lien of the typical first mortgage bond indenture also contains language intended to subject all of the hospital's property acquired after the issuance of its first mortgage bonds to the lien of the indenture. This is intended to provide additional security to the bondholders as the hospital's assets increase.

The lien of the trust indenture continues as long as any of the bonds remain outstanding. Often the indenture will provide for partial releases of property pledged to secure the bond issue. Typically, property that is no longer useful or is worn out may be released.

Releases

Complete release of the lien of the indenture occurs when all of the bonds are repaid. This may occur through redemptions or at the stated maturity dates. In either of these cases, the bonds themselves are paid and are no longer outstanding.

Some indentures will allow the hospital to deposit funds with the trustee that are sufficient to repay the bonds in their entirety. The indenture may have specific redemption provisions which will not permit the trustee to use the money deposited by the hospital immediately to repay the bondholders. In such cases, the indenture permits the trustee to release the lien of the indenture, hold the funds as security for the outstanding bonds, and pay the bondholders in due course according to the terms of the indenture. This arrangement is known as defeasance. The defeasance may be "net," or it may be "full cash." Net defeasance allows the hospital to deposit funds which will earn interest with the trustee. These funds, plus the earnings thereon, will be used to pay the principal and interest on the bonds to maturity. Full cash defeasance requires the hospital to deposit, in cash, funds equal to the full amount necessary to pay principal and interest on the bonds to maturity.

Chapter 15

Disclosure-Securities Law, The Official Statement, and Due Diligence

John Fenner, Thomas E. Lanctot, and Donna S. Wetzler

FEDERAL LAW

If the health care facility's bonds will be sold in a public offering, a prospectus (called an "official statement") for a tax-exempt bond issue is necessary for the offering. The official statement must disclose all material facts about the health care institution and the bond issue, just as a registered prospectus does for a for-profit corporation. (For-profit corporations sell their debt securities to the public through prospectuses registered with the Securities and Exchange Commission (the "SEC").)

Federal Statutes and Rules

Although tax-exempt hospital revenue bonds are exempt from the formalities of registration with the SEC by virtue of Section 3(a)(2) of the Securities Act of 1933, as amended (the "1933 Act"), the standard of disclosure is the same. Sections 10(b) and 15B of the Securities Exchange Act of 1934, as amended (the "1934 Act"), and Section 17(a) of the 1933 Act require the hospital and the underwriters[1] to disclose fully all material facts to the investing public.

For a number of political, practical, and constitutional reasons, governmental issuers of tax-exempt bonds are not required to register their securities with the SEC, but they are still subject to those antifraud provisions of Section 17(a) of the 1933 Act and Sections 10(b) and 15(c) of the 1934 Act.[2] Primary responsibility for disclosure rests with the hospital and the underwriters, but their attorneys and officers are also subject to liability for misstatements or failure to disclose.[3]

Rule 10b-5 under the 1934 Act[4] states the standard for disclosure in deceptively simple terms:

It shall be unlawful for any person, directly or indirectly, by the use of any means or instrumentality of interstate commerce, or of the mails, or of any facility of any national securities exchange,

(a) To employ any device, scheme, or artifice to defraud, or

(b) To make any untrue statement of a material fact *or to omit to state a material fact* necessary in order to make the statements made, in the light of the circumstances under which they were made, not misleading, or

(c) To engage in any act, practice, or course of business which operates or would operate as a fraud or deceit upon any person, in connection with the purchase or sale of any security.

Outright frauds or deceits are fairly rare, but the requirement not to omit any material fact leads to a great number of practical problems.

Material Facts

It is difficult to define in the abstract which facts are "material" to an offering. The usual formulation of "materiality" is that any fact to "which a reasonable man would attach importance in determining his course of action in the transaction in question" is material and must be disclosed.[5] An insight into this standard is contained in the statement: "I wish we did not have to disclose that to the purchasers. They may not want to buy the bonds."

It is vital that any such fact be disclosed to the potential purchasers of the hospital's bonds, completely and understandably. Because nonprofit hospitals do not usually make the well-publicized financial reports publicly owned corporations are required to make, the official statement is often the hospital's only introduction to the financial community and the bond-buying public. It must tell the hospital's full story, "warts and all."

Such a standard is easy to state, but harder to put into practice. Like most businesses, the hospital must cope with competition, rising prices for supplies, litigation, bad debts, pension funding, and employee relations. Unlike most businesses, the hospital is nonprofit, is heavily regulated by state and federal government agencies, often relies heavily on government reimbursement and has a number of imperatives in addition to accumulating a surplus.

Since liability and possible criminal penalties can result from any failure to include a fact later deemed to have been "material" at that time, all parties must take a conservative approach. Close cases are best resolved in favor of disclosure. It is relatively easy to include an item in the official statement, and potentially dangerous to omit a fact which a court may later decide was important. If an omitted fact is deemed material, questions as to whether the bond purchaser would have relied on that fact (if it had been disclosed) are moot. The omitted fact is presumed to have been "relied upon." [6]

The dangers inherent in any failure to disclose all material facts about a complicated entity such as the hospital operating in a changing and highly regulated environment have sometimes led to "overkill." Some official statements have become as thick (and as readable) as the Manhattan telephone directory. This is perfectly understandable, as conscientious counsel and other professionals strive to set forth anything about the hospital "which could go bump in the night." Fortunately, experienced underwriters, underwriters' counsel, bond counsel, and other experts have developed formats for disclosing the important facts about a hospital without requiring disclosure which is so detailed that it ceases to inform. [7]

It has become a standard part of the disclosure about the health care facility to include in the official statement both comparative financial statements and a financial feasibility study, in addition to a description of the hospital and of the legal documents used in the financing.

Financial Statements

At the heart of the official statement are the financial statements of the hospital. These include both audited statements for the three to five years preceding the offering, and unaudited statements for the period since the last audited figures, if this is more than three months prior to mailing of the official statement. The underwriters and the hospital's accountants use these statements to develop significant ratios and historical tables. These highlight important aspects of the hospital's financial condition and significant financial trends. Occupancy rates, the proportion of income derived from Medicare and Medicaid, and historical and pro forma debt service coverage ratios are some of the significant measuring rods of the hospital's financial condition. They give valuable clues about the hospital's ability to meet debt service payments in the future.

Because the participation of the hospital's outside auditors is critical to the success of an issue, they should be consulted at the earliest stages of a financing and retained on the "financing team" throughout the process. Even if the hospital will have recent audited financial statements at the proposed time of the offering, the auditors must verify or prepare the extracts from these statements. Continuing involvement helps to avoid the delays and extra expense of a last-minute rush, and makes it easier for the accountants to render their "cold comfort letter" at the closing.

Feasibility Studies

Another vital part of the official statement is the feasibility study. This is a report by an organization of independent experts of its projection of the hospital's future debt service coverage.

The feasibility consultant makes certain assumptions about the hospital, its market, state and federal regulations, general economic conditions, and other relevant matters. It then projects its estimate of the hospital's debt service coverage for the first two or three years after the project is finished. Of course, this estimate is carefully hedged and does not constitute a guaranty by the consultant or the hospital that this coverage will occur in those years, or even that the assumptions will prove to be accurate in the future. Nonetheless, the municipal bond market and the bond rating agencies have made feasibility studies a regular part of hospital official statements.

This practice has no ready analogy in corporate finance because the SEC has traditionally been cautious about allowing companies to make financial projections in prospectuses.[8] However, there would appear to be few abuses which have been connected to hospital feasibility studies by reputable and responsible feasibility consultants. As a practical matter, the municipal bond market and the bond rating agencies consider these studies to be important in evaluating a hospital's credit. Since a new project may dramatically affect both the earning power and the obligations of the hospital, even such an "educated guess" is useful and material.

Hospital management should work closely with the feasibility consultants and review their assumptions with great care, for many consultants state that the hospital is the principal source of these assumptions. Conservative, realistic assumptions make a study's conclusion more persuasive, particularly to the analysts and rating agencies that are an important audience for the official statement.

Description of the Hospital

This section of the official statement is the hospital's self-portrait. It covers matters such as the history of the hospital, its service area, special programs, medical staff, statistical comparisons with other hospitals in the area, brief biographies of senior administrators and the hospital's board, sources of patient revenues, accreditations, affiliations, the project, other properties, affiliates, and other planned major projects. The underwriters usually provide an outline of areas to be covered, and the hospital writes the first draft. The working group for the financing then polishes it to its final form. The result often is the most readable part of the official statement because it describes a unique, living institution—what it does today and its plans for the future.

Attorneys, Opinions, and Due Diligence

Aside from the financial statements and information (the province of the accountants) and the "business" terms of the issue (redemption and maturity schedules, etc.), lawyers tend to draft and review the balance of the official statement. This is probably inevitable, since the potential liabilities of the hospital and the underwriters for failure to disclose or misstatements of fact can be substantial. The bond purchase agreement usually requires counsel for the hospital and the issuer and bond counsel to give their opinions as to the completeness of the disclosure by the parts of the official statement prepared by them or their clients. Underwriters' counsel then generally furnishes its clients with its opinion to the effect that (after investigation, and relying on the opinions of other counsel where appropriate) nothing has come to its attention to indicate that the official statement misstates a material fact or fails to disclose a material fact which must be disclosed in order to make the official statement "not misleading."

In order to discover any facts which should be disclosed and to uncover any problems that should be solved before the closing, underwriters and their counsel conduct a "due diligence" review. Due diligence enables the underwriters to assert, if the need arises, that they used due diligence ("reasonable investigation" under Section 11(b) (3)(4) of the 1933 Act) to verify the statements made in the official statement and to discover additional material facts. Such investigations rarely turn up "the smoking gun," but they often uncover minor problems to be disposed of before the closing or matters which must be disclosed.

Particular Problems

Hospitals are highly regulated entities which must survive in an increasingly competitive environment. Government action has tended to hold down "medical costs" by restricting Medicare and Medicaid reimbursement, and by other measures. This leads to a unique set of potential problems that are of no concern to the average business corporation.

To remind investors of this dimension to hospital finance, underwriters, hospitals, and their counsel have developed language for a section of the official statement called "Bondholders' Risks." This section, sometimes informally referred to as the "Parade of Horribles," sets forth, in general terms, risks common to American hospitals in general and potential problems particular to hospitals operating in that state. A copy of a recent "bondholders' risks" portion of an official statement is attached as Appendix 15-A to this chapter.

Benefits from Disclosure

Complete and meaningful disclosure complies with the law and protects the participants in a financing from liability and possible criminal penalties. More importantly, full and exact disclosure creates a favorable impression with professional analysts working with the rating agencies and institutional investors, who review the hospital and its financing. These professionals tend to respond favorably to a hospital that understands itself and its problems, and is willing to confront these problems openly. Such a hospital will be better able to deal with the many uncertainties of the future.

STATE SECURITIES LAWS

In addition to federal securities statutes and regulation, every state in one form or another regulates the sale of securities. State securities laws are known as "blue sky" laws. These laws were first enacted in the early 1900s to restrain promoters who were, in the words of one judge, selling "lots in the blue sky." Blue sky laws are principally concerned with the prohibition of fraud, the registration of securities, and the registration of securities brokers and investment advisers. Only the antifraud provisions and securities registration requirements directly affect a hospital in raising capital. It seems unlikely that a hospital would sell its own securities directly and not through a securities broker or dealer, but if a hospital did engage in direct sales of its own securities, it would have to comply with any applicable broker and seller registration provisions.

Securities Fraud

Virtually every blue sky law provides that it is unlawful for any person, in connection with the offer, sale, or purchase of a security, to: (1) employ a device, scheme, or artifice to defraud; (2) make an untrue statement of a material fact or omit to state a material fact necessary in order to make the statements made, in light of the circumstances, not misleading; or (3) engage in an act, practice, or course of business that operates or would operate as a fraud or deceit upon a person. These standards are quite similar to the antifraud provisions under the federal securities laws.

The statutory remedies for a violation of blue sky antifraud provisions typically include rescission and criminal penalties. It is in part because of these antifraud provisions that lawyers for both the hospital and the underwriter will, through the due diligence process, attempt to verify statements made in any offering documents by examining hospital records and meeting with hospital officials to discover any omitted material information.

Securities Registration

Almost every state blue sky law requires that securities sold in that state be registered. However, every blue sky law exempts some kind of securities from the registration requirement. One of the most common exemptions from blue sky registration is the one for securities issued by governmental bodies. While general obligation state and municipal bonds are exempt from blue sky registration in every state, about 15 states have restricted in varying degrees the availability of such exemptions for revenue bonds issued by state and local governments on behalf of hospitals.

State regulatory interest in municipal bonds, and in revenue bonds in particular, has heightened in recent years because of New York City's financial problems and because of a general concern about the tremendous growth in the issuance of revenue bonds by state and local governments on behalf of private entities. Blue sky restrictions on publicly issued hospital revenue bonds take three forms: (1) requirements that such bonds be registered like any other nonexempt security; (2) requirements that any guaranty or other security arrangements issued or entered into by a hospital be registered; and (3) requirements that statutory exemptions be perfected through the filing of a description of the transaction, the official statement, the indenture, and the mortgage or loan agreement. Some states have required the review of otherwise exempt offerings by characterizing a guaranty or other security arrangement as a "separate security" requiring either registration or a separate exemption from registration. These guaranties or security arrangements are often automatically exempt because another typical blue sky exemption covers securities issued by not-for-profit corporations. However, several of these not-for-profit exemptions are conditioned on the perfection through the filing of various materials and review by the staff of the state securities administrator.

Some states will handle registration or exemption filings routinely, while others will scrutinize filings very carefully. A number of these states have promulgated regulations setting forth requirements for satisfying the exemptions. Blue sky authorities often will comment on the content of the official statement and other aspects of the proposed transaction and will impose additional disclosure or other requirements. A fee is sometimes required in connection with a filing.

The managing underwriter is typically responsible for complying with blue sky requirements in connection with a hospital revenue bond offering. Underwriters' counsel will survey the blue sky laws to determine whether a particular transaction complies with those laws, and, if not, to initiate the action necessary to achieve compliance. The blue sky survey is made and action initiated well before the mailing of the preliminary official statement. When the preliminary official statement is circulated, underwriters' counsel provides members of the underwriting syndicate with the preliminary blue sky memorandum, which, among other things, lists (1) the states in which the bonds may be sold to the public without registration; (2) the states in which action has been initiated so that the bonds may be sold to the public; and (3) transactions, typically sales to institutional purchasers, which are exempt from the blue sky laws of a particular state and thus do not require registration of the bonds. On the date that the bond purchase or underwriting agreement is signed, presumably the date upon which the underwriters also issue confirmations of sales of the bonds, a supplemental blue sky memorandum is delivered listing the states in which action was completed so that the bonds may be sold to the public. Occasionally a state in which a filing was made may refuse to allow registration, may deny an exemption, or will not have reviewed a filing by the time that the bond purchase agreement is executed. In such states, no sales may be made to the public. Sales may only be made in so-called "exempt transactions." Exempt transactions generally are sales to institutional purchasers, such as banks or other financial institutions, insurance companies, investment companies, or pension plans. The institutional purchasers who qualify for exempt transaction status are typically listed in the preliminary blue sky memorandum. It is sometimes possible to avoid the expense of lawyers' time and filing fees by not taking action in certain jurisdictions where the underwriters do not feel there will be a strong retail market, since the institutional market will almost always be available whether or not blue sky filings are made.

The purchase contract or underwriting agreement often provides that the hospital will defray some part or all of the expense of the blue sky qualification of the bonds sold on its behalf.

Legal Investment Laws

While not part of the actual blue sky laws, each state regulates by statute the legality of particular investments for savings banks, fiduciaries, and insurance companies. Underwriters' counsel is often called upon to provide the underwriters with a legal investment survey setting forth the eligibility for investment by such institutions of the particular securities being sold. In preparing such a survey, underwriters' counsel must examine the features of the bonds—the issuer, the security arrangements, interest payment features, and so on in order to determine the eligibility of such an investment. While a blue sky memorandum is always provided in connection with the sale of hospital revenue bonds, legal investment surveys are prepared at the managing underwriters' option. The legal investment survey assists the underwriting syndicate's sales force in determining whether the bonds may be sold to a particular type of institutional buyer, and also helps the underwriters in directing their marketing effort toward appropriate purchasers. However, the ultimate responsibility for determining whether a particular investment is permissible is with the purchaser and not with the underwriter. Each purchaser must decide for itself whether it is permitted to invest funds in particular securities.

DUE DILIGENCE

The term "due diligence" is one of the many mysterious bits of jargon bandied about during the initial meetings of any financing team. Its meaning and rationale are rarely, however, explained; rather, all a hospital generally learns about "due diligence" is that it creates pounds of photocopying, hours of phone calls, and days of visits by pesky young representatives of underwriters' counsel and bond counsel.

Rationale for Due Diligence

As discussed above, Section 11 of the 1933 Act provides that, in a transaction subject to securities registration, various parties may be subject to civil suit if the registration statement contains a material misstatement or omission. However, a sued party can interpose a defense to such actions if it can be shown that, after reasonable investigation, the sued party has reasonable grounds to believe, and did believe, that statements made in the registration statement were true and that there were no material omissions. This "reasonable investigation" is commonly known as due diligence.

Although tax-exempt financings are not registered under the 1933 Act and are therefore not subject to Section 11 liabilities, as discussed above, tax-exempt bond issues do remain subject to liabilities under Rule 10b-5 of the 1934 Act, under which rule it is unlawful "to make any untrue statement of a material fact or to omit to state a material fact necessary in order to make the statements made, in the light of the circumstances under which they were made not misleading." Underwriters and other parties undertake a due diligence investigation in tax-exempt transactions in an endeavor to assure themselves, through "reasonable investigation," that all material items have been accurately disclosed in the official statement (or in a private placement in the placement memorandum) and that no material disclosures have been omitted.

Practicalities of Due Diligence

Due diligence is done by the underwriters and their counsel and, in some cases, also by bond counsel and issuer's counsel. Due diligence with respect to hospital financings generally requires (1) participation in drafting sessions; (2) discussions with hospital administration, feasibility consultants, auditors, consultants, contractors, and architects (if a construction project is involved); (3) tour of hospital facilities; and (4) review of major contracts, operating permits, licenses, debt instruments, articles, bylaws, minutes, etc. Frequently, a formal "due diligence" meeting is held at which representatives of the underwriters, bond counsel, and the issuer are given an opportunity in a structured setting to question hospital representatives (usually, representatives of the hospital administration, staff, and board of directors, as well as accountants, feasibility consultants, architects, and contractors). A sample "due diligence" list of documents, which underwriters and other parties usually require the hospital to provide, is included as Appendix 15-B to this chapter.

Unfortunately, due diligence places fairly substantial time and labor burdens upon a hospital. Documents must be located and copies made; conferences must be scheduled; questions must be answered.

Equally unfortunate is the fact that due diligence investigations often do turn up problems that require attention and, in some cases, disclosure. It is in the interest of everyone on the financing team to identify these problems and to discuss them openly and honestly, since everyone involved in the transaction is subject to suit if full disclosure is not made.

Examples of Due Diligence "Finds"

In the course of doing due diligence, problems are often uncovered, including these "real-life" examples:

- *Defects in articles of incorporation.* In one financing, a review of the articles of incorporation showed that the corporate existence of the hospital was to terminate in 1990, ten years before the bonds to be issued were to mature. Obviously, there is a problem in an obligor disappearing midway through the performance of its obligations. It was a simple matter to amend the articles of incorporation and, since the discovery was made early, the deal was not delayed.

- *Defaults.* In one transaction, a review of outstanding debt instruments revealed that the hospital was in default under all of them. Even though these obligations were to be paid off with bond proceeds, a determination was made that these defaults were material and should be disclosed.

- *Litigation.* After inquiries from counsel, hospital administration and general counsel gave assurances that no major litigation existed. In order to be extracautious, counsel to the hospital's insurance carrier was contacted. Such counsel was less sanguine about the outcome of a malpractice case he was handling; he could not give an opinion that the damages claimed in the case would not be "material." Disclosure regarding this litigation was added to the official statement.

- *Bylaws.* It was learned in the course of due diligence that a hospital's bylaws prohibited directors from any business relationship with the hospital. The chairman of the board, however, was also general counsel to the hospital; he saw to it that the bylaws were quickly amended.

- *Staffing.* In a discussion of one hospital's efforts at nurse recruitment, the question of the hospital's current staffing needs arose. At that point, it was revealed to the financing team that 22 beds had been closed for a year because of insufficient nursing personnel. This was, of course, a matter that was disclosed in the official statement, as well as the hospital's stepped-up efforts to recruit nurses and other professional staff members.

- *Facilities.* In a routine discussion with a hospital as to any problems it might have that should be discussed, the hospital informed the underwriter that a portion of the hospital facility had serious structural deficiencies requiring immediate, expensive remedial action. This information, besides resulting in substantial disclosure, also caused the postponement of the financing.

Other Due Diligence Problem Areas

In addition to the "smoking guns" discussed above, underwriter's counsel also often discovered problems requiring remedies and disclosures in the following areas:

- *Certificate-of-need and health planning problems.* Frequently, the certificate-of-need and other health planning applications by the hospital will not have been adequate either in the amount requested or their inclusion of the financing costs associated with the bond issue. A due diligence review should reveal these problems and alert the hospital to the need for amendments. In addition, it is important to disclose the possibility that the actual construction cost may exceed the certificate of need amount and that an amendment would then have to be requested after the issuance of the bonds. Although such amendments are almost invariably granted, the risk that the project may not be completed must be disclosed.

- *Title problems and description of property.* Due diligence review occasionally will uncover title and property description problems that will have to be corrected prior to closing. The due diligence review should include a check to see that the proposed construction project will be situated on the property actually leased or mortgaged.

NOTES

1. Section 15B of the 1934 Act deals with the responsibility of underwriters and the establishment of the Municipal Securities Rulemaking Board (the "MSRB"). Section 15B was added in 1975 in the wake of the financial problems of New York City to regulate the sellers of tax-exempt municipal bonds. MSRB Rule 32 requires any underwriter to deliver a copy of the official statement to every purchaser of an initial offering of bonds.

2. *See* the excellent discussion by Judge O'Connor of the interrelationships between the various federal securities laws and tax-exempt finance in Woods v. Homes & Structures of Pittsburgh, Kansas, 489 F. Supp. 1270 (D. Kan. 1980).

3. *Id.* at 1278. Although Judge O'Connor applied and quoted the statements in Woodward v. Metro Bank of Dallas, 522 F.2d 84 (5th Cir. 1975), to the effect that a party not owing a specific duty to disclose may be required to have a higher degree of knowledge of improper disclosure before it is held liable, he remanded for further hearings the question of whether the trustee bank and the issuer's general counsel, both of which made no representations, should have known about (and disclosed) a fraud (Woods v. Homes & Structures, *id.* at 1279, 1283). *See also* Stolser v. Lokken, C.C.H. Fed. Securities Law Reptr. ¶98,209 (8th Cir. 1981).

4. 17 C.F.R. § 240 10b-5 (1980).

5. SEC v. Texas Gulf Sulphur Co., 401 F.2d 833 (2d Cir., 1968), quoting *Restatement of Torts* § 538(2)(a) and other authorities.

6. Affiliated Ute Citizens of Utah v. United States, 406 U.S. 128, 92 S.Ct. 1456, 31 L.Ed. 2d 741 (1972).

7. Daley, Joseph C. *A Guide to Municipal Official Statements* (New York: Law and Business, Inc./Harcourt, Brace, Javanovich, 1980); and *Disclosure Guidelines for State and Local Governments* (Chicago: Municipal Finance Officers Association, 1979).

8. SEC 1933 Act Release No. 5992 and 1934 Act Release No. 15305 (November 7, 1978); and 1933 Act Release No. 6084 and 1934 Act Release No. 15944 (June 25, 1979).

Appendix 15-A

Bondholders' Risks

The bonds are payable solely from the payments to be made by the corporation pursuant to the loan agreement and from certain moneys available under the indenture. The forecasts of future revenues and expenses are only for a limited period, and, while they are based upon assumptions the corporation believes are reasonable and appropriate, the operations of the corporation are subject to conditions which may change in the future to an extent that cannot be determined at this time. Thus, no assurance can be given that the forecasted results will be attained for the forecast period or any period thereafter.

GENERAL

The forecasts of future revenues and expenses of the corporation and the realization of such forecasts are subject to, among other things, the capabilities of the management of the corporation, the confidence of physicians in the corporation, receipt of grants and contributions, changes in the economic conditions of the corporation's service areas, the level and restrictions on federal funding of Medicare and federal and state funding of Medicaid, imposition of government wage and price controls, the demand for the corporation's services, competition, rates, government regulation and licensing requirements, and future economic (including the impact of inflation) and other conditions which are unpredictable and may not be quantifiable or determinable at this time.

NO CONSTRUCTION CONTRACTS YET SIGNED

No construction contracts have yet been signed for construction of the projects. Should the construction contract price amounts exceed the amounts approved through certificates of need and § 1122 approval letters, amendments to such approvals would have to be obtained prior to commencing those projects. There is no assurance that such amendments can be obtained.

PROJECT COMPLETION

If completion of the projects should be delayed beyond the period estimated therefor, the cost thereof could be increased, and "capitalized" interest could be depleted. This could adversely affect the ability of the corporation to receive revenues and to make the required payments under the loan agreement for project completion and debt service. Furthermore, increases in project costs due to modifications in any project as directed by the corporation or other causes within or beyond the control of the corporation could affect the ability of the corporation to complete the projects within the projected time or within the cost estimates presently contemplated. The corporation has not yet entered into a guarantied maximum price contract with a contractor for any of the projects. There is no assurance that such contracts could be entered into for the amount presently allocated to the projects or that, under some circumstances, a guarantied maximum price would not be increased.

GOVERNMENT REGULATION ON THE HOSPITAL INDUSTRY

Recent Enactments

On August 13, 1981, President Reagan signed the Omnibus Budget Reconciliation Act of 1981, Public Law 97-3982, which will reduce the funding for governmental health care programs over the next three fiscal years. The nature of the reductions is numerous and varied. The Congressional Budget Office estimates for fiscal year 1982 that these spending reductions for hospital reimbursement will be $187 million to $262 million under Medicare and $325 million to $347 million under Medicaid. Specific program modifications include, but are not limited to, a change in the Medicaid hospital reimbursement formula and a new limitation on reimbursement for outpatient hospital services under Medicare. Determinations as to the precise impact of this reduced governmental funding, if any, on the corporation will depend on the extent to which the corporation has specific services and programs directly affected by the areas of reduced funding. The Reagan administration has announced its intention to reduce Medicare and Medicaid reimbursement further. The precise form and amounts of those reductions is not now known.

Medicare, Medicaid, Blue Cross, and Other Reimbursement Arrangements

As noted above, for the fiscal year ended August 31, 1981, the corporation received ____ percent of its patient service revenue from the federal Medicare program, ____ percent from the state's Medicaid program, and ____ percent from Blue Cross and other insurance. The revenues of the corporation could be adversely affected should the federal government, the state, or Blue Cross substantially decrease the moneys available for these programs or alter the terms for reimbursement.

Changes resulting from the 1972 amendments to the Social Security Act permit the Secretary of Health and Human Services to set limits on the amount of costs to be reimbursed under the Medicare and Medicaid programs. Should a hospital's actual costs for these services exceed the specified limits, the hospital would not be reimbursed for such excesses unless it were eligible for an exception, exemption, or adjustment as permitted by the regulations. Additionally, the 1972 amendments limit reimbursement to the lower of reasonable costs or customary charges. If reasonable costs exceed customary charges, such excess costs may not be reimbursed under the Medicare and Medicaid programs. Medicare regulations permit retroactive adjustment to settlements made in prior years. Such action may result in reduced revenue in the year in which such adjustments are made. Based on the present scheduling of limits and the present relationship between the corporation's reasonable costs and customary charges, the corporation does not anticipate that its actual costs will exceed the applicable limits. The corporation cannot predict the effect, if any, that the future changes in the reimbursement system might have on its operations.

Other Federal Proposals

From time to time, bills are introduced into Congress which could result in limitations on hospital revenues or operations, including those of the corporation. Also from time to time, proposals have been introduced into Congress which would establish some form of national health insurance which, if enacted, could adversely affect the revenues and operations of hospitals, including those of the corporation.

OTHER CONSIDERATIONS

Competition and Factors Decreasing Utilization; Population Changes

Competition from other health care providers now or hereafter located in the corporation's service area could adversely affect the corporation's operations. In addition, development of health maintenance organizations, future medical and other scientific advantages resulting in decreased usage of inpatient hospital facilities, and efforts by insurers, employer-purchasers of health care insurance, and governmental agencies to reduce utilization of hospital facilities by such means as preventive medicine, improved occupational health and safety standards, and more extensive utilization of outpatient care could adversely affect the operation of the corporation. The corporation could also be adversely affected by economic trends and shifts of the population in the corporation's service areas.

Labor Relations

Nonprofit hospitals and their employees came under the jurisdiction of the National Labor Relations Board in 1974. At the present time the corporation has no union contracts. Any substantial increase in the federal minimum wage or shortage of qualified professional personnel could cause an increase in the corporation's payroll costs beyond those projected. The corporation cannot control the prevailing wage rates in its service area, and any increase in such rates will directly affect its costs of operation.

Malpractice Costs

The number of malpractice suits and the dollar amount of patient damage recoveries have been increasing nationwide, resulting in substantial increases in malpractice insurance. Changes in the availability and cost of malpractice insurance and the cost of paying self-insured claims directly could directly (and indirectly, by affecting the number of practicing physicians) adversely affect the operating results of the corporation.

Special Purpose Buildings

The hospital facilities are not general-purpose buildings and would not generally be suitable for industrial or commercial use. If it were necessary to foreclose a judgment lien on the hospital facilities under the "forced sale conditions'' that are present in a foreclosure context, the real property of the hospital facilities might provide less than full value to the trustee. In addition, the hospital facilities may be subject to restrictions limiting the use thereof to hospital purposes, and consequently it could be difficult to find a purchaser for these facilities.

Tax-Exempt Status; Federal Income Tax

Taxing authorities in certain jurisdictions have sought to impose or increase taxes related to the property and operations of nonprofit organizations, including hospitals, particularly where such authorities are dissatisfied with the amount of service provided to indigents.

At the federal level, the Internal Revenue Service has ruled in Revenue Ruling 69-545 that the tax-exempt status of nonprofit hospitals is not dependent upon their acceptance of patients who cannot pay. The corporation believes its service to indigents is adequate, but it is possible that future administrative or judicial proceedings will require the corporation to increase its services to indigent patients in order to retain its tax-exempt status.

Market for Securities

Subject to prevailing market conditions the underwriters intend, but are not obligated, to make a market in the bonds. There is presently no secondary market for the bonds, and no assurance that a secondary market will develop. Consequently, investors may not be able to resell the bonds purchased should they need or wish to do so for emergency or other purposes.

Issuance of Additional Securities

The indenture permits the authority to issue additional bonds and the corporation to issue parity debt.

Enforceability of Remedies

The practical realization of any rights upon any default will depend upon the exercise of various remedies specified in the indenture. These remedies, in certain respects, may require judicial action, which is often subject to discretion and delay. Under existing law, certain of the remedies specified in these documents may not be readily available or may be limited. A court may decide not to order the specific performance of the covenants contained in these documents. Also, certain judicial decisions have cast doubt upon the right of the trustee, in the event of the corporation's bankruptcy, to collect and retain accounts receivable from Medicare, Medicaid, and other government programs.

Recent revisions of the federal bankruptcy laws may have an adverse effect on the ability of the trustee and the bondholders to enforce their claim to the security in the corporation's gross receipts granted by the loan agreement and indenture. Federal bankruptcy law permits adoption of a reorganization plan even though it has not been accepted by the holders of a majority in aggregate principal amount of the bonds, if the bondholders were provided with the benefit of their original lien or the "indubitable equivalent." In addition, if the bankruptcy court concluded that the bondholders had "adequate protection," it could (1) substitute other security for the security provided by the loan agreement and the indenture for the benefit of the bondholders and (2) subordinate the lien of the bondholders (a) to claims by persons supplying goods and services to the bankrupt after bankruptcy and (b) to the administrative expenses of the bankruptcy proceeding. In the event of the bankruptcy of the corporation, the amount realized by the bondholders might depend on the bankruptcy court's interpretation of "indubitable equivalent" and "adequate protection" under the then-existing circumstances.

Appendix 15-B

Due Diligence Review—Basic Documents Required

1. a. Corporate bylaws
   b. Corporate articles and charter
2. Corporate minutes
   a. Resolution authorizing sale of bonds
   b. Any reference to planned construction
   c. Any reference to financial matters
   d. Any reference to labor problems or changes in administrative personnel
   e. Any other matter which might reflect on creditworthiness of hospital
   f. Any reference to outstanding bonds or other debt
3. Specimen signatures of officers
4. Corporate seal imprint
5. Architect's sketch or existing photographs
6. Project approval letters from health planning agencies
7. Any certificates of need (CON) and CON applications
8. State hospital license
9. Internal Revenue Service tax exemption letter
10. Health and Human Services, Medicare, and Medicaid participation letters
11. Construction contract
12. Construction bonds
13. Architect's contract
14. Accreditation letter
15. Certificate of Secretary of State stating that the hospital association is a nonprofit corporation in good standing
16. Insurance policies and proof policies are still active; all policies including
    a. Fire and other types of damage insurance

    b. Professional liability insurance
    c. Workers' compensation
    d. Business interruption insurance
17. Blue Cross contract
18. Any outstanding debt documents, including guaranties
19. Any affiliation or shared services agreement
20. Audit letters
21. Audited financial statements for last five years

Chapter 16

Tax-Exempt Financing for Nonsection 501(c)(3) Health Care Facilities

John Fenner

Much of the foregoing discussion has assumed that the hospital is an organization exempt from taxes under Section 501(c)(3) of the Internal Revenue Code of 1954, as amended (the "Code"). Section 501(c)(3) organizations may have tax-exempt bonds issued for their current capital projects without limitation on the total amount of the issue.

However, all other health care institutions financing capital projects with the proceeds of tax-exempt bonds are limited by Section 103(b)(6) of the Code. If these institutions have tax-exempt bonds issued for them, the bonds must qualify under this "small issue exemption." Bonds issued under this exemption are commonly referred to as "industrial revenue bonds" or "IRBs." Section 103(b)(6) restricts the size of bond issues for proprietary and other health care institutions to a maximum of $10 million under ideal circumstances, and may prevent many institutions from financing more than $1 million on a tax-exempt basis.

WHO MUST USE THE "SMALL ISSUE EXEMPTION"?

Nonqualifying Facilities

Even 501(c)(3) entities must use the small issue exemption for certain projects. Section 501(c)(3) corporations may issue tax-exempt bonds for their capital projects in unlimited amounts only if the facilities are used "with respect to a trade or business carried on by such organization which is *not an unrelated trade or business,* determined by applying section 513(a) to such organization."[1] If nonqualifying facilities amount to more than 25 percent of the bond issue, the Internal Revenue Service (the "IRS") will treat the entire bond issue as a small-issue IRB.

The most frequent nonqualifying facility is a physician's office building. The IRS has ruled that these are used in the trade or business of physicians, and not in the operations of the 501(c)(3) not-for-profit hospital.[2] Other "non-501(c)(3)" facilities which may not be financed with tax-exempt bonds in unlimited amounts are shared laundry facilities,[3] facilities earning unrelated business income, and facilities subject to long-term management contracts by non-501(c)(3) organizations where compensation is tied to "profitability" of the facilities.[4] In this last situation, the IRS has stated that proprietary management companies may be the "principal user of the facilities financed," and that the facilities may not be financed with tax-exempt bonds except under the small-issue exemption.

Other Nonprofit Entities

Since Section 103(b)(3) of the Code defines an "exempt person" as only a "governmental unit" or "an organization described in Section 501(c)(3) and exempt from tax under Section 501(a)," other nonprofit entities must use the small-issue exemption as well. Such nonprofit organizations include many health maintenance organizations or shared service organizations receiving their tax exemptions under other subsections of the Code.

Proprietary Facilities

Of course, proprietary or investor-owned health care facilities, hospitals, or nursing homes are restricted to the small-issue exemption for tax-exempt financing.

THE "SMALL-ISSUE EXEMPTION"

Capital Expenditures Limits

Section 103(b)(6) of the Code limits the amount of all industrial revenue bonds to an aggregate of $10 million for any "nonexempt" organization or its "related persons" for facilities within the same incorporated municipality. In addition, if the bonds to be issued are for more than $1 million, the "principal user" of the project is limited in the amount of the capital expenditures it has paid or incurred, or will pay or incur, within that incorporated municipality for the six-year period beginning three years before the date of the bond issue and three years after the bond issue. The total amount of "capital expenditures" (broadly defined) plus the amount of the bond issue may not exceed $10 million at any time during this six-year period. If it exceeds $10 million, the interest on the bonds becomes subject to federal income taxation.[5] (These restrictions apply to tax-exempt bonds for any manufacturing or commercial facility.)

These limitations only apply to capital expenditures in the same incorporated municipality. If the facility is not located in an incorporated area, the relevant area for determination is all the unincorporated areas of the county or parish in which the facility is located.

All capital expenditures must be counted if they were made with respect to facilities located in the same incorporated municipality if the principal user of such facilities is or will be the same person as (or a related person to) the principal user of the facilities financed out of the proposed bond issue. Capital expenditures or bonds issued for continuous or integrated facilities on both sides of a border between two or more political jurisdictions may also have to be considered in determining whether either limit has been exceeded.

Capital Expenditures

As noted below, certain capital costs that cannot be financed and many other expenditures not related directly to the project may also constitute "capital expenditures" for the purpose of this determination. Briefly, every expenditure which could be capitalized under any section or election under the Code must be included within the $10 million limit. Capital expenditures must be counted if they are paid or incurred within the six-year period, even though the hospital currently deducted them as expenses, and the face amount of outstanding bonds issued under the small-issue exemption must also be counted regardless of when such bonds were issued.

All capital expenditures may not be financed out of bond proceeds. Expenditures can be financed out of bond proceeds only if they are properly attributable to the project (and qualified under state law) and if:

1. they are properly capitalized as part of the basis of land costs or property of a character subject to the allowance for depreciation under Section 167 of the Code; or
2. under applicable Code provisions, they could have been capitalized as part of the basis of land or property of a character subject to the allowance for depreciation if the hospital had elected, or would have been so capitalized but for an election by the hospital to deduct such expenditures; or
3. they are incurred in connection with the issuance and sale of the bonds.

Principal User

The IRS has specified that a "principal user" is considered to be any person (or corporate entity) who uses more than 10 percent of either the area of the project[6] or 10 percent of the value of the project (which can be measured by rent[7]) in its trade or business. Consequently, there can be several principal users of the same project. The lessor of a project is usually a principal user, and major tenants may be principal users.

However, most capital expenditures of a Section 501(c)(3) nonprofit corporation are not considered in the $10 million limit even if the "not-for-profit" is a principal user of the project as owner.[8] This is because 501(c)(3) corporations are "exempt persons" as defined in Code Section 103(b)(3). This can be a significant benefit to a large hospital contemplating a nonqualifying capital project (such as a physicians' office building) for less than $10 million under the small-issue exemption. The hospital's other capital expenditures in the municipality can be ignored, particularly if the hospital owns or leases the project through a separate corporation. An exception to this exception is that the expenditures of the not-for-profit corporation at the project site must be included.[9]

Need for Early Official Action by the Issuer

A 1980 Revenue ruling on an exempt small issue provides that a facility may not be financed if the acquisition or construction thereof commenced prior to this adoption of a "bond resolution" or the taking of "some other official action" by the issuer.[10]

It is therefore vital that the issuer of the bonds adopt a resolution expressing the intent of the issuer to issue the bonds ("official action") before the hospital orders any equipment or materials or (if possible) signs a contract for the acquisition or construction of any part of the project.

If the acquisition of land has commenced, such as by execution of a contract (which is not subject to cancellation if tax-exempt financing is not obtained or is obtained with limited liability) prior to the date of the official action, it may not be possible to have the purchase cost financed. However, if the hospital has an option to purchase, or a contract to purchase where the hospital's liability is limited to a 10 percent down payment, the purchase cost may be financed if the closing occurs after official action.[11] Contracts subject to conditions should be examined on a case-by-case basis.

Even if it is determined that such costs, including land acquisition costs, cannot be financed, they constitute capital expenditures for purposes of the $10 million limitation.

COMPOSITE ISSUES

There is presently no overall national limitation on the total amount of IRBs which can be issued for one entity, and the $10 million capital expenditure limitation only applies to the facilities within a particular incorporated municipality. As a result, many proprietary chains of hospitals or nursing homes have been able to use IRBs successfully in a number of different areas in the country. Their facilities are generally smaller than those of major metropolitan hospitals so that their total financing needs and capital expenditures for each facility do not typically exceed $10 million.

The IRS has issued Proposed Regulations[12] restricting the ability of nonexempt persons (including chains of proprietary hospitals or nursing homes) from marketing several of these issues at once. These issues can still be marketed separately.

Choice of State Law

A health care institution interested in bonds issued under the small issue exemption often has some latitude in choosing between various state enabling acts and potential governmental issuers. Experienced bond counsel should be consulted to discover alternatives and to explore the advantages and disadvantages of any competing options.

Possible Federal Restrictions on IRBs

In recent years legislation has been introduced which would greatly restrict the use of IRBs for "commercial" projects.[13] Although some of this legislation explicitly exempts "nursing and personal care facilities" and "hospitals" from its initial cutbacks, it would permit no more IRBs to be issued after December 31, 1983.

The Reagan Administration has also proposed legislation to prevent users of small-issue IRBs from also using the accelerated cost recovery system (accelerated depreciation) for their projects and to limit the total amount of capital expenditures of the principal user and related persons to $20 million worldwide.[14] This proposal would not exempt health care projects. Other congressional representatives have also expressed an interest in restricting "private use" IRBs.

At this time it is impossible to say what the future of this type of tax-exempt bond issue will be.

IRB—COMPLICATED BUT USEFUL

The IRS has never been enthusiastic about the use of IRBs. As a result, the maze of IRB restrictions and regulations requires the guidance of experienced counsel. At the same time, IRBs are a versatile and flexible tool for solving a number of financing problems, even for a major 501(c)(3) hospital. For smaller proprietary health care institutions and many health maintenance organizations, they are an indispensable financing tool.

NOTES

1. I.R.C. § 103(b)(3)(B) (emphasis supplied).

2. Kirkpatrick v. U.S., 79-2 U.S. Tax Cases § 9582 (10th Cir., 1979).

3. HCSC Laundry v. U.S., 450 U.S. 1, 101 S.Ct. 836, 67 L.Ed.2d 1 (1981).

4. Rev. Procs. 82-14 and 82-15.

5. I.R.C. § 103(b)(6).

6. IRS Private Letter Rulings 7952184, 8042033, and 8124136.

7. IRS Private Letter Rulings 8112071 and 7938040.

8. Treasury Rev. Rul. 74-289 (1974) and Private Letter Rulings 8008221 and 8012090.

9. *Ibid.*

10. Treasury Rev. Rul. 80-227 (1980).

11. Treasury Rev. Rul. 81-167 (1981).

12. Proposed Treasury Regulation § 1.103-7(b)(6) and Examples (16), (17), and (18), published in the *Federal Register* on October 8, 1981.

13. H.R. 4420 (97th Cong., 1st Sess.), introduced on September 9, 1981 by Reps. Rangel, Gibbons, and Moore.

14. U.S. Department of the Treasury, "General and Technical Explanations of Tax Revisions and Improved Collection and Enforcement Proposals" (Washington, D.C., Treasury release, February 26, 1982).

Chapter 17

Credit Strengthening: Special Considerations

Geoffrey B. Shields

As financing for hospitals has matured, investment bankers and lawyers specializing in health care finance have developed a number of means to strengthen the credit, and thereby lower the interest rate, on the bonds of a particular hospital. It is likely that in coming years additional techniques will develop to improve credit strength of health care facilities. These credit strengthening techniques sometimes involve credit pooling through the "piggybacking" of a health care institution's credit on the credit of other health care institutions. In addition to these credit pooling techniques, there have developed third-party credit strengthening techniques such as insurance and letters of credit which, in essence, substitute, for a fee to the hospital, the credit of an insurance company or bank for that of the hospital.

A hospital should talk to its investment banker about methods of credit strengthening and credit pooling.

CREDIT POOLING

"Credit pooling" is a generic term used to describe techniques that bundle security from several institutions so that their combined creditworthiness is improved. For example, affiliation or merger with other hospitals can strengthen a hospital's credit. Partially because of the need to borrow substantial amounts of money in the cheapest available mode, some of the loose-knit affiliations of hospitals have moved to strengthen the central control over their member hospitals. (Generally, there have also been other reasons for the strengthening of control, including the ability to form better banking relationships, the ability to attract management, and the economies of centralized purchasing.)

One of the best known examples of merging fairly loosely affiliated hospitals under centralized control is the Adventist Health System structure which today has four regional groups of Adventist hospitals. The Adventist Health System/Sunbelt, for instance, includes the Adventist hospitals in Florida, Georgia, Kentucky, Tennessee, Texas, Oklahoma, and New Mexico. This particular system is noted for a very strong flagship hospital, the 919-bed Florida hospital in Orlando, and many other smaller hospitals which it owns or manages. These smaller hospitals range in size from 28 beds to 307 beds. Adventist Health System/Sunbelt, with the assistance of its investment bankers, decided in 1979 to merge its flagship hospital with six of its other hospitals, which ranged in size from 100 beds to 307 beds, together into one corporation. The reason for this merger was to strengthen the credit of the smaller hospitals to permit them to borrow through the issuance of tax-exempt bonds at an attractive interest rate. This method worked, and a number of hospitals that would have been unable to receive an investment grade rating before the merger benefited from the A-1 rating from Moody's Investors Service and the A rating from Standard & Poor's Corporation received by the consolidated corporation after the merger. Adventist Health System/Sunbelt has since merged into this central corporation several other hospitals as they have developed financing needs. The merged entity has retained its credit ratings.

By merging all or several of their facilities, a number of other multihospital systems have had similar success in obtaining investment grade ratings and correspondingly attractive interest rates for the financing of new facilities at hospitals which, on their own, would be unable to borrow money at attractive rates.

For a variety of reasons, some hospital systems are unwilling to enter into a complete corporate merger of their hospitals. In these instances, several techniques are available for strengthening the credit of the member hospitals.

GUARANTIES

Parent/Child Guaranties

If a central entity, such as a church or a religious order, has the ability to designate the board of trustees of each of the hospitals of its multihospital group, then a guaranty from that entity of the debt of each of the hospitals may be a credit-strengthening device. Through control of membership of the board of trustees of its member hospitals, the religious entity can, subject to various limitations, force money up to itself and reassign it to other hospitals over which it has control. Thus, its guaranty of the debt of its member hospitals is a credit pooling device.[1]

Brother/Sister Guaranties

Similarly, brother/sister guaranties by health care corporations that share services can be a credit-strengthening device. For example, in a recent life care financing the facility being financed shared a campus with two other health care institutions. A common religious entity controlled all three health care institutions. The brother health care institutions provided guaranties for their borrowing sister corporation's debt. Sometimes, brother/sister guaranties are incorporated into a master-indenture financing structure. Every system hospital that is a signatory to the master-indenture becomes a guarantor or co-obligor of the debt of the other signatories.

Affiliate Guaranties

Guaranties are also used as a mechanism for regulating transfer of assets to affiliated corporations. Frequently "transfer to affiliates language" contained in long-term debt documents provides for a guaranty from the transferee to the bond trustee in the amount of the transferred assets or the present value of these assets at the time of exercise of the guaranty, whichever is greater.[2]

Guaranties from a Major Tertiary Care Hospital

Guaranties are sometimes used to strengthen the credit of a particular hospital. Sometimes, a large, financially strong hospital will offer its credit umbrella as a way of attracting satellite or affiliated hospitals. This offer has taken a variety of forms. One model is the outright acquisition of the satellite's facility with a leaseback of the facility after the new project has been completed at a lease price equivalent to the debt service on the bonds for the new project.

A second model is a guaranty by the tertiary care hospital of all or a part of the debt service of the affiliate hospital. These guaranties range from all debt service payments when due, to lesser guaranties such as one year's maximum principal and interest on the bonds. The tertiary care hospital will often require that should it have to make payments on its guaranty it will be able to intervene in the management of the affiliate hospital. Such an arrangement can be very attractive for a small or start-up facility that cannot obtain an investment grade bond rating on its own.

Legal Considerations of Guaranties

In each type of guaranty (parent/child, brother/sister, and affiliate) certain legal conditions must be met to assure the enforceability of the guaranty.

A guaranty is simply a type or kind of contract in which one promises to answer for the debt, default, or miscarriage of another. It is an undertaking or promise on the part of one entity that is used as collateral to a primary or principal obligation on the part of another and that binds the promisor (guarantor) to performance in the event of nonperformance by such other, the latter being bound to perform primarily.

A transaction of guaranty necessarily involves at least three parties: a promisor; a creditor (the party to whom the promise is made); and a debtor (the party entering into the principal obligation). Since the guaranty is the collateral obligation, there must be two contracts—one being that of the principal debtor and the other that of the guarantor. Since the debtor is not a party to the guaranty and the guarantor is not a party to the principal contract, both contracts should meet all the requirements of contract law, each in its own right.

The principal requirement of contract law is that consideration must exist in order to have an enforceable contract. There may be some concern that, because a corporation may be guarantying debt that provides no benefit to the corporation, consideration may be lacking in the guaranty agreements.

Generally, any consideration that would be sufficient under contract law will sustain a guaranty agreement. For instance, the payment of money to the guarantor is sufficient consideration. A promise of guaranty from shareholders of a corporation is also supported by consideration because of the benefit the shareholders derive from the loan to the corporation. However, it is not necessary to have consideration or a benefit moving directly to the guarantor in order to have an enforceable guaranty.

The guaranty contract between the guarantor and the creditor can also be supported by the detrimental reliance of the creditor (and the resulting benefit to the debtor) in loaning the money. As a result of this detrimental reliance concept, rules specifically applying to guaranties have been developed in common law. A well-accepted rule now exists, and is best stated as follows:

Where the contract of guaranty is made before or at the same time as the principal contract, and both contracts form parts of the same transaction, one consideration is sufficient for both the principal and the collateral contract and there need not be any other consideration than that moving between the guarantee (creditor) and the principal contract; and in some jurisdictions this rule is prescribed by statute. *In accordance with this rule, where a guaranty of payment of a note is made before or at the time of the execution of the note, the consideration for the note is the consideration for the guaranty, and no further consideration is necessary.* . . .

Although a contract of guaranty is executed subsequently to the principal contract, it is regarded as being made at the same time so as to constitute a part of the same transaction and be supported by the same consideration, where it is executed pursuant to an understanding had before and is an inducement to the execution of the principal contract; or where it is delivered before any obligation or liability is incurred under the principal contract; or where it is made pursuant to some provision in the principal contract; or where the principal contract does not become operative until the execution of the guaranty; or where the contract of guaranty expressly refers to a previous agreement between the principal debtor and the creditor which is executory in its character and embraces prospective dealings between the parties.[3]

Thus, the requisite consideration in connection with a guaranty may be summarized as follows:

1. If executed on or before the execution of the primary debt obligation, the guaranty is generally enforceable if induced by and given in consideration of the primary debt obligation.
2. If executed subsequent to the execution of the primary obligation, it may be enforceable if supported by additional consideration or if an understanding existed prior to the primary debt execution.
3. Any detriment incurred by the creditor which is induced by the guarantor will support the guaranty.

Since the guaranties and the principal obligation are typically executed simultaneously, the guaranties of the corporations are almost always supported by consideration and are enforceable under contract law.

The question of whether a contract of guaranty is enforceable against a corporation also depends upon the power of the corporation to enter into such contracts. The general rule is that a corporation has implied powers to enter into contracts of guaranty only when the transaction can reasonably be said to be incidental to the legitimate furtherance of the corporation's purposes and business authorized by its articles of incorporation.[4] Whether, under the circumstances of a particular case, a contract of guaranty is within the scope of a corporation's legitimate purposes and business is a question giving a wide range to the exercise of judicial discretion. However, the case law provides some insight into this question.

It is well settled that corporations may guaranty the debts of their subsidiaries[5] since such guaranties may be necessary or appropriate to protect the parent's interest in the subsidiary. Therefore, such guaranties are within the parent's purposes and are enforceable obligations of the parent corporation. This also holds true for a guaranty from a controlling entity such as a health care system 501(c)(3) corporation that controls the board of a system member.

A corporation's guaranty of an "unrelated" entity presents a more difficult question. The general rule is that the agreement must be reasonably incidental to the corporation's business. It is more difficult to show a benefit resulting from the guaranty of another corporation's obligation if such corporation is unrelated.

The courts have considered many different circumstances in applying this general rule, and most of these cases arose during the early part of the century. It has been held that a brewing company may act as guarantor on a liquor bond for a saloon owner,[6] or may guaranty payment of the saloon owner's rent;[7] that a manufacturing company may guaranty the interest on railroad bonds where the building of the railroad is necessary to carrying on the manufacturing business;[8] and that a corporation may guaranty an employee's payment for furniture bought from another, since the employee is a valuable salesperson for the guarantor corporation.[9]

On the other hand, the courts have decided in some cases that the guaranty was not directly related or beneficial to the authorized business carried on by the company: a railroad company's guaranty of a hotel company to help the latter build a hotel on the railroad line, merely in the hope that the guests of the hotel would travel on the railroad, was invalid;[10] cross-guaranties by a railroad company and a streetcar company were not authorized by the fact that the operation of a railroad and streetcar line would each tend to increase the population of a city and the business of the road.[11] The difference between these cases and those discussed above is clear. In those cases in which the guaranty was valid, the contract was reasonably appropriate to the business, but, in those cases in which the guaranty was invalid, the contract was for the benefit of a company with a distinctly different business purpose than the guarantor.

Since the validity of the guaranty agreement depends upon all of the facts and circumstances involved, each situation must be considered separately, using the case law as a guide. In any event, the focus will always be on the purpose clauses in the articles of incorporation of the corporation executing the guaranty.[12] If a reasonable argument can be made that the guaranty is reasonably incidental to the guarantor's business, the contract will be a binding and enforceable obligation of that corporation.

Very few cases actually address the issue of cross-guaranties, and, therefore, there is very little law on the issue. As discussed above, the cross-guaranties will be enforceable obligations if it can be shown that each guaranty is reasonably incidental to the respective corporations' businesses.

There is some authority that cross-guaranties are generally within the corporate powers of each corporation. In *Gotshal v. Mill Factors Corporation*,[13] the district court held that the guaranties were not beyond the powers of the corporations, which were in the importing business, since the corporations were promoting their own best interests by executing the cross-guaranties. Two benefits were cited by the court:

> . . . (1) That of obtaining the benefit of the reduced (3½ percent) commission by the test of the aggregate sales of three corporations; and (2) that of inducing the defendant to make advances indiscriminately to the three corporations. Thus the three corporations were so dovetailed that the agreement with defendant was advantageous to each, enabling each to obtain the advantage of a more liquid cash situation. . . .[14]

Cross-guaranties may not always benefit all the corporations involved. One corporation may actually be lending its credit to others without a corresponding benefit to itself.

The Fraudulent Conveyance Problem

In examining the enforceability of cross brother/sister and affiliate guaranties the pitfalls of "fraudulent conveyance" doctrine should not be overlooked. Creditors of a guarantor generally raise this doctrine when payment of a guaranty would force the guarantor into bankruptcy. Under the doctrine of fraudulent conveyance there must have been "fair consideration" rendered to the guarantor in exchange for its guaranty. If fair consideration has not been paid, then a bankruptcy court may find that the conveyance of the guaranty was done to defraud the creditors of the now bankrupt guarantor.[15]

There is no clear legal standard for what constitutes "fair consideration."[16] Therefore, counsel will choose to qualify its opinion on the enforceability of a guaranty in the event of bankruptcy of the guarantor.[17] In response to the fraudulent conveyance problem, the best drafted master indentures provide a "guaranty cap," limiting the amount of each master-indenture signatory guaranty to an amount that is defensible as (a) fair consideration and (b) would not, if exercised, force the guarantor into bankruptcy as of the date it entered into the guaranty.

CENTRALIZED SERVICES

Any centralized management services provided by a multihospital system or management company or cooperative can be of assistance to a borrowing hospital in persuading the rating agencies and prospective purchasers of bonds that it will be able to offer efficient management and operations in difficult times. Thus, even evidence of participation in centralized services, such as purchasing, banking relationships, management consulting services, and shared hospital services with other health care institutions, can provide assistance to a hospital in its efforts to obtain a better rating and lower interest rates on its bonds.

MASTER INDENTURES AND MASTER DOCUMENTS

As a carryover from utility financing, some multihospital system financings and financings of reorganized hospitals with a number of affiliated corporations have been done with a "master indenture." The master indenture is an agreement entered into by all or some of the health care institutions and other affiliated corporations in a multicorporation group. In the master indenture each corporate entity within the group covenants that it will restrict its additional borrowings to amounts within certain designated limits and that it will also adhere to a variety of other restrictions on its operations. Thus, the "master indenture" becomes an umbrella agreement restricting the additional borrowing activities of all of the members of the multicorporation group. It provides a central source document which can be reviewed by any subsequent lender to any of the affiliated health care institutions. Review of this one central document permits the lender to know what restrictions govern the borrowing of all of the related health care institutions. Often nonborrowing provisions such as rate covenants, restrictions on mergers and acquisitions, and insurance provisions are also included in the master indenture. The cross-guaranty provisions of a master indenture provide "pooled" credit strength for the signatory hospitals.

A similar technique is to have a set of "master documents" governing the borrowing of all affiliated corporations in a multihospital system. Although there is not one "master indenture," standardized borrowing provisions permit the multihospital system to ascertain restrictions governing all of its hospitals easily and to give lenders assurance that all of the affiliated entities will follow identical restrictions with regard to their ability to enter into future borrowing.

POOLED DEBT SERVICE RESERVE FUND

Occasionally, affiliated health care institutions have established a "pooled debt service reserve fund" as security for either taxable or tax-exempt bonds. It is traditional to have a debt service reserve fund equal to one year's maximum annual principal and interest on the bonds in tax-exempt financings, and occasionally a debt service reserve fund is also established in taxable financings. In a pooled debt service reserve fund the amount of maximum debt service on each bond issue of each affiliated hospital is contributed to a common fund. The moneys in the common fund are then available to pay debt service, when due, on the debt of each hospital in the affiliated group of hospitals. Although simple in principle, in a tax-exempt financing this technique must be very carefully structured to meet the criteria of state law and the Internal Revenue Code Arbitrage Regulations.[18]

POOLING OF ASSETS

Another pooling concept which has been discussed is to have a number of hospitals transfer ownership of their plant and equipment to a common 501(c)(3) "property holding company." This property holding company would then lease back to each of the original 501(c)(3) corporations the assets each had originally transferred to the holding company. The holding company becomes the debtor or co-obligor on any bonds issued to build additions to any of its member hospitals. The leaseback to each member hospital provides for rental payments to the property holding company in an amount equal to the debt payments for the respective hospital's additional construction projects. In addition, the hospitals may pay some amount to the property holding company as a reserve to strengthen further the unified credit of the holding company. The concern of hospitals which have reviewed this structure is that each 501(c)(3) hospital would be responsible in a variety of ways for the debt of each other member of the holding company affiliated group of hospitals. All of the hospital facilities owned by the holding company would be subject to being seized in a bankruptcy proceeding against the holding company.

SALE OF A HOSPITAL TO A MULTIHOSPITAL SYSTEM

Another way of strengthening the creditworthiness and ability to borrow of a hospital is to sell or lease the hospital to another hospital or a multihospital chain with a better credit rating. The sales or lease agreement can require that the purchaser maintain a hospital in the community. If the hospital is tax-supported, such an arrangement can relieve the community of the responsibility of raising money through taxes to support the hospital.

The sale or lease will permit the hospital to benefit from the borrowing power of the purchaser. A large number of not-for-profit and proprietary multihospital groups are actively seeking acquisition of other hospitals. The seller of a hospital should be sure that it is represented by legal counsel experienced in sales of hospitals and by an investment banker. These experts will assist in structuring the sale in a form most advantageous to the seller and at the highest price.

OTHER CREDIT-STRENGTHENING TECHNIQUES

A hospital may find that it can increase its credit rating in a variety of other ways. Raising rates to provide for better debt coverage is an effective means of improving credit strength. Another method is to enter into a management consulting relationship with a strong, nationally known consulting firm. Such a relationship demonstrates to potential bond purchasers and to the rating agencies a commitment to modern management techniques.

A change in the hospital's mix of services may also be beneficial, particularly adding services that are in short supply in the service area and that will produce larger fund balances.

Other hospitals have sought to strengthen their credit by a concerted effort to attract physicians to the hospital or to enter into a teaching relationship, which will strengthen the perception of the quality of services offered by the hospital.

These, and other credit-strengthening techniques, should be discussed with the hospital's investment banker and should be initiated as early as possible so that they have begun to take effect prior to the completion of the financial feasibility study.

INSURANCE

It will sometimes be advantageous for hospitals to purchase bond insurance. Hospital bond insurance is sometimes available through American Municipal Bond Assurance Corporation ("AMBAC"). An AMBAC policy insuring the payment of principal and interest, when due, will carry a AAA rating from Standard & Poor's Corporation. Under recent market conditions, the value of the AAA rating for lowering interest rates has been sufficient to make it worthwhile for hospitals that cannot obtain an A− or better rating without insurance to seek insurance. Currently, insurance generally is not available (due to New York insurance laws) in financings that provide a mortgage as security for the bonds.

Recently, there has been sufficient insurance written on hospital bonds so that AMBAC has, from time to time, placed a moratorium on writing new hospital bond insurance in order to diversify its insurance portfolios with other types of risks. A number of other insurance companies have expressed an interest in getting into this market, and there may be a number of other issuers of insurance for hospital bonds in the coming years.[19]

Bond insurance is available for long-term bonds, including bonds out for 30 years or longer. The cost of insurance has varied from time to time, and a hospital should discuss with its investment banker the current advantages of purchasing hospital bond insurance.

LETTERS OF CREDIT

High long-term interest rates, contrasted with more attractive short-term rates, have led a number of hospitals to engage in short-term letter of credit ("LOC") backed financing.[20] LOC-backed loans are usually three- to seven-year bullet loans in which only interest is paid until the final maturity of the loan, when all principal is due. Generally, the hospital will intend to refinance this loan with a long-term level debt service bond issue when interest rates become more favorable. Irrevocable letters of credit also are used in some floating rate note financings as third-party security devices.

The irrevocable letter of credit is a technique analogous to insurance in that it substitutes a bank's credit (rather than an insurance company's credit) for that of a hospital. Through its letter of credit, a bank agrees that should the health care facility default on payment of the bonds it will pay the trustee on the bonds the full amount due the bondholders. Thus, the LOC provides bondholders with the comfort of knowing they will be paid whether or not the health care facility is able to refinance prior to the end of the LOC-backed bullet loan. In an LOC financing a bank, for a fee (now generally about ¾ to 1 percent of the dollar amount of the LOC as an initiation fee and ¾ percent to 1½ percent each year the LOC is outstanding), agrees to pay to the trustee on the bonds principal and interest, when due, up to the amount of the LOC, at such time as the hospital defaults on its payment of principal and interest or at such time as payments are accelerated for any reason. Typical letters of credit have run from three to seven years. However, there have been some ten-year letters of credit offered and a few of even longer duration.   Appendix 17-A is a "criteria letter" of an LOC issuing bank setting forth the typical conditions and cost of an LOC.

Rollover Letters of Credit

In addition, there have been a few financings which have permitted the hospital, at its option, to leave bonds outstanding for a period of time beyond the original LOC expiration date. This is permitted if the hospital is able to get an additional LOC which permits it to have the same rating on its bonds as the original LOC for some specified time period after expiration of the original LOC.

Sometimes the bank issuing the LOC will also enter into an agreement that it will offer a line of credit at the end of the term of the bond issue at a predetermined rate so that the hospital will be able to refinance its bond issue.

Lines of Credit

Recently several banks which have issued a substantial number of LOCs backing hospital bonds have reached the limit of outstanding LOCs permitted by the banks' management. Some of these banks have suggested to certain hospitals and investment bankers that they would be willing to issue, instead of an LOC, a line of credit to the hospital as security for its outstanding bonds.

While a line of credit will provide a hospital with a "bridge" for getting over short-term cash flow problems, it does not provide the irrevocable third-party credit security of an LOC. This is because the line of credit runs to the health care institution, not the bond trustee, and because the line of credit (unlike an irrevocable LOC) is cancellable upon bankruptcy of the hospital and upon the occurrence of certain other events.

Thus, lines of credit will not permit the hospital bonds to obtain the same rating as the rating on the bank's securities, as is the case with a properly structured LOC.

FHA—242 AND 232 MORTGAGE INSURANCE

Mortgages insured by the Federal Housing Authority (FHA) were made possible by the Housing and Urban Development Act of 1978, which added Sections 242 and 232 for hospitals and nursing homes respectively to Title II of the National Housing Act. These sections authorize the Secretary of Housing and Urban Development to insure mortgage loans used to finance the construction or rehabilitation of hospitals and nursing homes and the purchase of major movable equipment.

Defaults under the mortgage are defined as failure to make any payment due under the note or mortgage securing the project or to perform any other mortgage covenant. The insurance contract provides that the trustee or noteholder is entitled to receive mortgage insurance benefits after a default continues for 30 days. FHA has the option of paying mortgage insurance claims in cash, in FHA debentures, or in a combination of both in an amount equal to approximately 99 percent of the outstanding principal of the loan and interest in arrears from the date of default to the date of insurance settlement at the applicable debenture interest rate. FHA debentures are issued in the name of FHA's general insurance fund as obligor and are backed by the full faith and credit of the United States government.

Tax-Exempt Bonds Backed by an FHA 242 or 232 Insured Mortgage

A properly structured tax-exempt bond issue secured by an FHA-insured mortgage will allow the bonds to be rated AAA. The FHA/Tax-Exempt Bond program is available to any nonprofit health care institution that can obtain a mortgage loan insurance commitment from FHA. Proprietary institutions able to obtain an FHA mortgage insurance commitment are also eligible subject to limitations on the amount of tax-exempt bonds that can be issued in accordance with industrial revenue bond regulations.

The FHA/tax-exempt bond program collateralizes tax-exempt revenue bonds with FHA insurance benefits. The security in the form of an FHA-insured mortgage note is held by the trustee/FHA mortgagee and is pledged with the payments thereon as security for payment of the bonds.

Cost and Delays

The costs of the FHA 242 and 232 program are high enough that a health care institution which can obtain an A or better rating without the insurance will generally be better off without it. In addition, it takes a year or more from the time of the original application for the insurance until approval or disapproval is determined. Table 17-1 summarizes the advantages and costs of FHA-insured mortgage loans.

Table 17-1 FHA-Insured Mortgage Loans

Advantages	Disadvantages
1. AAA credit rating resulting in a lower interest rate on the loan.	1. Processing of the FHA application is time consuming.
2. Loan to value ratio can be as high as 90 percent. The value of the land, existing buildings, and major movable equipment may satisfy hospital's equity requirements.	2. Construction and design must conform to FHA/HHS standards.
3. Most preparation and application costs can be included in eligible costs.	3. Construction labor costs can be higher than other methods of financing because of strict government regulations.
4. The U.S. government full faith and credit insurance (FHA) allows the hospital to secure an attractive interest rate.	4. The hospital must pay an annual mortgage insurance premium of ½ of 1 percent of the unamortized principal amount.
5. The term of the loan can be as much as 25 years after completion of construction.	5. The hospital must pay front-end inspection and filing fees totalling .8 of 1 percent of the principal amount plus legal and other expenses.
6. Prepayment of 15 percent of the original principal amount is permitted in a calendar year without penalty. In addition, prepayment can be made in excess of this amount at any time for a negotiated penalty.	

FARMERS HOME ADMINISTRATION

The Farmers Home Administration ("FmHA"), a division of the Department of Agriculture, offers two programs for small rural hospitals serving communities of 50,000 or less. These are a direct loan program administered by the Communities Facilities Loan Division of FmHA and the Business and Industrial Loan Guarantee Program.

Under the direct loan program the borrower pays only 5 percent interest on the loan with up to 40 years to pay it back. The guaranty program guaranties 90 percent of a mortgage through a local bank or mortgage broker. The guarantied mortgage is then used as collateral on the bonds which, in a properly structured tax-exempt financing, generally will be rated AA.

NOTES

1. Joyce A. Dixon and Baldwin B. Tuttle, eds., *Third Party Guaranties* (New York: New York Law Journal, Law Journal Seminars—Press, 1981) (hereafter "Third Party Guaranties"); Richard E. Brennan and Christopher W. Burdick, "Does the Guarantor Guarantee? Lender, Beware," *Seton Hall L. Rev.* 11 (1981): 353.

2. *See* Chapter 5 hereto, "Corporate Restructuring and Other Planning Considerations," esp. Appendix 5-A.

3. 38 C.J.S. Guaranty § 26B, pp. 1163–1164 (emphasis added).

4. Pacific Industries, Inc. v. Mountain Inn, Inc., 232 F. Supp. 801 (1964); Walter E. Heller & Co., Inc. v. Cox, 343 F. Supp. 519 (1972).

5. Lumbermen's Trust Co. v. Title Insurance & Investment Co. of Tacoma, 248 F. 212 (1918); *In re Duncan & Goodell Co.*, 15 F. Supp. 550 (D. C. Mass. 1936).

6. Horst v. Lewis, 71 Neb. 365, 103 N.W. 460 (1905).

7. James Eva Estate v. Mecca Co., 40 Cal. App. 515, 181 P. 415 (1919).

8. Central Trust Co. v. Columbus Co., 87 F. 815 (1898).

9. M. Burg & Sons v. Twin City Four Wheel Drive Co., 140 Minn. 101, 167 N.W. 300 (1918).

10. Western Maryland Railroad Co. v. Blue Ridge Hotel Co., 102 Md. 321, 62 Atl. 351 (1905).

11. Northside Railroad Co. v. Worthington, 88 Tex. 562, 30 S.W. 1055 (1895).

12. Another possible means to avoid potential problems is to amend the guarantor's articles of incorporation so that there is no question that the guaranty is within the guarantor's purposes.

13. 289 F. 1005 (2d Cir., 1923).

14. *Ibid.* In Gotshal, the three corporations were controlled by the same individual; however, the court considered this fact to be of "slight importance."

15. Robert J. Rosenberg, "Intercorporate Guaranties and the Law of Fraudulent Conveyances: Lender Beware," 125 *U. Pa. L. Rev.* 233 (Dec. 1976); Rubin v. Manufacturers Hanover Trust Co., *et al.*, F.2d (2d Cir., 1981); 8 BCD 297 (1981).

16. *Ibid.*

17. This language concerns two brother/sister guaranties in a life care facility financing. The language is taken from the official statement on the $10.6 million Illinois Health Facilities Authority Revenue Bonds, Series 1980 (Covenant Health Care Center, Inc. Project). Ziegler Securities, Inc. was the lead underwriter, Chapman & Cutler of Chicago was the bond counsel, and Gardner, Carton & Douglas of Chicago, the underwriters' counsel.

> While Messrs. Chapman and Cutler are of the opinion that the Covenant Home Guaranty and the Holmstad Guaranty have been duly authorized and are valid and binding, their opinion will state that it is questionable whether such Guaranties could be enforced in accordance with their terms if the Guarantor thereunder is insolvent at the time of realization thereon or subsequently becomes insolvent. In addition to the general effects on the enforcement of the Guaranties of bankruptcy, reorganization, insolvency, moratorium or other similar laws affecting creditors' rights and of applicable principles of equity if equitable remedies are sought, under the so-called "fraudulent conveyance" provisions of both Illinois law and Federal bankruptcy law, a court dealing with the property of an insolvent Guarantor or a Guarantor which would be rendered insolvent by performing under its Guaranty could refuse to enforce either of such Guaranties or require repayment by the Trustee or the Bondholders of amounts paid on either of such Guaranties if it determined that the consideration to Covenant Home or the Holmstad, as the case may be, for its respective Guaranty must have a reasonably equivalent value (calculated as of the date of realization on such Guaranty) to the amount paid on such Guaranty. It is unlikely that such reasonable equivalency would be found to exist where the Corporation's financial condition necessitated performance on the Covenant Home or Holmstad Guaranties. Messrs. Chapman and Cutler believe that such equivalency should be judged as of the date of execution of such Guaranties. If this were done, the Illinois and Federal bankruptcy "fraudulent conveyance" provisions should not apply since it would appear that neither Covenant Home nor the Holmstad would be rendered insolvent as a result of realization upon their respective Guaranties were such realization to occur on the date of execution thereof given (a) the current market value of the Corporation's assets, and (b) the fact that the Covenant Home and Holmstad Guaranties are guaranties of collection (as contrasted with the Church's guarantee of payment) such that they would be enforced only after the Corporation's property subject to the lien of the Mortgage had been liquidated. However, no reported cases have been discovered which support a conclusion that the determination of reasonable equivalency would be made on the date of execution of the Covenant Home and Holmstad Guaranties."

18. Frederick R. Blume, "Must Liberalize Covenants to Ease Hospital Corporate Restructuring," *Modern Healthcare*, April 1980, p. 108.

19. *Third Party Guaranties supra* note 1, at p. 67.

20. "Letters of Credit," *Third Party Guaranties, supra* note 1, at p. 1; L. Simpson, *Handbook on the Law of Suretyship* (1950); "Standby Letters of Credit—True Letters of Credit or Guaranties," Republic National Bank v. Northwest National Bank, *S.W.L.J.* 33 (1980): 1301; H. Harfield, *Bank Credits and Acceptances* (5th ed., 1974).

SUGGESTED READINGS

Dixon, Joyce A., and Tuttle, Baldwin, eds. *Third Party Guaranties*. New York: New York L.J., Law Journal Seminars—Press, 1981.

O'Halloran, J. *The ABC's of Commercial Letters of Credit*. (7th ed.). 1973.

Reade, H. Ryan, Jr., *et al. Letters of Credit*. New York: Practising Law Institute, 1981.

Appendix 17-A

Criteria Letter

DATE

Dear _____ :

Pursuant to your request for Bank _____ criteria in establishing a letter of credit facility to backstop a bond issue for your member hospitals, I have prepared an outline of the structure and basic credit requirements which is presented below.

FACILITY: Letter of credit to support a five-year bond anticipation note or series of notes with a maximum tenor of five years.

TERM: Five years on initial credit, to fund a term loan or second letter of credit for up to an additional five years.

FEES: *Years 1-5*
Commitment fee: ½ percent at closing plus any mortgage filing fees.
Annual fee: 1½ percent per annum

Years 6-10
Commitment fee: ½ percent at rollover for term loan or new BAN.
Annual Fee: 1½ percent per annum
Term Loan (should we not be able to refinance tax-exempt or be taken out): 1-½ percent over p.a. bank base fluctuated p.a.

BOND
AUTHORITY: To be determined.

DEBT SERVICE
RESERVE FUND: Up to 15 percent of issue or the amount of
                    borrowing by the weakest participant.

PARTICIPATIONS: To be determined.

The documentation supporting this facility will include a refunding agreement which anticipates that the participants will obtain 20–30 years financing at either a taxable or tax-exempt rate (documents will have a rate floor at which refinancing will occur) but should interest rates remain too high or long-term money not be available for any reason (other than the financial weakness of the hospitals), six–twelve months prior to the expiry date of the letters of credit, the hospitals will be able to choose one of two bank refinancing vehicles.

   a. Rollover the BANs with a renewal of the clean credit. At the sixtieth month, all cash collateral including debt service reserve fund would be applied to the then outstanding BANs—less any newly required debt service reserve requirements. The anticipated new rollover would be approximately 50 percent of the original issue. During the second five-year period the participants would make debt service payments or sinking fund contributions which would be applied against the outstanding debt. These payments plus the debt service reserve fund would result in the complete repayment of the BANs at the end of the ten-year term.
   b. Fund out the BANs in a bank five-year term loan.

The participants will each sign a five-year bullet maturity note equal to their share of the deal simultaneous to the bank providing a clean letter of credit. This note will have a three-year refunding provision providing no calls for price prior to the thirty-sixth month. But the bank will have the ability to request a call by the trustee for violation of a covenant or misrepresentation. There will be (1) master bond resolution, (2) master bond indenture, (3) private placement agreements with the local state authority having jurisdiction over each of the hospitals, (4) construction loan agreement, (5) refunding agreement. Bank counsel will prepare items 4 and 5, and bond counsel will draft items 1, 2, and 3, but counsel will have full input into whatever is drafted by bond counsel. The BANs will be secured on a project basis through each authority assigning its interest in the documents and collateral to the bond trustee who will represent the interests of the bondholders and the bank.

Collateral will consist of:

1. gross revenue pledge and pledge of accounts receivable;
2. all temporary investments during construction, including the construction fund, unexpended project funds, arbitrage interest, debt service reserve fund;
3. mortgage on hospitals; bank will be in second position unless bonds fund, when we will automatically move to first position;
4. negative pledge of assets.

We would perfect our interest in the collateral by lending $10,000 simultaneous to the issuance of the clean credits on a grid note which will enable us to move up to a fully secured position if the credit funds without a new 90-day perfection period. (This procedure depends on local and state regulations.) We file a mortgage. The bondholders automatically relinquish their interest when paid out, by issuing a satisfaction, and our refunding agreement as well as bond documents will prevent the hospitals from pledging any assets. The bank needs the ability to cause the trustee to call bonds at any time for a breach of covenants, including misrepresentation of warranties, material adverse change, and loss of 501(c)(3) status.

Included in the bank's documentation will be several financial tests:

1. current ratio
2. minimum profitability
3. long-term debt: none without bank permission; working capital: same
4. leasing: cap will be set
5. capex: cap will be set
6. construction project
   - full payment and performance bonds on general contractor by A-1 bonding company acceptable to bank
   - approval by bank-designated engineer of plans and specs including full cost analysis to determine validity of contractor's guaranteed maximum price
   - review of contract by bank engineer
   - guarantied maximum price on each project
   - monthly inspection by bank engineer (first four months semi-monthly) who will determine beneficial occupancy
   - cost overrun and change order approval with concurrence of bank engineer/$10,000 individual/$100,000 aggregate
7. trustee: must be approved by bank
8. standard construction loan covenants

9. all letter-of-credit fees due to be escrowed (for three years) to be held and advanced quarterly by the trustee.
10. minimum long-term rate floor at which hospital must refinance
11. letter of credit cannot be called if the authority defaults (we are backstopping hospitals only)
12. negative pledge on all assets

All of the above assumes that each institution you are asking to participate individually meets the bank's minimum requirements for completing the transaction.

I look forward to sitting down with you and discussing the transaction contemplated herein at your earliest convenience.

Chapter 18

Special Considerations of Financing Life Care Facilities

Robert C. Liden and Arthur J. Simon

The history of care for the elderly parallels changing social mores as well as changing demographics and economic conditions. It was not too many years ago that the elderly admitted to an acute care hospital for treatment of a chronic disorder would later be discharged into the home of the eldest "child" for further rehabilitation and recovery. The eldest child and the extended family commonly provided financial support and nursing care to enable the elderly to be at least "comfortable." Prior to World War II, the commonly available options for care of the elderly were the county ("poor") farm or a limited number of private "homes," to both of which negative stigmas were attached. Only in the most severe circumstances were these options of care selected.

Since World War II, the likelihood of the family unit directly caring for the elderly has decreased substantially due, in part, to the increasing number of two-income families and the development of other options for the care of the elderly to which negative stigmas are not attached. Since the early 1950s, a number of nursing home facilities have been constructed to provide, as the name implies, nursing care for the chronically disabled elderly.

The current approach to providing care for the elderly embraces the concept of a "continuum of care" or "life care" that recognizes the need for facilities that provide all services required by the elderly, not just nursing facilities.

THE CONTINUUM OF CARE OR LIFE CARE CONCEPT

The continuum of care concept recognizes the differences in the continually changing physical and emotional status and well-being of elderly individuals. As a consequence, a contemporary life care facility typically provides, on a single campus, facilities to accommodate these differences.

Today, a life care facility will likely include (1) independent residential facilities (apartments, townhouses, or duplexes) that may include laundry and housekeeping services, (2) assisted living facilities that provide limited nursing care (such as assistance in dressing, administering medication, and providing meals), and (3) skilled nursing facilities, together with common dining, recreation, and, perhaps, convenience (shopping, boutique, laundry) facilities. As a further extension of the continuum of care concept, life care facilities are often located near and affiliated with or owned by acute care hospitals. In a very real sense, a contemporary life care facility is a "community" for the elderly. Applying the analogy of a community, such facilities are commonly located in areas that enable the life care residents to interact with other segments of society. Regular programs include activities involving the community.

If properly managed, the orientation of a dynamic community is toward "well residents"; the facility residents are not viewed as being a static population, but rather, if one is admitted to the skilled nursing facility, the objective is to return the resident to the residential facility after treatment.

FINANCING LIFE CARE FACILITIES

The traditional source of financing nursing homes (as opposed to life care facilities) was conventional mortgage loans. Such loans generally provided long terms at fixed rates and were obtained through local banks, life insurance companies, and, to a lesser extent, savings and loan associations. However, in recent years, conventional long-term mortgages have become either unattractive or unavailable as a source of capital. As a result, the life care industry has been required to examine other long-term financing alternatives, including tax-exempt financing.

The first tax-exempt nursing home bond was issued in 1965, but it was not until the last few years that a market has existed for tax-exempt life care revenue bonds. Since 1965, tax-exempt revenue bond financing has emerged as one of the most significant alternatives available for life care capital.[1]

Although many of the business and legal factors involved in financing hospital construction from tax-exempt bond proceeds are also present in financing life care facilities, certain business and legal characteristics of life care financing exist that distinguish life care financing from acute care financing.

Business Characteristics

While most acute care financings involve renovation, expansion, and improvement of an existing hospital, the majority of life care financings involve the construction of a completely new facility. Consequently, the project's preplanning and planning process assumes even greater significance. The planning process prior to the development of a financing plan contains several crucial elements.

Board of Directors and Management

Most life care facilities financed on a tax-exempt basis are owned by private, not-for-profit corporations. Since most life care facilities are start-up ventures, the composition of the board of directors is extremely important. While visionaries are needed to begin anything new, pragmatists are also needed to make a project work. The success of a project, in large part, will depend upon the efforts of the directors. In addition, the board is the link between the project and the community, and, because community support is crucial to the project, the board should be representative of the surrounding community.

The day-to-day operations of life care facilities are generally the responsibility of a private, for-profit management firm selected by the board of directors. There are a number of nationally recognized, professional firms that specialize in this activity. Regrettably, there are also a number of less than professional management firms and individuals who can seriously jeopardize the project. It is crucial to engage competent, and preferably experienced, management that can anticipate and adapt to changing demographics and the needs of elderly residents.

Market Research

In addition to usual demographic studies that identify a significant eligible elderly population within a given area, it also must be determined directly if such eligible individuals will elect to participate in a life care facility in the community. This involves far more than the identification of an eligible population base and includes direct contact with the population to determine community appeal of the project, as well as potential utilization and potential residents' ability to pay and actual willingness to buy.

Architects and Contractors

The sequence of events in developing a life care facility effectively involves juggling a number of balls simultaneously. Typically, the not-for-profit corporation must initially sell the concept of life care in a given community. Once interest has been identified, it is necessary to have a project to sell.

In order to develop the project, the not-for-profit corporation must acquire, preferably by option, a parcel of property and engage a capable architect willing to work on a contingency basis. Once plans have been prepared, the project must be bid on a guaranteed maximum price basis. Bids must be held for a minimum of 60 days (or interim construction financing must be in place to ensure that the project can be completed as anticipated). After bids are available, the actual cost of units can be ascertained and actual presales can occur. Only after significant presales have been consummated can bonds be issued.

Presales

While preplanning of a life care facility may involve years, the actual financing of a project generally occurs within a very concentrated period of time, usually a 60–90 day period culminating in the sale of bonds. One of the most critical aspects of the project during this period is the sale of commitments for the life care units (presales) since both the feasibility study and, consequently, the ability to finance the project are dependent on such presales. A life care presale involves a cash investment of 10 percent to 20 percent of the actual cost of the unit to be occupied (upon completion of construction). Such payment, paid in conjunction with entering into a residency agreement, constitutes a portion of the "initial endowment." The underwriters generally require presales of 60 percent to 70 percent of all residential units before bonds can be offered.

Initial Endowment

While some life care facilities are offered on a rental, condominium, or cooperative basis, the majority of not-for-profit facilities are financed, at least in part, on an endowment basis. Under this approach, the future resident of a life care facility purchases the right to use a residential unit for life and is given preference in the use of health care facilities located on the campus, generally for an additional per diem fee. The endowment represents the equivalent of a life estate interest in the residential unit, the cost of which represents a significant percentage of the actual cost of construction of the unit. The resident then pays an additional monthly fee to cover the costs of operations and maintenance, including the management fee, of both the residential unit and the life care facility at large.

Life care facilities financed on an endowment basis are essentially "double financed" over time. During the start-up period, the tax-exempt bond proceeds are used to construct the project. As both initial residents and subsequent residents occupy the facility, endowments are received and held in a restricted, trusteed escrow account. Over time, generally a seven- to ten-year period, these endowment funds, together with the interest earnings thereon, are amortized as a source of payment of debt service on the bonds (together with a modest, if any, debt service component of monthly fees). It is assumed that the turnover of residents will cause the facility to continue to generate endowments sufficient to pay debt service; this assumption is the basis of the period of endowment fee amortization.

Actuarial Assumptions and Admission Requirements

The annual amortization of endowments as "income" is determined based upon assumptions of attrition commonly developed from standard insurance mortality tables. Since the ability to pay debt service depends in large part on the realization of projected attrition, it is paramount that such attrition assumptions are conservative and that the amount of the endowment is significant. Sponsors of life care facilities should engage (directly or indirectly, through the feasibility consultant) an actuary particularly familiar with the demographic mix of residents anticipated to occupy the facility to be assured that, in fact, attrition assumptions are conservative.

The actual mix of residents is also significant and must be considered in establishing admission requirements. Residents of life care facilities have a longer life expectancy than the population at large, in part due to the quality of care provided at the life care facility. While not meaning to sound morose, this factor must be considered, along with financial requirements, in developing admission standards to the facility. Generally, individuals less than 62 years of age are not eligible for admission in life care facilities.

In addition to admission requirements pertaining to age, most life care facilities require prospective residents to (1) demonstrate their financial ability to pay monthly maintenance fees, (2) pass a preadmission physical examination, and (3) provide proof of adequate health insurance.

Feasibility Study

The necessity of a feasibility study and its importance to the life care financing is, again, based principally upon the fact that most life care facilities are start-up facilities, and, as noted, the success of the project is dependent in part upon the operating assumptions made.

While in most acute care financings, projections are based in large part on historical operating results, this is not the case in life care financing. This lack of historical performance is also a major reason why Standard & Poor's Corporation and Moody's Investors Service do not rate life care issues (as discussed below). Therefore, potential investors in life care bonds are left with the "opportunity" to invest in a life care facility that is generally yet to be constructed and, therefore, has no operating history.

Engagement of a feasibility consultant of exceptional repute, together with engagement of competent management, takes on even greater significance to the investor in nonrated life care bond issues and serves to differentiate the quality of one life care bond issue from another.

Ratings

Standard & Poor's Corporation and Moody's Investors Service do not rate life care issues per se. However, both services will consider rating issues where there is additional third-party security, such as an irrevocable letter of credit, for the bonds. In effect, the rating agencies are rating the third-party credit as the principal credit, not the life care facility.

The lack of historical ratings may be one of the major reasons Standard & Poor's Corporation and Moody's Investors Service do not rate such issues. While it is not possible to speak for the rating agencies, it is understandable, given the historical negative image of the "nursing home" industry, to expect some seasoning, some passage of time (as was the case in the issuance of acute care ratings), before Standard & Poor's Corporation and Moody's Investors Service will be willing to rate life care bond issues.[2]

Fitch Investors Service, however, does rate certain life care financings that meet very stringent requirements. Anyone considering a life care issue is well advised to consider meeting these requirements in developing a life care financing. As previously suggested, all of the positive factors that can differentiate a given transaction from others available in the market (including, as previously discussed, the selection of an experienced management group and the feasibility consultant) should be explored. Regrettably, without such positive distinctions, the major distinction differentiating one life care financing from another in the marketplace is the interest rate borne on the bonds.

Third-Party Reimbursement

The financial operation of the skilled nursing care component of a life care facility may rely, in large part, on third party payers, principally Medicare and Medicaid. Medicaid reimbursement varies significantly from state to state and is a matter that must be investigated thoroughly and included in the projected operating assumptions of a given facility. Because of the rate of reimbursement in some states, this source of financial support is potentially so deleterious that a number of life care facilities have elected not to become eligible for Medicaid reimbursement, but rather limit use of the health care facility component to those individuals who are either self-pay or who carry private insurance. In any event, the feasibility study should address reimbursement factors and include appropriate assumptions.

Legal Characteristics

The legal documents drafted in connection with the issuance of tax-exempt bonds for life care facilities must take into account characteristics unique to life care institutions. Although in many respects the key terms of the legal documents relating to tax-exempt bonds for hospitals are the same as those in life care facilities, the discussion below summarizes certain differences that do exist.

Mortgage Security

The focus of the financing of hospitals is typically on the income that is or can be generated by a hospital. Generally, hospital facilities are not multiple-purpose buildings and are not suitable for industrial or commercial use. Consequently, although a mortgage is often placed on the real estate owned by a hospital, the mortgage is not the principal security of a potential investor. In fact, in the case of a hospital with a strong operating history, a mortgage may not be necessary.

The principal property of a life care facility, however, can provide important security for bondholders. In most cases, the facilities consist of multiunit structures and may include several single unit structures that are easily convertible for general residential use. Therefore, a mortgage is both common to and required in virtually all life care financings.

Subordination of Management Fees

The management of a life care facility is a crucial factor in its profitability, and generally an organization experienced in the operation of the facilities is contracted to manage the operations. The fees paid pursuant to the management agreement may be considerable in comparison to the income of the life care facility. As a result, the legal documents should subordinate such management fee payments to the payments of principal of and interest on the bonds. In addition, special care must be taken in drafting the management contract, particularly in terms of duration and basis of compensation, to assure eligibility for tax-exempt financing.

Third-Party Guaranties

Many life care facilities are affiliated with hospitals, other life care institutions, religious organizations or management consultants. In consideration of developing the strongest possible financing credit to finance a particular life care institution, it is often helpful or necessary to rely on affiliations with others to improve and differentiate the credit of a particular life care facility.

One means of improving the credit of the life care institution, in addition to those previously discussed, is to have an affiliated organization guaranty the debt created pursuant to the bonds through the execution of a guaranty. The affiliated organization guaranties either the payment of the bonds or the underlying obligations of the payments pursuant to a lease or loan agreement.

There is an important legal consideration that exists if the guarantor-obligor is not a parent-subsidiary relationship, but rather an affiliated corporation through a common parent corporation. In addition to the general effects on the enforcement of the guaranties of bankruptcy, reorganization, insolvency, moratorium, or other laws affecting creditors' rights, and of applicable principles of equity, the so-called "fraudulent conveyances" provisions of the federal bankruptcy law and state bankruptcy laws may be applicable. A court dealing with property of an insolvent guarantor or a guarantor that would be rendered insolvent by performing under a guaranty could refuse to enforce the guaranty if it determined that the consideration given to the guarantor for the execution of the guaranty was not of "reasonably equivalent value" to the amount paid on the guaranty.[3] The possibility for such a decision certainly should be disclosed to prospective bondholders and may limit the strength of such third-party guaranties.

Additional Bonds

Indentures generally permit the issuance of additional bonds in the future for certain purposes that will rank on a parity with all bonds issued under the indenture. The requirements for the issuance of additional bonds consist principally of ratio tests of either historical or pro forma debt service coverage. Frequently, the historical coverage test requires that the net income available for debt service (and funds that may be available from certain reserved funds) for the preceding one or two years be not less than 110 percent of the maximum annual debt service on all long-term debt, including the additional bonds proposed to be issued. Alternatively, the life care facility must show a 110 percent historical coverage ratio excluding the additional bonds proposed to be issued and a pro forma coverage ratio of 120 percent generally for five years following the issuance of additional bonds.

Funds and Accounts

In connection with the issuance of hospital bonds, the indentures typically establish various funds including the principal, interest, and optional redemption funds. The indentures also establish a debt service reserve fund and require that the institution maintain a balance in this fund generally equal to the maximum amount of principal and interest to be paid in any year. Indentures drafted in connection with life care bond issues require these same funds; however, additional funds and accounts are also required in order to increase the security of bondholders.

Unlike hospitals that rely heavily on federal and state reimbursement payments, life care facilities (other than perhaps the health care component of such facilities) rely principally upon endowment fees, monthly fees, and interest on such moneys to fund the operation of the facility. The endowment fees are required to be paid to a corporate trustee under the indenture and are maintained for payment of debt service. In addition, such endowments may also be used to make up deficiencies in other funds maintained under the indenture, to fund certain costs incurred in connection with constructing, equipping and improving the facilities, or to refund moneys to residents due to early termination of a residency agreement.

Finally, other funds and accounts also may be established which may or may not be maintained by the trustee. For example, some indentures require a facility to maintain an account for the purpose of paying the monthly fees of those residents who are no longer able to do so. Another fund that is often required maintains a percentage of the entrance fees for the purpose of refunding the fees in the event the residency agreements are terminated. Again, the amount maintained in those funds varies with each financing.

Rate Covenant

Life care facilities are generally required to maintain rates, consisting of entrance and monthly fees, so that the facilities' net income is at least some percentage of the maximum annual debt service required in any year. This percentage is typically between 110 percent and 130 percent and has varied, in some instances, from year to year, depending upon the funds maintained in any account, with respect to entrance fees.

Permitted Indebtedness

A critical provision in the documents relating to a life care financing defines the restrictions on the nature and terms of indebtedness the life care facility may incur in the future in addition to additional bonds. Permitted indebtedness provisions vary widely, and the life care facility should consider the restrictions and its future plans in order to ascertain that the facility will be able to operate under the indenture for the term of the bonds.

Indebtedness, as commonly used in permitted indebtedness provisions, includes short-term bank borrowings, rental payments, purchase money mortgages, and capitalized leases. In addition to the restrictions applicable to additional bonds, the indenture typically restricts additional indebtedness to a percentage of the gross or adjusted operating revenues of the life care facility.

Residency Agreement

The success of the life care project depends to a significant extent on the institution's ability to meet the assumptions established in the feasibility study. The residency agreement and the related documents should be drafted in accordance with those underlying assumptions.

For example, assumptions are made with respect to the level of endowment fees and monthly rates that are necessary to maintain the facility and make the debt service payments. The commitments entered into by the life care institution should conform to those assumptions. Also, the residency agreement should not guaranty payment of future health care costs if the provision of such services is not within the organization's financial means. Because important characteristics vary with each life care project, it is impossible to list all of the provisions that should be reviewed. However, the parties to the financing should make sure that the legal documents are consistent with the underlying premises established in the feasibility study.

In addition to the special business and legal characteristics common to the financing of life care facilities discussed here, there may be other considerations, notably individual state enabling legislation, that must be considered with respect to a proposed life care facility. As in acute care financing, it is most prudent to engage competent professionals, including bond counsel and underwriters, in developing a sound financing plan.

NOTES

1. From 1965 to 1969, the life care industry expanded the total stock of beds by more than 50 percent, from 462,000 to 704,500 (U.S. Senate, Special Committee on Aging, Subcommittee on Long-Term Care, *Nursing Home Care in the United States*, 94th Cong., 1st Sess., 1975, pp. 20–21). It raised a substantial portion of the necessary capital for the expansion through the sale of public stocks and bonds.

2. In the early 1960s, hospital bonds were unrated; however, in 1980, hospitals issued more than $3 billion in bonds, most of which were rated by the rating agencies.

3. R.J. Rosenberg, "Intercorporate guaranties and the law of fraudulent conveyances: Lender beware," *U. Pa. L. R.* 125 (December 1976): 235–236.

Chapter 19

Financing in the Future

Frederick R. Blume

THE CHANGING CAPITAL FORMATION

In order to prognosticate about future financing vehicles, it is necessary first to address the environment in which hospitals will be raising or attempting to raise future capital. Unlike many fields where history typically provides indications of upcoming events, the future of health care will be undergoing sufficient change to render historical evaluations of limited use. The industry is facing change of the magnitude of the implementation of the Medicare and Medicaid programs in 1966. The financial community is aware of the pressures on hospitals, receptive to change by the industry, and anxious about the ultimate resolve underlying the transformation the industry is attempting to undertake—consolidation, competition, and corporate restructuring. The present view of these changes by the financial community is favorable in that it represents a maturation by the heretofore cottage industry to a more businesslike posture.

There are several factors causing significant increases in the need for capital among the acute care provider sector of the health care industry. Three factors acting in unison greatly magnify the need. These factors are inflation, reduced federal budgets, and inadequate growth in equity capital from internally generated sources (albeit beyond many hospitals' individual control). In part, the private, nonprofit hospitals are now starting to feel the less attractive effects of accepting, without unified rebellion, 15 years of government's less-than-full-cost reimbursement and the disincentive for efficient business operation created by the regulations that evolved.

The health care industry, the patients, and the health payers will suffer over a long period of time the effects of our recent inflationary costs that have been the focus of recent national attention. Unfortunately, the in

289

flationary growth in the cost of construction and in the cost of high technology equipment will impact the health care industry for the coming decades. Hospitals will have to raise an estimated $150 billion to cover the forecasted capital expenditure requirements (new capital demands) between 1981 and 1990.[1] The range of current estimates for capital requirements in the industry journals is from $150 billion to $190 billion. The low end of the scale represents a tripling of historical demand which averaged $5.3 billion per year during the 1970s. The high end of the estimate is just short of four times the historical demand for capital.

Not only is the hospital industry increasing its demand for capital, but so is every other segment of the economy. The well-publicized government budget deficits and resulting funding needs represent only a portion of the increased capital requirement. The steel and auto businesses require major recapitalization, to name some examples of other industries' appetites. Municipal governments will be faced with increased funding obligations. The heightened demand for capital means increased competition for scarce resources, increased cost of either debt or equity, and different decision-making criteria to be applied by the prospective investor. These three results have already started to emerge. They are noticed in the more limited use of the highest-quality rating categories by the nationally recognized bond rating services. The recent cycles of tight money and high-cost credit were accompanied by periods when lower quality hospital bonds could not attract investor interest virtually at any price.

In addition to sharing in the problems of a generally tougher capital market environment, hospitals have increased their reliance on the tax-exempt revenue bond dramatically over the past ten years. Concomitant with a growth in hospitals' use of revenue bonds has been substantial increase in their reliance on debt. Thus, the primary source of capital has become the tax-exempt revenue bond. That fact by itself is not a problem. The problem comes from the mounting pressure in Washington, D.C., to restrict greatly, if not eliminate, the tax-exempt revenue bond as a source of capital available to hospitals (among others). There have been two recent assaults on the legality of hospitals' issuing tax-exempt bonds. Thus, the financing vehicle which constituted about 75 percent to 80 percent of the borrowed funds for hospitals over the past five years is endangered. Hospitals may, therefore, have to seek record amounts of capital at the same time they are confronted with intensified competition and with the forced usage of new or less familiar higher-cost taxable debt instruments.

Unfortunately, the intensely competitive environment for hospitals in the capital market will be faced at a time the inequities in rate review and in cost-based reimbursement from both Medicare and Medicaid have caused nonprofit hospitals to realize little equity growth. Moreover, the tax-exempt debt markets have accepted debt leverage ratios well over those other markets are accustomed to seeing. The overall impact of the government's squeeze on equity will cause the nonprofit hospitals to need substantial amounts of internally generated fund balances to support their demand for debt during the next ten years.

Prior to 1970, the borrowing requirements of the industry had been provided primarily by the life insurance companies and banks. Banks currently are not as interested in long-term fixed income as a matter of policy. Life insurance companies, like other fixed income investors, have become both more credit conscious and concerned over inflation's impact on fixed income securities. The life insurance companies do, however, have a vested interest in health, wellness, and the appropriate delivery of acute care. Thus, it is likely there would be a major purchaser of taxable debt if and when excellent hospital credits used such funds.

CHANGES WITHIN THE INDUSTRY

Hospitals are changing their corporate structure in response to the need to preserve assets to build equity and to develop new revenue sources. Hospitals are creating different corporate structures to avoid ill-conceived government regulation. They are joining systems to increase their capital base and corporate size for cost containment and a competitive edge. In short, the corporate form of the hospital is changing. The hospital is becoming part of a diversified corporation seeking either a broader share of the health market or a bigger share of the geographic area served. Moreover, the major hospitals and hospital systems are joining regional or nationwide networks of systems or groups to gain further strength in the size and scope of services which may be undertaken.

These consolidations and corporate restructurings alter the nature of the financing needs and borrowing capacity of the hospitals involved. It is expected that these trends will continue, if not accelerate, especially if the capital markets reflect both an understanding and an appreciation of the consolidation and businesslike approach being taken by hospitals. In fact, successful diversification may become a significant contributing factor in the ability to attract borrowed capital.

The credit quality is affected by the changing corporate structure in two ways. The separation of function and assets to avoid regulation makes borrowing slightly more complex if a reduction in underlying credit strength is also to be avoided. Although there will undoubtedly be improvements and refinements to the present covenants and structures that provide for asset transfer, corporate restructuring, and merger and consolidation, the present covenants are quite flexible. The real pressure on hospitals that have undertaken the new corporate structures is to demonstrate they have, in fact, run the new entity as an integrated successful business. The capital markets are particularly interested in the performance of the unbundled and new health-related ventures. The pressures of price competition, the reduction of the barriers to competition by this unbundled selling activity, and the risk of reduced margins all will affect an investor's interest in a credit. The key to the ability to attract capital will be financially successful operations.

The trend toward networks or "super groups" as they are being called will accelerate. The super groups represent a dynamic potential, even broader than the multihospital systems that started the trend, to increase dramatically the asset base, revenue support, and risk diversification. More important in the eyes of the capital market, a truly coordinated and tightly knit super group represents a better credit in that its size will enhance toe-to-toe competition with proprietaries, major health maintenance organizations, or other similar systems or super groups. The management capacity, the broader market base, and the competitive edge will clearly give super groups a credit preference.

A concomitant pressure for capital that will affect the nonprofit hospital, system, or network will come from the proprietary hospital chains. Heretofore, the proprietaries in general have concentrated expansionary efforts in the area of ownership or management of hospitals principally in the regions with less onerous regulations and favorable population trends. The major proprietary chains are now poised to take advantage of their capacity virtually countrywide to diversify into the sale of unbundled ancillary services and a broader range of health services and levels of care. The proprietaries are poised for this market diversification with the singular advantage of superior capacity to attract capital—both equity and debt. During the 12 months ending November 30, 1981 the five largest proprietary hospital chains raised $1.2 billion of capital, as shown in Table 19-1. By virtue of their ease of access to capital, the proprietaries will prove to be awesome competition.

CAPITAL VEHICLES FOR THE FUTURE

Predicting future capital-raising vehicles could be a separate book unto itself. The hospitals' demand for capital and the changes discussed previously will necessitate efforts for new sources of equity as well as debt

Table 19-1 Financial Comparison of Proprietary Systems

(Dollars in Thousands)

	Charter Medical Corporation 9/30/81	National Medical Enterprises 5/31/81	Humana 8/31/81	Hospital Corporation of America 12/31/81	American Medical International 8/31/81
Net Revenues	$288,027	$892,407	$1,342,906	$2,063,637	$913,536
Net Income	11,570	51,779	93,177	111,131	50,807
Cash Flow	18,654	72,781	162,393	199,328	86,965
Total Assets	204,656	867,497	1,502,232	2,958,156	984,149
Capitalization:					
Long-Term Debt	108,171	282,572	733,060	1,648,836	328,640
Preferred/Convertible	7,219	5,141	63,925	—	51,820
Common Stock Equity	39,616	376,150	297,314	767,600	326,619
Net Income/Net Revenues	5.07	5.80	6.94	5.39	5.56
Net Income/Common Stock Equity	29.2	13.8	31.3	14.5	15.6
As of May 11, 1982 (Most recent 12 months)					
Market Value of Common Stock	197,939	708,210	1,423,614	1,683,805	740,554
Price Earnings Ratio	15.5	10.5	13.6	14.5	12.2
Market Value as a Multiple of Book Value	5.00x	1.88x	4.79x	2.19x	2.27x
% of Market Value Shares That Equate to Book Value	20%	53%	21%	46%	44%

Source: Blyth Eastman Paine Webber Health Care Funding Database.

capital. An example of how one health-related company used equity capital may in fact help explain both its advantage and the importance of operating performance when considering equity capital.

A single family started and built a highly successful, regionally based automated reference laboratory business. The operating earnings of the company were both sizable and on an upward trend. The capitalization was appropriately balanced between debt and equity. After the initial capitalization of the firm, the company's profit performance was approximately 20 percent of sales and 36 percent of equity. The enterprise was enjoying consistent growth. Given that performance, the owners were able to sell to the public 40 percent of the common stock for 2.8 times the then-book value of the company. Thus, they had recaptured more than their original investment and still owned 60 percent of the shares of the company on which they were receiving a 36 percent return (on the remaining book value of equity). I should comment that the 36 percent return is based on profit accumulation. Since there was and continues to be no dividend payment, all of the net profits have been reinvested and represent equity growth through retained earnings. Having recaptured the original capital, the family has an opportunity to invest in a new venture with reduced risk of failure since the income stream from the original enterprise is still available and control of that enterprise remains absolute, even though there are now minority shareholders. To reiterate ad nauseam, the key to this type of equity capital generation is successful financial performance.

CAPITALIZATION OF CORPORATE VENTURES

As an extension to the access-to-capital concept, hospitals, systems, or super groups may wish to invest in for-profit corporate ventures in order to diversify and improve their income stream. To capitalize start-up or underdeveloped opportunities properly, an injection of permanent equity funds will be necessary to realize expected financial promise in the future. However, the public stock market generally is not receptive to supplying equity capital to new companies without a track record or a demonstrated proprietary product in an explosive growth industry. Still, the amount of moneys needed or the extent of the business risk involved may warrant such hospital, system, or group to seek an outside investment partner. A venture capital firm becomes a logical candidate under these conditions.

By way of definition, venture capital's main thrust is the early-stage financing of relatively small, rapidly growing companies. More explicitly it is a source of "seed capital," and as such it is start-up and initial-phase development financing. It also can provide several rounds of funding for expansion to companies which have already demonstrated the viability of their businesses, but are not seasoned enough to gain access to the public stock market or credit-oriented lending institutions. It must be stressed that venture capital generally is a high-risk endeavor. As a result, it has the following characteristics:

- It has an active, ongoing involvement with the management of the enterprises in which it has invested. From the formulation of business plans to the installation of control procedures, a venture capital firm becomes an integral part of the activities of its portfolio companies. This fact is definitely to the advantage of the subject hospital, system, or group because the venture capital partner can provide a broad spectrum of industry knowledge and business discipline in support of the investment.

- It has a long-term investment horizon of five to ten years for the realization of significant return (significant being multiples of 3 to 10 times the original investment). This aspect is important in that venture capital firms will only make commitments to enterprises with exceptional business promise commensurate with the risk. To underscore this point, the targeted annual rates of return for institutional venture capital range from 35 percent to 115 percent. Thus, the willingness of a venture capital firm to participate in an investment serves as an excellent screening signal regarding the potential for success.

A venture capital firm typically structures its investment in a company to balance its rate of return and liquidity objectives. Within this context, it will be useful to review the major investment vehicles employed in venture capital financing.

- *Common stock* (or equivalents, such as warrants) is the most frequently used instrument for purchasing an ownership interest in a company. It carries the right to vote on certain corporate decisions, and it can receive dividends, although it rarely does in venture investments. In liquidation, however, common stockholders are the last to share in the assets of the corporation. If the company is successful, shares can be sold through a registered public offering. Stock may be sold without registration under Rule 144 of the Securities Act of 1933. Rule 144 states that purchasers of privately issued common stock (not registered with the Securities and Exchange Commission) must hold such stock two years before selling. After this holding period expires and if there is a public market for the stock, restricted investors may sell in any three-month period up to the greater of 1 percent of the total outstanding shares of the company or the average weekly trading volume for the four prior weeks. In an attempt to avoid Rule 144 constraints, investors generally will insist that registration rights accompany the common stock purchased in a venture capital financing.

- *Preferred or convertible preferred stock* (convertible into common) provides the investor with rights that the common shareholder does not have. Business covenants are negotiated for each financing and can establish financial tests that, if not met, provide for control of the board of directors to shift to the preferred investors. Investor liquidity is improved by virtue of the fact that many preferred stock purchase agreements possess scheduled mandatory dividend or redemption features, which provide an investment return even if conversion to common stock does not take place.

- *Senior, subordinated, or convertible debt* (either convertible or with warrants) is used in venture financing situations in which the investor wants the security and yield of a debt instrument, and the company does not want to restrict its ability to borrow from banks or insurance companies. If subordinated debt does not dominate the capital structure, it will be viewed as equity by senior lenders. Senior and subordinated debt gives the venture capitalist more options than does a straight equity position. If the company defaults on the loan, the investor can accelerate repayment, and if the company cannot repay, the venture capitalist (now a creditor) has strong leverage to influence management decisions.

Because of the interrelationship between return and liquidity objectives, a sophisticated venture financing approach to an enterprise will utilize a mixture of the various securities discussed above. By aligning itself with a professional venture financier, the subject hospital, system, or group can gain direct assistance in formulating its investment structure to meet its goals. Thus, apart from being just a provider of outside equity, a venture capital firm can represent a source of business and investment expertise that can be most beneficial and rewarding to the subject hospital, system, or group in the pursuit of new business opportunities.

CHANGES IN BORROWED CAPITAL

In addition to equity capital, the demand for debt will be insatiable. Notwithstanding the potential change in the government's allowance of tax-exempt bonds, the demand for borrowed capital will increase for both taxable and tax-exempt debt, as previously mentioned. The investors in such debt instruments will demonstrate a preference for shorter maturities and floating or much higher fixed interest rates, a tendency exhibited in other debt market segments. The higher interest costs will exacerbate the problem of scarce capital and the investors' increased concern over credit strength.

The presently volatile capital markets reflect a narrowing of the cost differential between taxable debt and tax-exempt revenue bonds. Even though that narrowing probably will not continue, systems and groups may look to taxable debt as being more suitable due to the ability to raise working capital, the avoidance of jurisdictions of issuance problems, and the broader market represented by taxable bonds and notes. It should be reemphasized here, however, that the taxable debt market has traditionally mandated more conservative borrowing limits and more stable operating performance.

In response to the demand for capital, the industry is also making two distinct changes that will undoubtedly continue and accelerate. The major hospitals, systems, and groups are increasing their rapport with the banking community. Some are keeping investment bankers on retainer, in addition to their auditors and attorneys, for ongoing use as a resource to the corporation. The need to develop strong commercial banking ties for working capital lines and other short-term capital needs is just beginning.

There are several financing vehicles that, although not novel, will also increase in popularity. Tax-exempt commercial paper started increased usage in 1981 and then the Internal Revenue Service increased the restrictions relative to arbitrage of those funds. It is expected use of tax-exempt commercial paper will increase, but so will the use of taxable commercial paper for or on behalf of major systems and networks. The use of commercial paper will depend on the creditworthiness of the institution and commercial papers' cost relative to taxable or tax-exempt commercial bank borrowings. Convertible (to equity) debt securities that have been used by proprietaries and industry for some time will begin to appear within the major providers' capital alternatives, especially given the restructuring of profitable services.

For the hospital that has restructured, unbundled, spent its capital resources and not generated a bottom line result, the lack of access to capital resulting from those limited results may be the harbinger of a decline or worse. For the banking, accounting, and legal communities the transformation of the hospital providers from a cottage industry to big business has substantial rewards. The entrepreneurial manager among the health care providers will be on the cover of the trade journals and recognized as the dynamic executive required. It is expected that for the financial managers who are successful in 1990, the 1980s will be most rewarding. For the programs in health care management, the business and finance curriculum will expand dramatically. For the trade group "clubs" that used to meet to swap ideas on marketing, management, finance, pricing, and competition, the meeting rooms of the latter part of the 1980s will be quiet, if not empty. For the successful, well-managed hospital, system, or network that can meet the coming competitive challenge, the 1980s will be an exciting time.

NOTE

1. Speech by Thomas W. Reed, American Hospital Association Convention, August 30, 1981.

Chapter 20

Financing Outpatient and Prepaid Health Care Facilities

James J. Unland

THE GROWING IMPORTANCE OF OUTPATIENT HEALTH CARE

Many health care professionals believe that outpatient health care and prepaid health care will dominate the American health care industry by the turn of the century. Thus, it will become more important for the investment banking community to find ways of providing access to the capital markets for health maintenance organizations (HMOs), physicians' office buildings, surgicenters, emergicenters, and other outpatient or prepaid treatment programs.

Two factors argue in favor of accepting the hypothesis that outpatient care will become the dominant form of health care treatment over the next two decades. First, improvements in medical technology now make it possible to deliver treatments unheard of on an outpatient basis even a decade ago. The concept of treating people on an ambulatory basis is now not only possible from a technological standpoint, but also profitable for the medical community, and any analysis of changing medical trends must take into account the need for physicians and facilities to make money. The profit margin of outpatient treatment can be lucrative, while at the same time overall costs per medical incident are held far below costs of inpatient hospitalization.

A second factor creating new trends in medical treatment will be continued cost containment pressures upon the entire health care industry. These pressures will come not only from government, but also from private insurers, employers, and consumers. The recent trend in Washington toward repealing some health care regulations and encouraging "free enterprise" in the health care industry will accelerate pressures toward new treatment modalities.

The traditional hospital complex with which we are now familiar may be a thing of the past by the year 2000. By then, a typical community hospital operating with 250 beds could very well be a 30- to 50-bed facility providing acute care, with adjacent satellite physicians' office complexes, outpatient centers, day surgery centers, and convalescent facilities in which patients can be treated at a much lower per diem cost. It is encouraging to the investment banking community to see some of the leading hospitals moving in this direction already. They are realizing that massive complexes with huge bed towers are becoming a thing of the past.

One of the most important factors arguing in favor of the development of outpatient treatment facilities is the fact that these facilities are not nearly as capital-intensive as hospitals. HMO clinics, surgery centers, emergency clinics, and physicians' office buildings can all treat a large number of patients for an initial capital investment of a few million dollars, as opposed to tens of millions of dollars for hospital facilities. It is almost unheard of for an outpatient center to spend as much as $10 million on plant and equipment, whereas it is common for hospitals to spend anywhere from $20 million to $50 million on modernization projects and bed-replacement projects.

The figures become even more astounding when comparing the "per episode" amortized facility cost between hospitals and outpatient centers. Because they can see more patients in less time, outpatient centers providing relatively sophisticated care have a large competitive advantage, for the per visit capital cost of such care becomes minute when compared to that of a hospital.

ACCESS TO THE CAPITAL MARKETS

Even though it is difficult to bring outpatient facilities into the capital markets, such financings are becoming more common. While the challenge to the investment banker is to introduce a new type of facility to the capital markets, the relatively low fixed costs of such facilities plus the efficient operations and potentially large profit margins will, over time, overcome most barriers of access to the capital markets for these new health delivery programs.

One of the challenges in giving these new types of facilities access to the capital markets is to create a relevant measurement system so that such facilities can be measured relative to one another and relative to the rest of the health care industry. One of the most important developments in giving hospitals access to the capital markets more than a decade ago was the emergence of financial feasibility studies that could measure the historic performance of institutions and make projections for the future.

These feasibility studies give nonhealth care professionals, and especially the financial community, a consistent way of comparing one hospital to another. They also give the bond rating agencies, bond insurance agencies, and ultimate purchasers of bonds the same advantage. Therefore, it will be important for outpatient and other new delivery systems to involve the financial feasibility community in planning for capital development.

FINANCING HMOs AND OTHER PREPAID HEALTH PLANS

For nearly a decade, the federal government has encouraged the development of HMOs. At the end of 1981 there were approximately 250 such organizations throughout the United States. In addition, there were also a number of prepaid health plans not exactly defined as HMOs, but roughly organized along the same concept.

In the 1982 fiscal year budget, the Reagan Administration reduced the commitment of the federal government to the HMO industry. This created a funding crisis for many HMOs desiring expansion. It has become important to give HMOs access to the capital markets, especially the debt markets, where at all possible.

From a financial standpoint, there are some advantages to a prepaid health care plan. The most important advantage is obvious; the prepayment by a population for health care services creates a consistent revenue stream. Another advantage is that prepaid health care systems do not require a large capital investment in plant and equipment. They generally operate from clinics, physicians' office complexes, or even the individual offices of physicians (known as an individual practice association).

The fact that HMOs collect their revenue over a consistent time period for their covered population means that they are not as vulnerable as hospitals to swings in utilization. Therefore, HMOs with an adequate population base can remain financially sound through seasonal changes in utilization. In addition, because HMOs operate out of outpatient facilities, they have an incentive to treat people on their feet rather than to hospitalize them. It has been the experience of most HMOs throughout the United States that their patient populations, on average, occupy hospital beds approximately one-half as much as the rest of the population. This is a dramatic statistic which points to the potential of outpatient care in the future.

The problem with the prepaid health care plan is getting the plan off the ground and building up a membership sizable enough to create an adequate revenue base and to construct physical facilities. Financing a not-for-profit start-up HMO is nearly impossible without the assistance of the federal government or a private corporation. Many large insurance companies and private corporations, even including some hospitals, have provided seed money for the development of HMOs and other prepaid health care plans.

Start-up HMOs do not need to construct or purchase physical facilities. They can lease offices or even use the offices of existing physicians. However, when an HMO reaches a membership of roughly 30,000 families, it is important to consider buying or constructing a physical facility or satellite facilities, so that a capital base and a marketing base can be established. In addition, many HMOs today have their main medical complex in a clinic which provides a wide variety of diagnostic and treatment services; they also have smaller satellite clinics scattered throughout their marketing area. This can be effective, because people have demonstrated the desire to seek medical treatment close to where they live.

A "mature" HMO which has a significant enough population base should be able to finance the construction of additional facilities with the proper financial feasibility study and other groundwork. However, because HMOs are a new industry, the rating agencies have not granted them ratings, and most purchasers of bonds and other debt are unfamiliar with HMO financing. Therefore, even a financially healthy HMO will have trouble accessing the capital markets until those markets become more familiar with the HMO concept. Still, there are ways to strengthen an HMO to give the organization access to the tax-exempt bond markets or other debt markets if, as a free-standing organization, the HMO is unprepared to enter the debt markets without a bolstering of its credit. These credit-strengthening techniques include:

- HMO physicians can provide a guaranty of the incurred debt to finance a physical facility. This is usually done by permitting the physicians to own the building and lease it back to the HMO for a period of seven years, at which time the building reverts to HMO ownership under certain conditions. This permits the physicians to take advantage of tax benefits during the initial years and permits the HMO to own the facility eventually.

- A hospital can guaranty the debt of an HMO. This is especially appropriate in cases where a hospital has contributed in a major way toward the formation of the HMO and where the hospital can benefit from the HMO through patient referrals.

- An HMO can obtain a bank letter of credit giving the organization a vote of confidence in the financial community. Bank letters of credit generally are difficult to obtain unless an organization has been in business for several years, has established a proper membership base, and has a good financial track record.

Because physicians play such a key role in the development of an HMO, they may be willing to assume the ownership of a building and provide the personal guaranties and equity financing necessary to enter the capital markets. Physicians can gain significant tax advantages through the use of the investment tax credit, depreciation, the ability to deduct interest payments, and other benefits common to the ownership and leasing of an office building. The actual financing of a facility owned by physicians can be undertaken either on a tax-exempt basis through industrial revenue bonds in most states, or on a taxable basis.

Having physicians involved in the capital development program of an HMO or other prepaid health care plan gives those physicians a vested interest in the success of the overall organization and motivates them to behave accordingly. It is probably true that the more ownership and control physicians have over outpatient facilities, the more outpatient utilization we will have in the United States, because physicians still do control the decision process of how and where patients are treated. If physicians have a direct economic incentive to provide prepaid and outpatient health care, they will tend to do just that. Such an economic incentive can be created by the direct ownership of buildings and equipment.

Many state health authorities do have statutory authority to finance HMOs, physicians' office buildings, and other programs as long as they are not-for-profit 501(c)(3) corporations. Proprietary corporations as well as those in states without health authorities must seek financing through banks, insurance companies, or private corporations, or through tax-exempt industrial revenue bonds.

For the new not-for-profit HMO, access to the capital markets is difficult without the support of the government or another organization. Recently some HMO chains and consortia have been formed to help the newer HMOs get started. These groups can also help the mature HMOs into the capital markets and can provide lobbying muscle, sharing of technical services, and many other benefits.

PHYSICIANS' OFFICE BUILDINGS

The office building in which a number of physicians own or lease space and are otherwise separate in terms of operations is becoming a thing of the past. More often, physicians are joining together to purchase major equipment, to centralize accounting programs, and to deliver a more sophisticated level of patient care. Such groups do not rely upon the prepaid health care concept; rather they simply rely on patients' other insurance programs. Many national insurance companies now encourage outpatient care by reimbursing such care 100 percent or to a very large degree. They realize that it is prudent to reimburse for outpatient care, especially when such care can prevent hospitalization.

The physicians' office complexes which are growing around the United States involve a range of services depending upon the specialties of the member physicians. Many of these facilities contain x-ray equipment, scanning devices, fluoroscopic equipment, outpatient surgery capability, and other diagnostic and treatment facilities. Some of these facilities even have an "emergency room" capability.

As an investment banker, I generally like to see the office complexes that offer a multifaceted type of patient care and have a diverse group of physicians owning and operating the facility. When physicians own an outpatient office complex, they are generally willing to guaranty the debt of such a complex personally and, in this way, give it access to the capital markets. Physicians' office complexes of this type have been financed either through taxable bank financing or through tax-exempt debt, usually in the form of industrial revenue bonds. Either way, the capital markets still consider the guaranties of physicians to be a strong asset, because many physicians have high net worths and because their future earning power is significant.

There are many ways in which a group of physicians can get together to own an office complex. Some of the financial structures and financing mechanisms are:

- *Limited partnerships*. In a limited partnership each physician contributes a specific amount of "equity capital" in return for a specific percentage of ownership in the partnership. A general partner manages the complex and assumes more liability than the limited partners. The limited partners use their equity investment as a whole to leverage themselves into the debt markets or into the tax-exempt bond markets, especially in areas where tax-exempt industrial revenue bonds are possible. All of the tax benefits of owning real estate accrue to the various limited partners on a pro rata basis, depending upon their original equity contribution.

- *A stock company*. In some cases it is wise for physicians to form a corporation and issue stock. The stock is sold for equity dollars which are then, in turn, used to leverage the company into the debt markets to finance physical facilities. A stock corporation is especially useful if more than one facility is owned or being financed, or if the group of physicians is quite large. The liability of corporations is limited, and there are certain tax benefits to the corporate structure.

- *Bank financing*. Commercial banks still consider physicians an excellent credit risk, and many physicians' office complexes are financed conventionally through taxable or "conventional" mortgages. The major disadvantage of conventional financing is, of course, the higher interest rates relative to tax-exempt financing. However, in many areas industrial revenue tax-exempt financing cannot be undertaken for a proprietary corporation or partnership, leaving no other option than to enter the conventional debt markets. As with the other alternatives, bank financing usually requires a pool of equity and a sharing of the liabilities as well as the tax benefits.

• *Industrial revenue bonds.* Industrial revenue bonds are tax-exempt bonds that are generally issued through an industrial development authority, an economic development commission, or a similar local agency. Tax-exempt industrial revenue bonds are not always available for proprietary corporations. Their availability depends upon state laws and upon the inclination of local authorities. Furthermore, there is generally a $10 million limitation upon industrial revenue bond financing. This limitation applies not only to the amount being financed, but also to a three-year period before and a three-year period after the project itself. In other words, no more than $10 million can be spent upon "capital acquisition" during that six-year period. However, most physicians' office complexes fall well below the $10 million level, and this limitation should not present a barrier to most projects.

It is clear that continuing progress in medical technology, in addition to health cost containment pressures, will lead to broader, more efficient outpatient services in the years ahead.

The investment banking community will need to meet two important challenges in the future as the trend toward outpatient and prepaid health care increases. First, investment bankers will need to make certain that traditional hospitals are planning for the future in their capital development programs. Hospitals will need to factor into their planning the trend toward outpatient care, and, if possible, they should attempt to take a leadership role rather than simply focus upon the traditional inpatient setting.

Second, the investment banking community will need to devise ways of financing outpatient and prepaid health care systems. In the early years venture capital, the guaranties of physicians, support from hospitals, and other credit-boosting mechanisms will be important in giving these new modalities access to the capital markets. Later, as proper feasibility measurement systems are devised and as a successful industry track record emerges, access to the capital markets should become easier for these important new health facilities.

Bibliography

American Bar Association. *Forum on Construction of Health Care Facilities.* Chicago: American Bar Association, 1980.

Ballard, Frederick, L., Jr. *Tax Problems in Tax-Exempt Financing.* Series Number 141, Tax Law and Practice Course Handbook. New York: Practising Law Institute, 1980.

_____. *XYZ's of Arbitrage.* Packard Press, 1980.

Berriman, W. Thomas; Essick, William J., Jr.; and Bentivegna, Peter. *Capital Projects For Health Care Facilities.* Germantown, Md.: Aspen Systems Corp., 1976.

Cain, Daniel M., and Gilbert, R. Neal. "Capital Financing," *Topics in Health Care Financing* 5:1. Germantown, Md.: Aspen Systems Corp., Fall 1978.

Dixon, Joyce A., and Tuttle, Baldwin, eds. *Third Party Guaranties.* New York Law Journal, Law Journal Seminars—Press, 1981.

Eden, C. Gregory, ed. *Tax-Exempt Municipal Lease Financing: A New Look.* New York Law Journal, Law Journal Seminars—Press, 1980.

Fritch, Bruce E., and Reisman, Albert F., eds. *Equipment Leasing— Leveraged Leasing* (2d ed.). New York: Practising Law Institute, 1980.

Lamb, Robert, and Rappaport, Stephen P. *Municipal Bonds.* New York: McGraw-Hill, 1980.

Public Securities Association. *Fundamentals of Municipal Bonds* (1st ed.). New York: Public Securities Association, 1981.

Reisman, Albert F., ed. *Equipment Leasing 1981.* New York: Practising Law Institute, 1981.

Ryan, Joseph, ed. *Hospital Financings Through The Use of Tax-Exempt Securities, Financings For The 1980's.* New York Law Journal, Law Journal Seminars—Press, 1980.

Ryan, Reade H., Jr., ed. *Letters of Credit.* Course Handbook No. 251. New York: Practising Law Institute, 1981.

Strickler, Matthew M., and Ballard, Frederic L., Jr. *Representing Health Care Facilities*. New York: Practising Law Institute, 1981; *esp*. Ch. 6, "Taxable and Tax-Exempt Financing of Hospital Facilities" by Lee R. Voorhees, Jr.

Glossary of Health Care Finance Terminology

Accrued Interest—Interest earned on a security since the later of the last coupon payment date or the dated date.

Basis Point—Yields on securities are usually quoted in increments of basis points. One basis point is equal to $1/100$ of 1 percent.

Basis Price—The price of a security expressed in yield or percentage of return on the investment.

Bearer Security—A security that has no identification as to owner. It is presumed to be owned, therefore, by the bearer or the person who holds it. Bearer securities are freely and easily negotiable since ownership can be quickly transferred from seller to buyer.

Bond—An interest-bearing promise to pay a specified sum of money—the principal amount—due on a specific date.

Bond Anticipation Notes (BANs)—Usually tax-exempt, BANs are issued to obtain interim financing for projects that will eventually be funded long-term through the sale of a bond issue.

Bond Funds—Registered investment companies whose assets are invested in diversified portfolios of bonds.

Brokers—In the securities markets brokers play an important role in the secondary market by buying from and selling to dealers.

Callable Bonds—Bonds that are redeemable by the issuer prior to the specified maturity date at a specified price at or above par.

Competitive Underwriting—A sale of securities by an issuer in which underwriters or syndicates of underwriters submit sealed bids to purchase the securities. This is contrasted with a negotiated underwriting.

Concession—The allowance (or profit) that an underwriter allows a nonmember of the account; sometimes referred to as dealer's allowance.

Confirmation—A written document confirming an oral transaction in securities that provides pertinent information to the customer concerning the securities and the terms of the transaction.

Coupon—The part of a bearer bond that denotes the amount of interest due and on what date and where the payment is to be made. Coupons are presented to the issuer's designated paying agent or deposited in a commercial bank for collection. Coupons generally are payable semiannually.

Coverage—This is a key factor used in determining creditworthiness of a particular bond issue. It indicates the margin of safety for payment of debt service, reflecting the number of times by which earnings for a period of time exceed debt service payable in such period.

Current Yield—The ratio of interest to the actual market price of the bond stated as a percentage. For example, a $1,000 bond that pays $80 per year in interest would have a current yield of 8 percent.

CUSIP—The Committee on Uniform Security Identification Procedures, which was established under the auspices of the American Bankers Association to develop a uniform method of identifying municipal, U.S. government, and corporate securities.

Dated Date—The date of a bond issue from which the bondholder is entitled to receive interest, even though the bonds may actually be delivered at some other date.

Dealer—A securities firm or department of a commercial bank that engages in the underwriting, trading, and sales of securities.

Debt Service—The payments required for interest on and repayment of principal amount of debt.

Default—Failure to pay principal or interest promptly when due or failure to adhere to certain other covenants and conditions specified in the financing documents.

Denomination—The face amount or par value of a security that the borrower promises to pay on the maturity date. Most tax-exempt bonds are issued in a minimum denomination of $5,000, although a few older issues are available in $1,000 denominations. Most taxable bonds are issued in a minimum denomination of $1,000. Notes generally are available in a $25,000 minimum denomination.

Discount—The amount by which the purchase price of a security is less than the principal amount or par value.

Dollar Bond—A bond that is quoted and traded in dollar prices rather than in terms of yield.

Double-Barreled Bond—A bond secured by the pledge of two or more sources of repayment, such as the unlimited taxing power of the issuer as well as revenues generated by the health care facility.

Double Exemption—Tax-exempt securities that are exempt from state as well as federal income taxes are said to have double exemption.

Face Amount—The par value (that is, principal or maturity value) of a security appearing on the face of the instrument.

Financial Adviser—A consultant to the health facility or to the governmental issuer of tax-exempt securities who provides the issuer with advice with respect to the structure, timing, terms, or other similar matters concerning a new issue of securities.

Funded Debt—Long-term debt of the health care facilities corporation, generally debt maturing in more than one year from the date of computation of the corporation's debt.

General Obligation Bond—A tax-exempt bond secured by the pledge of the governmental issuer's full faith, credit, and, usually, taxing power.

Indenture—This is the instrument appointing a trustee (usually a bond trust department) and charging that trustee with receiving payments from the health care facility sufficient to pay to the bondholders principal and interest on the bonds when due. The indenture also charges the trustee with the power to declare the bonds in default should the health care facility violate certain terms and conditions including failure to pay principal and interest on the bonds when due.

Industrial Revenue Bond—A security issued by a state, certain agencies or authorities, a local government, or a development corporation to finance the construction or purchase of industrial plants and/or equipment to be leased to a private corporation including proprietary health care corporations; and backed by the credit of the private corporation rather than the credit of the issuer.

Interest—Compensation paid or to be paid for the use of money. Interest is generally expressed as an annual percentage rate.

Issuer—For tax-exempt bond issues a state, political subdivision, agency, or authority that borrows money through the sale of bonds or notes.

Legal Opinion—For tax-exempt bond issues an opinion concerning the validity of a securities issue with respect to statutory authority, constitutionality, procedural conformity, and usually the exemption of interest from federal income taxes. The legal opinion is usually rendered by a law firm recognized as specializing in public borrowings, often referred to as "bond counsel."

Marketability—A measure of the ease with which a security can be sold in the secondary market.

Maturity—The date when the principal amount of a security becomes due and payable.

Municipal Securities Rulemaking Board (MSRB)—An independent, self-regulatory organization established by the Securities Acts Amendments of 1975, which is charged with primary rulemaking authority over dealers, dealer banks, and brokers in tax-exempt securities. Its 15 members are divided into three categories—securities firms representatives, bank dealer representatives, and public members—each category having equal representation on the board.

Negotiated Underwriting—In a negotiated underwriting the issuer of securities chooses one underwriter or a group of underwriters to sell its bonds to investors. There is no competitive bid for the issue.

Net Income Available for Debt Service—This is the amount of money available to the corporation to pay debt service on its bonds. It is computed by determining the adjusted annual operating revenues of the corporation minus its total operating expenses (other than interest, depreciation, and amortization).

Net Interest Cost—The traditional method of calculating bids and proposals to purchase new issues of securities. The other method is known as the True Interest Cost.

Noncallable Bond—A bond that cannot be called either for redemption by or at the option of the issuer before its specified maturity date.

Notes—Short-term promises to pay specified amounts of money, secured by specific sources of future revenues, such as taxes, federal and state aid payments, and bond proceeds.

Offering Price—The price at which members of an underwriting syndicate for a new issue will offer securities to investors.

Official Statement—Document prepared by or for the issuer that gives in some detail security and financial information about the issue.

Par Value—The principal amount of a bond or note due at maturity.

Parity Debt—Debt ranking equally and ratably with other debt of the corporation.

Paying Agent—Place where principal and interest are payable. Usually a designated bank.

Permitted Indebtedness—The section of the loan agreement setting forth the types of debt, in addition to the outstanding bonds of the corporation, which the health facilities corporation may have outstanding.

Premium—The amount by which the price of a security exceeds its principal amount.

Primary Market (new issue market)—Market for new issues of bonds and notes.

Principal—The face amount of a bond, exclusive of accrued interest and payable at maturity.

Ratings—Designations used by investor's services to give relative indications of credit quality.

Refunding—A system by which a bond issue is redeemed by a new bond issue under conditions generally more favorable to the borrower.

Registered Bond—A bond whose owner is registered with the issuer or its agents, either as to both principal and interest or as to principal only. Transfer of ownership can be accomplished only when the securities are properly endorsed by the registered owner.

Revenue Bond—A bond payable solely from net or gross nontax revenues of the health care corporation borrower. Almost all 501(c)(3) health care bond borrowing is through revenue bonds.

Secondary Market—Market for issues previously offered or sold.

Serial Issue—An issue or portion of an issue that has maturities scheduled annually or, in some cases, semiannually over a period of years.

Sinking Fund—A fund accumulated by a borrower over a period of time to be used for retirement of debt, either periodically or at one time.

Spread—(1) Difference between bid and asked prices on a security. (2) Difference between yields on or prices of two securities of differing sorts or differing maturities. (3) In underwriting, difference between price realized by the issuer and price paid by the investor.

Subordinated Bonds—These are bonds that rank behind the other bonds outstanding or to be issued in order of priority in bankruptcy. They generally bear a higher interest rate than "parity bonds," which rank equally and ratably with other first priority bonds in level of security.

Syndicate—A group of investment bankers and commercial banks who buy (underwrite) a new issue from the issuer and offer it for resale to the general public.

Takedown (sometimes referred to as takedown concession)—The discount from the list price allowed to a member of an underwriting account on any bonds it sells.

Term Issue—An issue or portion on an issue that has a single stated maturity.

Transcript of Proceedings—Documents relating to a bond issue.

True Interest Cost—A method of calculating interest cost for new issues of securities that takes into consideration the time value of money. Also see Net Interest Cost.

Trustee—A bank designated by the issuer or borrower as the custodian of funds and official representative of bondholders. Trustees are appointed to insure compliance with the contract and represent bondholders to enforce their contract with the issuers.

Underwrite—To purchase a bond or note issue from the issuing body to resell it to the general public.

Unit Investment Trust—A fixed portfolio of bonds sold in fractional, undivided interest (usually $1,000).

Yield to Maturity—A yield concept designed to give the investor the average annual yield on a security. It is based on the assumption that the security is held to maturity and that all interest received over the life of the security can be reinvested at the yield to maturity.

Index

About the Editor

GEOFFREY B. SHIELDS is a partner in the law firm of Gardner, Carton & Douglas in Chicago, Illinois, specializing in the areas of health care and educational financing and not-for-profit corporations law. He is a graduate of Harvard College and Yale Law School and is the author of numerous law review and journal articles. He has served as underwriters' counsel or counsel to the borrower in more than 40 financings of hospital and educational facilities.

About the Contributors

THOMAS ARTHUR is a partner in the Chicago law firm of Gardner, Carton & Douglas, where he specializes in health law and securities transactions, including public and private sales and acquisitions. In recent years he has been most active in public utility mortgage bond transactions and sale of tax-exempt hospital bonds, serving as hospital counsel, underwriters' counsel, and bond counsel. His publications include: "Rule 146 Under the Securities Act of 1933: A Significant Codification," published in the *Chicago Bar Record* in 1974; "Financing of Pollution Control Facilities Through Tax-Exempt Bonds," cowritten with James R. Richardson and published in the *Chicago Bar Record* in 1977; "Federal and State Regulation of the Public Distribution of Securities—Its Effect Upon Sources of Financing," a 1979 *Business Planning Institute* publication; and, with coauthor Ray Garrett, Jr., "Corporate Bond Financing," published in 13 Corporate Practice Series (BNA, 1979). Mr. Arthur holds a B.A. from Hamilton College. He was awarded a J.D. from Northwestern University School of Law in 1958. He is a Citizen Fellow of The Chicago Institute of Medicine and former President of the Chicago Lung Association.

FREDERICK R. BLUME is an Executive Vice President at the Chicago office of Blyth Eastman Paine Webber Health Care Funding, Inc., where he has national responsibility for marketing and developing service programs for multihospital systems. Mr. Blume has been active in health care finance for more than a decade and has had in-depth experience in public and private financing. He has arranged taxable and tax-exempt financings aggregating more than $1 billion for numerous health care clients. Before joining Blyth Health Care, Mr. Blume was associated with another major investment banking firm; he has also headed the hospital lending activity for a major bank. The author of articles published in *Trustee Magazine, Modern Healthcare,* and *Health Care Finance,* Mr. Blume has guest-lectured on health care finance at several major universities. Mr. Blume did undergraduate work at Stanford University and University of the Pacific; he holds a Master's degree in business administration from Stanford University.

RICHARD J. BRASHLER, JR., is President of Ziegler Securities, Inc., Rolling Meadows, Illinois, which specializes in tax-exempt health care finance. Mr. Brashler received his A.B. degree in economics from Duke University in 1967.

ROBERT G. DONNELLEY is Vice President and Division Head of the Health, Education and Services Division of the First National Bank of Chicago. This 17-person division is responsible for providing financing and financial services for health care, educational, and other major service-related organizations on a national basis. Mr. Donnelley received his B.A. from Yale University; his M.B.A. from Harvard Business School; and a J.D. from Illinois Institute of Technology, Chicago-Kent College of Law. He is Director of Health Care Service Corporation (Illinois Blue Cross-Blue Shield); Trustee, Michael Reese Medical Center Foundation; and Trustee of Lake Forest Hospital.

JOHN FENNER is a partner of Gardner, Carton & Douglas, working in the health care finance area and as bond counsel. He chaired the 1981 Bond Attorneys' Workshop Panels on Health Care Finance and Disclosure, and has testified before the House Ways and Means Oversight Subcommittee on Industrial Revenue Bonds. A graduate of Wesleyan University and the University of Pennsylvania Law School, he has written articles on municipal finance.

WILLIAM D. GEHL is Vice President and General Attorney, B. C. Ziegler & Company, West Bend, Wisconsin. Mr. Gehl is a member of the State Bar of Wisconsin and the Florida Bar. He received his A.B. degree in economics from the University of Notre Dame in 1968 and was awarded a J.D. from the University of Wisconsin Law School in 1971. He also received a M.B.A. from the University of Pennsylvania's Wharton Graduate School of Business in 1974.

HARVEY J. GITEL is an executive of the national office of Ernst & Whinney, providing assistance in forecast consulting services. His responsibilities include control review and clearance of engagements, which include forecasted financial statements. He is a member of the Hospital Financial Management Association, the Illinois CPA Society, the American Institute of Certified Public Accountants, and the Municipal Finance Officers Association. Since 1973, he has directed more than 25 hospital financial feasibility studies.

WILLIAM J. GRAY is a Senior Vice President in the Chicago office of Blyth Eastman Paine Webber Health Care Funding, Inc., where he specializes in investment banking to health care institutions. Prior to entering the banking area, he was a health care consultant with Coopers & Lybrand, where he performed financial feasibility studies for hospital tax-exempt bond issues.

THOMAS E. LANCTOT is associated with the law firm of Gardner, Carton & Douglas. He attended the University of Pennsylvania, received his B.A. degree from Northwestern University, and graduated from the University of Chicago Law School. He practices in the areas of federal and state securities law, and, in addition to his experience in the tax-exempt hospital and general obligation bond area, he has worked with real estate limited partnerships, public utilities, and general corporate issuers.

ROBERT C. LIDEN is a Senior Vice President—Acquisitions/Underwriting of Ziegler Securities, Inc. He has been responsible for coordinating all of the firm's acquisition and underwriting activities and for directly originating and processing approximately $600 million in health care issues. He has a Bachelor's degree in state and local government from the University of Illinois and an M.A. in public administration from Northern Illinois University.

EARL L. METHENY received a B.A. from Reed College in 1973 and graduated from New York University School of Law in 1978. While in law school he was articles editor of the *New York University Journal of International Law & Politics*. Mr. Metheny has served as counsel to not-for-profit and proprietary hospitals and professional medical corporations with respect to corporate, tax, employee benefit, and reimbursement matters. He has also served on the Hospital Review Committee of the Chicago Health Systems Agency. He is associated with the Baltimore, Maryland, law firm of Venable, Baetjer and Howard.

ARTHUR J. SIMON is associated with the law firm of Gardner, Carton & Douglas, where he practices in the areas of general securities law and corporate and health care finance. He received his B.S. degree from Vanderbilt University in 1975 and a J.D. from Northwestern University School of Law in 1979. He is a member of the American and Chicago Bar Associations.

JAMES J. UNLAND is the Director of Public Finance at William Blair & Company, Chicago's largest regional-based investment banking firm. Mr. Unland came to William Blair & Company in January 1981 after serving as a Vice President for health care finance with A. G. Becker, Inc. in Chicago, where he specialized in originating and executing tax-exempt health care financings. Prior to that, he acted as President and was the founder of Chicago Health Care Associates in Chicago. That firm specialized in consulting and financial feasibility analysis for hospitals, nursing homes, retirement centers, and physicians' office facilities. Mr. Unland also worked with hospitals and nursing homes needing assistance with internal financial management systems and financial planning. He is a member of the American Hospital Association, the Hospital Financial Management Association, American Homes for the Aging, and the Chicago Lung Association.

DONNA S. WETZLER is a partner in the firm of Gardner, Carton & Douglas, where she practices in the areas of tax-exempt finance, general securities law, and health law. She received her B.A. degree from Yale College in 1972 and her J.D. from Harvard Law School in 1975. She is a member of the American and Chicago Bar Associations and has lectured at the Rush-Presbyterian-St. Luke's Medical Center School of Health Systems Management.

JAMES R. WYATT is a Vice President of Ziegler Securities, Inc., Rolling Meadows, Illinois, and a Vice President and Assistant to the President of B. C. Ziegler & Company, West Bend, Wisconsin. He has been the investment banker on scores of taxable and tax-exempt health care financings.